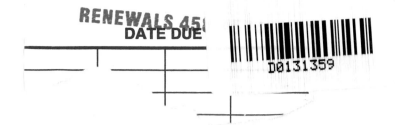

Safety in Numbers

A VOLUME IN THE SERIES

The Culture and Politics of Health Care Work

Edited by Suzanne Gordon and Sioban Nelson

Safety in Numbers

NURSE-TO-PATIENT RATIOS AND THE FUTURE OF HEALTH CARE

Suzanne Gordon,

John Buchanan, and

Tanya Bretherton

ILR Press

AN IMPRINT OF
CORNELL UNIVERSITY PRESS
ITHACA AND LONDON

Copyright © 2008 by Suzanne Gordon, John Buchanan, and Tanya Bretherton

All rights reserved. Except for brief quotations in a review, this book, or parts
thereof, must not be reproduced in any form without permission in writing from
the publisher. For information, address Cornell University Press, Sage House,
512 East State Street, Ithaca, New York 14850.

First published 2008 by Cornell University Press

Printed in the United States of America

Library of Congress Cataloging-in-Publication Data

Gordon, Suzanne, 1945–
    Safety in numbers : nurse-to-patient ratios and the future of health care / Suzanne Gordon,
John Buchanan, and Tanya Bretherton.
        p. cm. — (The culture and politics of health care work)
    Includes bibliographical references and index.
    ISBN 978-0-8014-4683-2 (cloth : alk. paper)
    1. Nursing services—Standards—California.   2. Nursing services—Standards—Australia—
Victoria.   3. Nursing services—California—Personnel management—Statistical methods.   4.
Nursing services—Australia—Victoria—Personnel management—Statistical methods.   5.
Hospitals—California—Administration—Statistical methods.   6. Hospitals—Australia—
Victoria—Administration—Statistical methods.   7. Ratio analysis.   I. Buchanan, John.   II.
Bretherton, Tanya.   III. Title.   IV. Series.
    RT85.5.G67 2008
362.17'30683—dc22   2007045442

Cornell University Press strives to use environmentally responsible suppliers
and materials to the fullest extent possible in the publishing of its books. Such
materials include vegetable-based, low-VOC inks and acid-free papers that
are recycled, totally chlorine-free, or partly composed of nonwood fibers. For
further information, visit our website at www.cornellpress.cornell.edu.

Cloth printing   10   9   8   7   6   5   4   3   2   1

Contents

Acknowledgments

This book has been a transcontinental collaboration that has required contact and communication across time zones, oceans, and land masses, as well as family ties and friendships. As we've hashed out ideas, discussed, and refined, our communication have been structured by the fact that John and Tanya are either just waking up when Suzanne is going to sleep or just going to sleep when Suzanne is yawning and struggling to get up. Even in the age of the Internet getting Sydney and Boston together is a feat that requires as much strategic planning as patience.

This collaboration would never have happened without the assistance of a grant from the Australian Nursing Federation's Victorian Branch and the support of Lisa Fitzpatrick, its secretary. Although the ANF gave us the seed money to embark on this book, we accepted it only with the understanding that we were doing an objective analysis of ratios—warts and all. We believe that the result shows not only the benefits of ratios but also the problems and limitations associated with them.

We would also like to acknowledge the help of Vicki Bermudez of the California Nurses Association. Vicki provided us with a great deal of documentation that has helped us grasp the complexity of the California story. We are grateful to the comments and insights of Sean Clarke and Sioban Nelson. Holly Bailey offered us invaluable editorial assistance. We are also deeply grateful to Kristin Elifson for her help in compiling, analyzing, and drafting material on the many studies that have been done on nurse staffing, nursing and patient outcomes, and nurses' health.

Our analysis of the experience of nurse-patient ratios in Victoria, Australia, has only been possible because of the generous cooperation of many individuals. Prime among these are the members and job representatives of the Victorian Branch of the Australian Nursing Federation. Since 1999 they have contributed to countless focus groups, filled in questionnaires, and provided important insights through extended, semistructured interviews. Many nursing managers and directors of nursing also helped us understand the impact of ratios. There are hundreds, indeed thousands, of nurses who have agreed to give so openly to help us (as health industry outsiders) understand the complex workload issues faced by nurses. There are too many people to name individually, and in many cases we have agreed to use pseudonyms to preserve the confidentiality of the nurses who agreed to participate. We extend our personal thanks and appreciation to these nurses, who often agreed to give up their own personal time to be interviewed before or after long and stressful shifts (in some cases at dawn, or very late in the evening). Important information about the origins and development of the ratios has been provided by Belinda Morieson, Lisa Fitzpatrick, Yvonne Kelly, Bob Burrows, and Nick Blake. Special thanks also to Terese Garreffa and Robyn Asbury for help in locating resources and contacts in the industry. Commissioner Wayne Blair of the Australian Industrial Relations Commission (AIRC) provided particularly important insights that only an arbitrator can provide. The registrar of the AIRC was very cooperative in making full transcripts of all arbitral proceedings available to the research team. Our analysis of the experience in Victoria has benefited from research and advice from our colleagues at the Workplace Research Centre (formerly ACCIRT) at the University of Sydney. Jill Considine assisted in the design and analysis of the first two evaluation surveys and Sarah Wise helped on the most recent ones. At various times over the years Sue Bearfield, Stephen Jackson, and Nick Harrington have contributed to the analysis that is contained in this book.

We also want to thank our families for putting up with the demands of the international effort. Suzanne would like to thank her husband, Steve Early, for his help in illuminating issues of labor law and for his many editorial suggestions. John owes his wife, Kylie Nomchong (and their children, Ben and Isobel) a huge debt for giving up their claims on his "free" time to get his sections of the manuscript finished. Tanya extends thanks to family—Jason, Clare, and Laura Anderson—for their patience and support. Both Tanya and John have [SG1]only been able to work on this project because of support provided by their colleagues at the Workplace Research Centre.

Finally, we would like to thank Fran Benson for supporting this project and for her patience as we extended deadlines and begged once and again for just that extra time that turned not only into weeks but months. We also want to thank Katy Meigs for her editorial help and many, many thanks go to Ange Romeo-Hall for her vigilance and polish and for tolerating the authors' many last minute changes and delays.

We would also like to add a note about citations, names, and spelling. Because this book is published by an American press, we have used American spelling and idioms rather than Australian in the sections on Australia. We trust that Australian readers will not be offended by this choice. When quotations are used but not followed by an endnote it means that, following a more journalistic practice, this material is taken from interviews that the authors conducted. In some cases, we have used pseudonyms indicated by asterisks to protect the anonymity of our sources. This interview protocol allowed participants to speak frankly and openly to us about their experiences, without fear of retribution by managers. Because we want to reach the widest possible audience on this important subject, we have attempted to write in a journalistic rather than traditional academic style while not compromising scholarly standards. We hope readers both inside and outside the academy will appreciate our mission to be more inclusive and that this book will help all concerned with the future of nursing and health care to understand the conditions and dilemmas nurses face as they do their critical work.

Safety in Numbers

Introduction

In February 2005, three hundred members of the British Columbia Nurses Union gathered in a Vancouver hotel for their Provincial Bargaining Strategy Conference, just days before negotiations were scheduled to begin on a new four-year contract. As the nurses finalized their bargaining agenda, their highest priorities were not just wage and benefit improvements but what they considered intolerable and unsafe patient workloads. Since the mid-1990s, nurses in British Columbia had been asked to care for an increasing number of patients, who, as a group, had more intense nursing needs than the patients they had cared for previously. More hospitals were filled with seriously ill patients, because less-ill patients were now likely to be treated in an outpatient setting. Nurses said they had asked their managers for additional staff on their units to meet the increased demands—to no avail. Hospital administrators insisted that new computerized staffing systems (known as patient acuity systems) or other formulas designed to measure nurses' performance and productivity would accurately calculate how many nursing hours were needed for particular groups of patients on each shift. Yet, from the perspective of bedside nurses, patient loads were not becoming more manageable.

By 2005, union activists at the British Columbia gathering argued that there was only one way to protect registered nurses from the stress of excessive workloads and their patients from a growing number of preventable complications and deaths due to understaffing. Their proposed solution was provincewide mandated safe nurse-to-patient staffing ratios that, they insisted, would reduce stress and enhance patient safety. As one bone-weary RN commented as he swiveled around to address his colleagues, his gaze sweeping across the room, "I have to go in to work tomorrow. I never know how many patients I will have to take care of. I can barely make it through the day. How

1

can I make it? How can we make it through the next five years without some relief?" After listening to many comments both pro and con, the delegates voted to petition the provincial government for mandatory nurse-to-patient staffing ratios.

At the same time that nurses in British Columbia were demanding government action to address excessive workloads, the twenty-four-thousand-member Massachusetts Nurses Association (MNA) union was lobbying, for the eleventh straight year, for a bill that would legislate minimum nurse-to-patient staffing ratios for hospitals in Massachusetts. Patients, staff nurses, and many consumer groups had long rallied behind the MNA's ratio bill. Year after year, nurses had presented state legislators with studies and surveys documenting the impact of cost-cutting on nurse recruitment and retention as well as the connection between nurse-staffing levels and patient outcomes and mortality. The Massachusetts Hospital Association (MHA) and other industry groups opposed the legislation and lobbied equally hard against it.

During this protracted debate, the Massachusetts hospitals had initially argued that there was no nursing crisis or patient harm resulting from existing staffing practices. Later, the MHA acknowledged that something did need to be done to enhance recruitment and retention and to protect patients, but it argued that the market—not government—was the best guarantor of patient-care standards. The MHA created a website on which hospitals voluntarily posted "easy to understand" charts of average annual staffing on its varied units.[1] Patients considering admission to a particular hospital could consult the website to decide whether that hospital had safe staffing. The hospital association also worked with a state senator who crafted a bill that would require hospitals to formulate and post—but not adhere to—staffing plans. Hospitals that did not formulate such plans could be fined.

As the annual staffing ratios debate wore on in Massachusetts, the union and the hospital association engaged in an advertising war in the pages of the *Boston Globe*, the state's leading newspaper. MNA ads insisted that ratios were the answer to the nursing-and-patient-care crisis, while the hospital association predicted that ratios would, like an earthquake, cause the entire Massachusetts health-care system to collapse. As of fall 2007, lawmakers had taken no final action on the MNA bill.

The staffing-ratio issue is of global interest and import. In April 2006, the Japanese Nursing Association succeeded in pushing through an improvement in staffing ratios—from one nurse to ten patients to one nurse to seven patients in Japanese hospitals. Hospitals that meet the one-to-seven ratios will receive more money per day than those that do not. (It should be noted that this ratio is quite low because the average length of hospital stay is longer in Japan and therefore the average acuity level of patients is considerably lower than that which prevails in most of the English-speaking world.) Hospitals everywhere in Japan are busily trying to recruit nurses. So desperate are hospitals for nurses that well-known institutions have persuaded physicians to be the ones to implore or entice nursing school students to work in their institutions.

All over the globe nursing shortages are a critical topic of discussion. Wherever public officials, academic experts, hospital managers, and health-care workers argue about the increasingly dire situation of nursing and patient care, the subject of mandated minimum nurse-staffing ratios is inevitably raised. In this context, the experiences of the states of Victoria in Australia and California in the United States are invariably cited.

For example, when the Royal College of Nursing (RCN) in the United Kingdom was recently pondering the country's perennial nursing shortage, it commissioned a report analyzing the U.S. and Australian precedents of staffing ratios. At its 2007 congress, delegates overwhelmingly passed a resolution seeking United Kingdom–wide legislation mandating appropriate staffing levels.[2] When the College surveyed its members, the results showed that "most members believe the move is the best way to improve patient care and safety."[3] The Canadian Federation of Nurses Unions, in considering its response to the problem of nursing workload and patient care, published a similar report highlighting the models established in Australia and the United States. In response to membership requests, the International Council of Nurses sent a researcher to California to prepare a report about ratios.

In the United States, fourteen states have proposed some sort of legislative action on staffing ratios. When state legislators hold hearings on these proposals, representatives of the California hospital industry often testify to describe the problems they insist ratios have created, while union representatives laud their success. Victoria and California also figure prominently in articles by nurse workforce researchers in major health-care publications such as *Health Affairs* and the *Journal of Nursing Administration* (JONA) as well as in presentations to local, national, and international conferences on the nursing workforce crisis.

The experiences in Victoria and California have been the subject of so much curiosity because until recently, when they were joined by Japan in 2006, they were the only two places in the world with legally mandated nurse-to-patient staffing ratios on all the units in their hospitals. In 1999, after a decade-long battle between the state's hospital industry and the state's most powerful nursing union, the California Nurses Association (CNA), the California Legislature passed AB 394—a bill mandating the state's Department of Health Services (DHS) to determine appropriate minimum staffing ratios for all units in the state's hospitals. Three years later, the department set ratios of one nurse to six patients on medical/surgical floors, effective January 1, 2004. The ratio went down to 1:5 on January 1, 2005. On January 1, 2008, the ratio on step-down units (where patients receive less monitoring than on ICUs but more than on a regular unit) will go to 1:3, and on telemetry (in-patient units that provide continuous cardiac monitoring for patients at risk for heart attacks and other cardiac problems) and specialty units, it will go to 1:4. Different ratios were phased in for other units.

In 2000, the Victorian Branch of the Australian Nursing Federation (ANF) won mandated staffing ratios in all public-sector hospitals. Its "enterprise bargaining agreement" (EBA) with the Victoria state government requires ratios of five nurses to twenty patients on medical/surgical units and other minimum ratios on other hospital units. (While this averages to a 1:4 ratio, managers have the flexibility to assign some nurses more patients who are less intensely ill and some nurses fewer patients who have more intensive nursing needs.) The state government immediately made money available to cover the cost of the ratio requirements. The ratios, which have the force of law, were renewed in the EBAs negotiated in 2004 and 2007.

For nurses all over the world, ratios have both a concrete and symbolic significance. In very practical terms, many nurses believe that mandated ratios are the only way to exert professional control over workloads that can otherwise jeopardize the health and recovery of patients, as well as the health of the nurses who care for them. On a more symbolic level, for many bedside nurses ratios mean that society takes nurses and nursing seriously. Ratios are a way of addressing the paradox of a society that increasingly frets about recruiting new candidates to nursing while failing to improve working conditions that drive them away from the bedside.

In this book we summarize what is known about the history, promise, and problems of ratios in Victoria and California. The book describes the working conditions that led RNs in these two states to conclude that ratios were the best form of relief for understaffing in hospitals. It discusses how the campaigns for ratios were waged and explains the process through which specific ratios were determined and implemented. It reviews and evaluates the arguments against ratios. In this book we also analyze what we know about the important links between working conditions for nurses and patient-care outcomes as well as nurses' health, and consider the limits of current knowledge on these issues.

Although ratios do not and cannot deal with many of the problems that have led to the current nursing crisis, we conclude that ratios are an essential step in any multifaceted effort to deal with the challenges facing hospital nursing now and in the future. We also consider what lessons those working in other occupations can learn from how nurses have dealt with the problems of understaffing and work overload.

Why Ratios?

No matter where it occurs, the ratio debate is generated by developments that have produced a global nursing shortage. Throughout the industrialized world, the nursing workforce is getting older, and many nurses are nearing retirement age. This comes at a time when patient populations are aging and needing more nursing care. In addition, younger patients are living longer with conditions that require constant nursing monitoring and intervention. Today there may be more recruits to nursing than there were during the years of hospital restructuring and nursing layoffs in the 1990s, when nursing school applications fell dramatically, but many of today's applicants are not able to get into nursing schools because professors and instructors are either retiring or in short supply. Moreover, it is not clear, even if the demand for nursing school slots were met, that there would be enough new graduates to satisfy the coming demand for nurses.

What is equally troubling is that many of those recruits who do enter the field often leave the hospital bedside as quickly as possible because working conditions are so stressful. Many hospitals report turnover rates in the double digits. All across the globe, government payers or private insurance companies have targeted nursing when they initiate efforts to cut costs. That is because nurses are the largest profession in health care and the largest single workforce in the hospital industry, and they represent more than 50 percent of a hospital's labor budget.

Throughout the 1990s, hospitals restructured or reengineered their workforces to reduce that percentage of the labor budget devoted to nursing. More highly paid, experienced nurses were laid off or encouraged to accept management buyouts. Vacant positions were not filled when nurses changed jobs or retired. Cheaper, poorly trained aides replaced more experienced and educated—and thus expensive—nurses. Nurses who remained at the bedside were forced to take care of more patients, sometimes ten, twelve, or even twenty patients at a time, depending on the shift. Because many hospitals also laid off janitors, housekeepers, unit secretaries, transport, and other workers, nurses had fewer support staff to assist them in their daily work.

Health-care payers also tried to cut costs by reducing the amount of time patients spend in hospitals—what is known as "average length of stay" (ALOS). Even before the rise of managed care in the United States and cost-cutting elsewhere, the average length of hospital stays was gradually diminishing. Some of this was due to technological advances. Improvements in surgical techniques such as the use of fiber-optic laparoscope, for example, allowed surgeons to perform operations with much smaller incisions and shorter recovery times.

Staying in hospitals for shorter periods has the advantage of reducing patient exposure to hospital errors and injuries. For example, patients who stay in a hospital longer than necessary might fall from a hospital bed, suffering a hip fracture. Hospitals are also notorious breeding grounds for drug-resistant bacteria. Patients whose immune systems are already compromised may pick up infections ranging from surgical-wound infections to pneumonias and other serious infections that are resistant to high-powered antibiotics that they wouldn't have caught at home. According to a 2002 report by the U.S. Centers for Disease Control and Prevention, almost two million Americans a year acquire infections in the hospital, contributing to 99,000 deaths each year.[4]

Because hospitalization is one of the most expensive components of health care, reducing hospital length of stay is a major focus of cost cutting. In everything from cardiac bypass surgery to hip replacements to mastectomies for breast cancer to childbirth, length of stay shortened dramatically. For bypass surgery, for example, hospital stays of two or more weeks were common in the late 1980s. By the mid-1990s, in the United States at least, insurers considered four days to be the goal. In the 1980s, women having mastectomies for breast cancer spent more than a week in the hospital. At the height of the managed-care revolution, insurers in the United States were trying to make mastectomy an outpatient procedure. Women having babies were hustled out of the hospital after only twenty-four hours for a normal vaginal delivery, and some insurers wanted to cut length of stay to only eight hours.[5] Although not in as drastic a manner, the same phenomenon occurred in Australia.

Shortened length of patient stays, particularly when combined with increased use of technology and invasive treatments, has created a very different mix of patient acuity (intensity of patient need) in hospitals. A decade ago, a patient having surgery would be admitted to the hospital the day before his or her operation for tests, observation, and perhaps some education. After surgery, the patient could convalesce before being discharged. This meant a nurse might be taking care of one patient who needed little monitoring or pain and symptom management—the patient admitted the day before surgery or the patient fully stabilized and about to be discharged. The nurse might also be taking care of several patients who were acutely ill following surgery or an acute admission. The caseloads of nurses were more balanced between high- and low-acuity patients.

Today, however, surgical patients are admitted the same day as their surgery. Once the patient leaves the operating room (OR), the hospital's goal is discharge as soon as the patient no longer has a temperature or a tube in his or her body. Even when less invasive surgical techniques are used, the patient population in the hospital is extremely high maintenance and in need of intense nursing care. The patients who would have been on an intensive care unit (ICU) in 1970 are now on regular medical/surgical floors. As one attending physician at the Brigham and Women's Hospital in Boston observed, "In order to get in the door here, you have to have not one but maybe three or four major things wrong with you. People here on general medical floors are really, really sick."

As patients are cycled through the hospital more quickly, some hospital units today have a patient turnover of up to 40 or 50 percent in an eight-to-twelve-hour period. Thus, the cumulative workload of nurses also increases, as does speedup on each unit. If a nurse comes to work at 7 a.m. and is taking care of eight patients in the morning, four of them may be discharged at noon. However, four more may be admitted at 1 p.m. Although a manager who comes onto the unit at 1:15 p.m. may see a nurse caring for eight patients, the nurse's caseload has actually been twelve. Admitting and discharging patients also requires much more work. There are more tests and procedures to do, more charts to read and prepare, more medications to administer. Moreover, the nurse has to get to know the patient and the patient's response to his or her illness and its treatment very quickly. When patients are discharged with more complicated home-care needs, they and their families require instruction about how to take medications or use medical equipment, how to adjust life to facilitate recovery, and how to access community services and follow-up care.

When more patients move through the system more quickly, nurses also have to interact more frequently and more rapidly with a variety of doctors and other personnel such as social workers and physical or respiratory therapists. In teaching hospitals, the cast of characters expands to include more interaction with interns, residents, fellows, and attending physicians—all of whom have increased patient loads. With more admissions and discharges, activity also escalates and the atmosphere in the unit is more chaotic.

Throughout the world, nurses complain about the impact of similar cost-cutting measures combined with increases in patient acuity. They say they are having great difficulty providing basic care, medications, and treatments in a timely fashion. They report they have less time to get to know their patients and address their social and emotional needs. They contend that patient outcomes are compromised and that preventable complications are increasing. They believe that patients may even die because nurses are too busy to rescue them.

Nurses report that when they ask their managers for relief, managers are unable or unwilling to supply extra nurses or ancillary staff. In fact, managers have themselves faced significant cuts and work intensification. Directors of nursing have seen their workloads escalate, seen their power erode due to cost cutting, or have even lost their positions during hospital restructuring. Many bedside nurses say that they have lost whatever trust they had in nursing management.

As Roy J. Lewicki and Caroline Weithoff have written, trust—"an individual's belief in, and willingness to act on the basis of words, actions, and decisions of another"—is the "glue" that holds relationships together and allows people to work through conflict. Without trust, "parties no longer believe what the other says, nor believe that the other will follow through on commitments and proposed actions." In a workplace context distrust can lead to "confident negative expectations," which lead to "fear of the other" and "a tendency to attribute sinister intentions to the other, and desire to protect oneself from the effects of another's conduct."[6] As we will see in later chapters, this distrust affects both nurses and their managers and shapes the debate about ratios.

Since the late 1990s, survey and quantitative research by nursing unions, professional organizations, and researchers has documented nurses' continued disaffection not only nationally but also internationally. A 2001 study conducted by Linda Aiken, Julie Sochalski, Judith Shamian, Anne Marie Rafferty, and several other researchers that was published in *Health Affairs* reported on the working life of nurses in the United States, Canada, England, Scotland, and Germany. Despite the different systems of health-care financing and delivery in each country, nurses who were surveyed voiced similar complaints and cited "similar shortcomings."[7]

Data from forty-three thousand nurses from more than seven hundred hospitals confirmed the deterioration of working conditions and the erosion of the quality of patient care.[8] Nurses reported job dissatisfaction, burnout, and a widespread desire to leave nursing. In two distinct categories, the United States led the world: 41 percent were dissatisfied with their current jobs, and 43 percent felt burned out. In Canada, the numbers for dissatisfaction and burnout were 32.9 percent and 36 percent, respectively; in England, 36 percent and 36 percent; in Scotland, 38 percent and 29 percent; and in Germany, 17 percent and 15 percent.

Many nurses reported that their workloads had increased: in the United States 83 percent said the number of patients assigned to them had risen; in Canada it is 64 percent, and in Germany, 44 percent. They reported a reduction in number of nurse managers (58% reported this in the United States, 40% in Canada, 14% in Germany). Many also reported the loss of a chief nursing officer without replacement (17% mentioned this development in the United States, 25% in Canada, and 23% in Germany). An alarming number also reported declining quality of care and an increase in patient harm. In all countries, only about a third—between 29 and 36 percent—reported that the quality of care on their unit was excellent. In Germany, a startling 11.7 percent of nurses said that their unit delivered excellent care. Nurses also reported that patients were "not infrequently" receiving the wrong medication or dose, getting hospital-acquired infections, and experiencing more falls with injuries. They said that there were more complaints from patients and more verbal abuse directed at nurses. The authors concluded, "Nurses feel that they are under siege and hospitals cannot find enough nurses willing to work under current conditions in in-patient settings."[9]

In a study on the nursing shortage in the United States, the researcher Julie Sochalski found that many nurses were no longer working in nursing. "The most common reasons given for working in other fields were better hours, more rewarding work, and better pay."[10]

Nurses outside Europe and North America echoed, and continue to echo, these sentiments. Nurses have become more dissatisfied and burned out. Studies report higher levels of speedup and stress in hospital work. As a result, nurses—whose jobs already put them at risk for back, neck, and shoulder injuries—are suffering from even more musculoskeletal injuries. They are also experiencing higher levels of stress-related illnesses, such as depression, hypertension, heart disease, and strokes, and they are at greater risk for needlestick injuries. As today's nurses approach retirement, some discourage new recruits from entering nursing; student nurses who work in hospitals before graduating quickly get the message that they too should flee the hospital bedside.

Work Intensification and the Global Nursing Workforce

Work intensification was central to the push for staffing ratios in Victoria and California. Indeed, it is the key to understanding the debate about staffing ratios throughout the industrialized world. Work intensification is not, of course, unique to nursing. Throughout the 1980s and 1990s initiatives to improve labor-productivity growth went by several names: lean production, reengineering, best practice, total quality management. Throughout this period, countries with national health systems were encouraged to adopt the market-based system known as "new public management" (NPM) with its consuming focus on cost containment.[11] As E. J. Schumacher has documented, advocates of NPM focus on cost containment and operational efficiency by hospital administrators.[12] They argue that the private sector always delivers goods and services more cheaply and efficiently than the public sector. This was a pivotal belief driving work intensification in health-care provision.[13] Government services were encouraged to adopt private-sector market-based approaches and to heed the advice of a raft of consultants who imported business theories into health-care delivery.[14]

Although the public-management approach may vary among nation states and state governments, several key principles always apply. These include a greater emphasis on productivity and measurement of individual worker output, a schedule of annual accountability that is enforced rigorously and for which individual hospitals are expected to take primary responsibility, and health-care environments that are judged on "efficiency" criteria. Some studies have even noted that this public-management model specifically impacts nurses more than other occupational groups, including those outside health care.

As in the United States, Australian health-care administrators hired consultants using Tayloristic "scientific management" monitoring techniques to assert greater control over nursing work and then to restructure it.[15] Although consultants claimed they were applying revolutionary principles, their templates, in fact, applied early twentieth-century industrial models to health care. As Simon Head puts it, consultants integrated health and human services into the "new ruthless economy" of the 1990s by updating the theories of a host of early twentieth-century "scientific" managers such as Frederick Winslow Taylor, John Hall, William S. Knudsen (who worked for and became president of General Motors), and William Henry Leffingwell.

Today, what Head terms "the four pillars of industrialism"—standardization, measurement, monitoring, and control—are guiding health care. Rather than controlling the labor of unskilled workers on the assembly line, the new industrialists "invaded the territory of the skilled worker, with the re-engineer trying to impose factory discipline on the work of even those classified by economists as 'very skilled.' "

The goal of the scientific manager was to "achieve machine-like standards of speed and reliability with the routines of the workforce whether of laborers, machinists, inventory clerks, purchasing agents, supervisors, or managers" and to "study the routines of all these employees, work out the simplest and fastest way for each to be done, and, finally, set a standard time for its performance."[16] The vehicles that allow Taylor's principles to be applied to the nursing workforce are patient acuity systems, clinical pathways, and benchmarking, all of which, critics argue, initiate a widespread deskilling of nurses' work.

Under both new public management and reengineering, services such as cardiology and oncology become product lines, and hospital units are advised to compete with one another. Patients are turned into "clients" or "customers," and clinicians into "providers." All are urged to take responsibility for producing better outputs with fewer inputs.

Although advocates of such cost-cutting restructuring assure greater efficacy and efficiency in the delivery of health-care services, underlying all these efforts is one fundamental reality: employers lay off more of their employees and ask those remaining to achieve more with fewer staff.

Reviews of the work-organization literature document how the increased amount of work each individual worker is asked to perform creates, among other things, escalating levels of workplace stress. Jeffrey Johnson of the University of Maryland School of Nursing explains that in the European Union since the 1990s work has dramatically intensified. According to the European Agency for Safety and Health at Work, an estimated 50–60 percent of all lost working days were related to stress.[17] In the United Kingdom alone, the prevalence of occupational stress doubled between 1990 and 1999, and, more recently, the number of days lost due to stress has increased from sixteen to twenty-nine days lost per affected person.[18] A 1988 report from the U.S. National Institute for Occupational Safety and Health (NIOSH) describes that what has changed for the majority of American workers is that they are not only working longer hours than workers in the rest of the industrialized world, including Japan, but also they work harder. Work intensification increases because of high performance/lean production worker systems, as well as "increased worker responsibility and accountability for production management and meeting production goals; increased vigilance (process monitoring) and problem solving demands and increased electronic monitoring; and increased speedup and reduction in idle time," among other factors. Workers are encouraged to overwork through fear of being replaced by temporary workers or because of "staffing reductions following organization downsizing." The report points out that even efforts to enhance worker control and learning opportunities can increase work intensification and job stress.[19]

Because of such pressures, most U.S. national surveys now indicate that over 25 percent of workers report high work stress.[20] Although equivalent data do not exist in Australia, the Australian Bureau of Labor Statistics reports that the median absence period for work-stress cases is twenty-three days—more than four times that for injuries and illnesses not caused by stress.[21]

Although workers all over the world complain about increased stress, nurses' concerns about work overload have some unique features. When a nurse doesn't have time to turn a patient in bed, that patient can develop an excruciating and costly bedsore. When a nurse can't give prescribed medication on time, a patient may develop a serious infection or suffer from unremitting pain. When a nurse is running among eight different rooms, that nurse will not have time to notice a subtle change in a patient's condition that indicates a catastrophe about to happen. Recent research on "failure to rescue" confirms that without enough educated eyes on patients enough of the time, that is, nurses monitoring what are often very subtle changes in patient status, hospitals cannot catch serious problems that could be prevented. When this happens patient mortality rises, and expensive complications add to total hospital and health-care costs.[22]

For patients, the consequences of nurse-work overload can be dire. In hospitals, nurses are responsible for admitting, processing, and discharging patients. They administer medications and deliver whatever treatments physicians order. They monitor medications' effectiveness and evaluate the patient's response to them. Nurses are also the ones who provide pain relief as well as prevent complications. They plan, monitor, and manage all aspects of a patient's illness from acute to long-term and palliative care. They also represent the front line of patient care in the most direct and intimate way. Nurses lift patients; hold bedpans; clean, shave, and dress patients. They notice problems and prevent them not only because they monitor and report a patient's condition but because their close contact with patients allows them to establish relationships of trust that encourage patients to confide information that may be critical to recovery. And, of course, they comfort and support patients and their families when they are feeling most vulnerable or alone.

The nurse-patient interaction is the cornerstone of a well-functioning health-care system, and for patients the nurse is the public face of that system. While doctors of all types obviously play critically important roles, nurses mediate and manage far more of patients' experiences of the hospital. Contrary to the impressions left by TV and films, hospital patients may see a physician only a few moments a day. Anyone staying in a hospital ward spends most of his or her time negotiating and dealing with nursing staff members. Patients are not, in fact, admitted to hospitals unless they need nursing care, which means, of course, that hospitals are primarily nursing institutions.

Doctors, as well as patients, are dependent on nurses. Although many people believe that nurses are a mere extension of a physician, physicians rely heavily on RNs for much of what they know about their patients. Physicians depend on nurses to collect, interpret, and prioritize the information and data on which they make diagnoses and treatment decisions. Without sufficient nurses, doctors cannot admit patients to hospitals. Consequences of nursing shortages include cancellations in elective surgeries, intensive care unit bed closures (which happens when although an actual bed is available, it is closed to new patient admissions because there are not enough nurses available to care for such a patient), and emergency room closures, both temporary and permanent. In an era when there is more open reporting of hospital and physician mortality rates and when more patients sue their doctors for poor outcomes, members of the medical profession may be blamed for problems that are, in fact, the result of understaffed units. Whether many recognize it or not, physicians, no less than their patients, have a major stake in the outcome of nurse-staffing debates.

In almost every nation, nursing is the single largest health profession. In the United States, nurses outnumber physicians four to one and constitute the largest profession in health care. In Australia, nurses represent roughly half of the entire national health-sector workforce. If nursing has a problem, the whole system has a problem.

Victoria and California: Differences
and Similarities

To make sense of the ratios mandated in Victoria and California, it's important to understand the different contexts in which these efforts took place. Both struggles for ratios involved powerful trade unions, opposition from hospital administrators and government officials, public mobilization, the media, and some form of government regulation. Because of the way health care is financed and labor law is structured, and because public attitudes about workers' rights and public obligations all vary, these struggles had very different dynamics and outcomes that nonetheless share a striking number of similarities.

The ratios in Victoria were a product of a publicly funded health-care system in a society in which labor is a major political force. The Australian health-care system is a tax-supported national health system in which the private sector plays a subordinate role, primarily providing faster service for those rich enough to have private health insurance. Most hospitals in Victoria are independently owned and operated nonprofit facilities that are funded by the government. Thus, the government does not own the hospitals but provides their funding. While private hospitals exist, these generally perform only simpler procedures.

All the training of nurses, physicians, and other health-care professionals takes place in public facilities, which makes them pivotal to the system. Even when Victoria's citizens have private supplementary health insurance, they will go to a public-sector hospital when they have a serious illness, because most specialist physicians work in these institutions and they are the only ones equipped to give high-level specialist care. Well over 50 percent of Victoria's nurses work in public-sector facilities and pride themselves on being public employees primarily concerned with caring for the community—not for profit. When public-sector services are eroded, it is not only the poor who suffer. Middle-class and even upper-middle-class Australians also suffer, which is why, as we shall see, the erosion of quality nursing care in public-sector hospitals became an issue that led many citizens to support nurse-staffing ratios.

In Victoria, unions play a very different role in the health-care system than they do in the United States. Within each state there is only one organization for nurses that deals with both their bread-and-butter as well as their professional interests. These organizations have formed a federation—the Australian Nursing Federation. Over the last three decades they have shifted from being relatively placid organizations that primarily voiced nurses' professional needs to becoming far more active within the health-care industry. In doing so they now combine concerns about professional nursing standards with highly effective techniques that involve stop-work meetings, bans, and work limitations (such as temporary bed closures), along with advocacy and lobbying as means to advance nurses' collective interests.

ANF affiliates represent and bargain for "registered nurses" (division 1 nurses) and "enrolled nurses" (division 2 nurses), as well as nurse unit managers, supervisors, and directors of nursing. To be licensed, a registered nurse in Australia must complete a three-year university education, while an enrolled nurse has a two-year technical school education. In hospitals, the union also represents nurse unit managers (NUMs) and even chief nursing officers (CNOs), often referred to as directors of nursing (DONs). In larger hospitals, when the union represents higher-level nurse executives, these executives often make supplementary agreements for higher pay and better benefits with the government.

The Victorian Branch of the ANF—whose members make up between 70 and 75 percent of the nurses in public-sector hospitals—was the key player in the ratio fight. Even though not all nurses in public-sector hospitals in Victoria choose to belong to the ANF, it bargains with the government for all nurses in the public sector. In Australia, union membership and participation in union activities is entirely voluntary, and by law there are no union security provisions or a union or agency shop (which, in the United States, require that all employees in a particular unionized workplace pay dues or the equivalent in "agency fees" to the union that negotiates for them).

Bargaining in Victoria takes place every four years and produces an enterprise bargaining agreement. For a period of six months, the union negotiates with an industrywide group called the Victorian Hospitals Industrial Association. All the public-sector hospitals appoint representatives to the negotiating committee. Negotiations will often include a director of nursing or chief executive officer of one of the major metropolitan hospitals, who also participates around the negotiating table. In 2004, for example, a member of the Nurse Policy Planning Unit within the Victoria Department of Human Services (the government agency overseeing the health system), also was involved in the bargaining.

If the union and government cannot come to an agreement, the union can resort to what is called "industrial action." In Victoria, rather than all nurses engaging in a strike, nurses will hold stop-work meetings and decide to come to work but selectively "close beds" on their units. If there is a twenty-bed unit, the nurses will announce, through a system of advance warning, that they will perhaps take care of patients in only sixteen beds and close the other four to any new admissions. Beds in maternity and cancer units and at the Royal Children's Hospital are legally exempt from such industrial actions. If the dispute is not settled, the unresolved issues can go to the Industrial Commission, a quasi-judicial institution established more than a century ago to help prevent and settle industrial disputes by conciliation if possible and by arbitration if necessary.

Nurses' salaries in Victoria are paid through a process of hospital budgeting. When staffing ratios were implemented, they were thus a funded mandate.

Health care in California is structured quite differently. The United States is the only industrialized nation that has no publicly funded national health system. If they are employed, most people in the United States have some form of employer-provided health insurance. Employers are not required to provide this job benefit. If the workers are unionized, health-care benefits are a subject for collective bargaining. Since only 9 percent of private-sector employees belong to unions, employers are free to change or even terminate job-based medical benefits or to require workers to pay more for them at any time. For citizens sixty-five years old or older and some (but not all) low-income Americans, there are two public insurance plans. Medicare, which is federally funded, is for those over sixty-five, and Medicaid, which is funded by a combination of state and federal money (which also covers nursing home care), is for low-income citizens. The number of uninsured people in the United States—those who are not covered by their jobs and are under sixty-five or who don't qualify for Medicaid or a state program for children—has increased to about forty-seven million, or 20 percent of the population. This number seems to increase annually and does not include the percentage of people in the United States who are underinsured, those who would be bankrupted by a major illness.

Of the 4,936 hospitals in the United States, 1,110 are public, 2,958 are nonprofit, and 868 are private.[23] The for-profit hospitals are generally owned and operated by large stockholder-owned hospital chains such as Tenet and the Hospital Corporation of America (HCA). Although there are fewer and fewer publicly owned hospitals, hospitals do receive a high portion of their revenues from the Medicare and state Medicaid programs. This money does not come in the form of block grant funding for the hospital's overall budget but rather in the form of fees for various services. Although nursing is bundled into these services, bills for hospital services do not separate out nursing costs. Because multiple private, state, and federal payers reimburse hospitals, there is no federal or state funding mechanism to finance mandates such as ratios, which require additional staff and add to a hospital's total labor costs.

On the union front, the picture is equally fragmented. There is no single national nursing union in the United States, nor is there a state nursing union in every state. Literally dozens of labor unions represent nurses. Those affiliated with the United American Nurses (UAN) are also members of the American Nurses Association. The UAN affiliates represent only registered nurses—a category in the United States that can include a registered nurse with a two-year degree from a community college, a four-year degree from a university, or a three-year diploma from one of the few remaining hospital-run nursing schools. Some nurses belong to the Service Employees International Union (SEIU), which represents RNs and licensed practical nurses (LPNs) or licensed vocational nurses (LVNs), as well as other hospital workers. What are referred to as LPNs on the East Coast of the United States are called LVNs in California. These are the equivalent of enrolled nurses in Australia. Although they are licensed, they tend to have approximately one year of technical school education that is generally provided through the community college system.

Many of the other trade unions that represent nurses also represent other workers as well. Examples include the SEIU, the American Federation of Teachers (AFT), American Federation of State County and Municipal Employees (AFSCME), the Communications Workers of America (CWA), and the International Brotherhood of Teamsters. In California, the most important unions involved in the ratio battle were the California Nurses Association (CNA), the SEIU, and the United Nurses Association of California (UNAC, which is an affiliate of AFSCME and represents only registered nurses in Southern California). The CNA was the most vocal and persistent in the fight for staffing ratios.

Before 1994, the sixty-five-thousand-member CNA, which represents only registered nurses, was a state affiliate of the American Nurses Association and had about twenty-seven thousand members. The ANA has both individual members and state affiliates with collective bargaining units (now linked together in the ANA and AFL-CIO–affiliated UAN). Its members include nurses giving direct care as well as educators, managers, and nurses working in other areas. The CNA had a separate collective bargaining arm, and the majority of its members—over 20,000—were involved in collective bargaining. Because of disputes about the way the ANA dealt with cost cutting in the early 1990s, the CNA split from the ANA and became a stand-alone labor union.

In California, academics and managers formed a smaller ANA state affiliate. Nurse managers and nurse executives may be members of the Association of California Nurse Leaders (ACNL), which is affiliated with the American Organization of Nurse Executives (AONE). Both groups consistently oppose any government regulation of hospitals and have been fierce opponents of ratios. The American Nurses Association also opposes mandated fixed-staffing ratios and prefers to ask state legislatures to mandate that hospitals create and publicly report nurse-staffing plans. It has underwritten studies and the development of a consensus set of "report card" measures that can be used to measure how hospitals fare on providing quality nursing care. It has also developed a benchmarking system, the National Database of Nursing Quality Indicators.

In the U.S. system, nursing unions do not bargain collectively with a statewide coalition of health-care employers as they do in Australia. Instead, unions bargain for individual contracts that cover only one hospital or, at best, all facilities in a particular nursing home, hospital chain or system, or health maintenance organization (HMO) such as Kaiser in California. To win bargaining rights nurses must sign union authorization cards and then gain legal certification based on a secret-ballot vote in a government-supervised representation election or through voluntary employer recognition after a third-party count of the union representation authorization cards. A union may represent just RNs and other workers in bargaining units of their own.

In the private sector, no nursing union represents managers or directors of nursing because the National Labor Relations Act (NLRA) legally excludes them from collective bargaining. Recent decisions by the National Labor Relations Board, the federal agency that regulates and rules on labor-management disputes, have even excluded working nurses whose job duties, such as being a charge nurse, are deemed to be supervisory. In a case decided on October 4, 2006, the NLRB created a new precedent by stating that charge nurses at a Michigan hospital could not be represented by a union because they did some supervisory work. The decision—known as the *Kentucky River* decision—was based on a 2001 U.S. Supreme Court case in which the Court decreed that nurses at a community-care facility in Kentucky could not be union members because they coordinated the care of less skilled personnel. In spite of the fact that they have no hiring and firing power, do not earn any more money in their temporary capacity as charge nurses, even a nurse who acts as a charge nurse only 10 percent of the time can be considered a supervisor and thus ineligible for union representation.[24]

Despite these significant differences in health-care systems and labor-management relations, the nurses and unions in California and Victoria faced very similar situations when they began their push for staffing ratios. In the early 1990s, state and federal governments in both the United States and Australia were trying to trim health-care costs. In Australia, from 1992 to 1999, a Liberal–National Party coalition government ruled in the State of Victoria. The most aggressive of a new breed of conservative governments to appear in Australia, it was explicitly modeled on the New Right philosophies of Margaret Thatcher in the United Kingdom and Ronald Reagan in the United States. Under this government, more than eighteen hundred nurses were fired in mass layoffs, and health-care budgets were slashed more drastically than in other states. When nurses pressed the state's conservative government for relief, Premier Jeff Kennett would not budge. It took years of public debate, media attention, political lobbying, favorable publicity, and industrial action to usher in staffing ratios. Ultimately, the voters moved for a change and elected a government led by the Australian Labor Party (ALP) in 1999. This created the political opening for the introduction and implementation of ratios.

In California, nurses faced similar cost cutting. There, the primary mechanism was "managed care." Under managed care both government and private payers micromanage clinical practice, usually via HMOs that set strict limits on hospitalizations, length of hospital stays, and physician services. As explained later in this book, California was the state hardest hit by managed care cost cutting and hospital restructuring. It has the highest penetration of managed care and employer-forced HMO participation in the country.

As in Victoria, CNA members and nurses in other unions began to protest the erosion of nursing care as soon as its impact was felt. With little initial success, they raised the issue of understaffing with state and federal legislators. When they finally developed enough political support to get a ratio bill passed in the state senate and assembly in 1998, the Republican governor, Pete Wilson, quickly vetoed the legislation. Only the election of a more labor-friendly Democratic governor, Gray Davis, enabled the CNA to get the same measure reintroduced, passed again, and signed into law in 1999.

At this point, however, the narratives in the two countries diverge. In Australia, the ratios were defined and settled as part of an arbitrated settlement to an intense industrial dispute. Before this settlement both parties agreed to abide by the arbitrators' decisions. Once made, the award (i.e., the legal instrument outlining the terms of settlement) was enforceable under Australian labor law and could not be changed by legislation at the state or federal level. Because ratios have the force of law, which the governing party agreed to respect, their implementation has been relatively smooth. The problems that have arisen since the ratios were introduced have occurred in rural and remote hospitals or on occasions when nurses ask for more staff to supplement ratios. Even after public-hospital managers (with state government support) unsuccessfully tried to jettison ratios in 2004, managers did not try to subvert them, and they continue to be effective in dealing with the critical issue of work overload.

In California, industry foot-dragging and efforts to undermine ratios significantly complicated and delayed their implementation. This reflects the unequal balance of power between organized labor and corporate interests in the United States. In 2003, the antiratio forces gained an additional ally in the form of newly elected Republican governor Arnold Schwarzenegger. The intervention of his administration prolonged the phasing in of the ratios for months.

Such rearguard action has a long history in lawmaking related to labor-management relations, working conditions, and patient safety in the United States. In 1935, Congress enacted the National Labor Relations Act—or Wagner Act—which forced private-sector employers to accept collective bargaining if their employees chose to be represented by a union. In appeals, which took two years to reach the Supreme Court, some employers argued that the NLRA violated their private property rights and prerogatives. During the same New Deal era, employers also resisted federal legislation establishing the eight-hour day and minimum wage standards on the grounds that it would drive them into bankruptcy.

Throughout the ensuing years, U.S. management has continued to fight—without exception—any expansion of job safety and health protection. As Michael Silverstein of the University of Washington has pointed out:

> Every significant workplace safety and health rule proposed at the federal or state level since the Occupational Safety and Health Act was passed in 1970 has met strong opposition from the business community. In virtually all such cases business representatives have argued that there was insufficient scientific evidence of risk; that the rule would interfere with business operations; and that compliance costs would be prohibitive. In many cases OSHA rules were adopted only after petitions, litigation and court orders. In other cases, Congress directed rulemaking. Most OSHA rules were challenged in court after adoption.[25]

Industry opposition has also stalled patient safety legislation in the form of efforts to better regulate managed care and the hospital industry.

This familiar scenario played out in California before and after the passage of AB 394. Rather than complying with the state's rule making, the hospital industry sponsored tutorials that implicitly encouraged nurse executives to derail the ratios. The industry challenged a key provision of the staffing-ratio regulations in state courts and lined up a friendly legislator to file a bill to revoke them. After making campaign contributions to governor-to-be Arnold Schwarzenegger, the California Healthcare Association (CHA)—the association that represents the hospital industry in California and that is affiliated with the American Hospital Association (AHA)—convinced him to issue an executive order suspending the implementation of the ratio phase-in. This created a chaotic stop-and-go legal situation that led to recalcitrance by hospitals that were preparing to implement ratios as required. Only by 2005, after extensive—and expensive—legal wrangling, were ratios finally implemented as intended.

In Australia, because of the high rate of unionization, workers were able to frame the debate about ratios in terms of quality public health care, patient safety, and nurses' well-being. There, the need for ratios was not judged only on their impact on patient care but also on how they affect nurse retention, recruitment, and health. In California, as we shall see, the focus on patient safety, while paramount, has overshadowed considerations of nurses' health, the nursing shortage, and working conditions.

Our presentation of the California and Victoria studies reflects these contextual differences as well as the authors' respective experiences. Because the ratios in the system in Victoria are more advanced and have been fully implemented, there is more material—especially statistical evidence—on their operation, impact, and how they work in practice. Much of this work has been done by the authors Tanya Bretherton and John Buchanan, who are based at the Workplace Research Centre in the University of Sydney's Faculty of Economics and Business. They undertake applied research on the changing nature of work for employers, unions, governments, and the nongovernment sector in areas as diverse as coal mining, engineering, retail, banking, and higher education. They have conducted several studies of the health workforce, especially of temporary doctors in public hospitals and labor shortages in the elder-care sector. Their most extensive studies in health have been about the recruitment and retention problems of nurses.

Since the late 1990s Buchanan and Bretherton, along with other colleagues at the Centre, have conducted a series of large-scale surveys of working conditions for nurses employed by the Victoria public-hospital system. The first survey predated the introduction of ratios and identified the need and strong support for their introduction among members of the Victorian Branch of the Australian Nursing Federation. Three subsequent surveys have examined how the ratios have operated in practice. This work has involved the conduct of focus groups and semistructured interviews with ANF (Victorian Branch) members. Insights from these sources have informed the development of comprehensive survey instruments that have been distributed to random samples of ANF (Victorian Branch) members. In addition, their insights about the evolution and operation of ratios is based on interviews with key informants (managerial as well as union) involved in their development and implementation, scrutiny of publicly available material (e.g., arbitration decisions), and consideration of limited circulation documents, especially working papers and material associated with collective bargaining about the ratios. All of these sources are used in their description and analysis of ratios in section 2.

Author Suzanne Gordon is a journalist and expert on nursing workforce issues. She has spent the past twenty years chronicling nursing practice, the impact of contemporary nursing shortages, and the changing image of nursing. Her account of the ratios in California, which appears in section 1, includes personal interviews and analysis of scientific studies, court documents, confidential memos, media reports, state and federal reports, and other data.

In their discussions of arguments for and against ratios, all three authors have also analyzed virtually all the published scientific studies that link nurse staffing to patient outcomes and consider a variety of other solutions to the global nursing shortage.

This book is a collaborative effort that considers staffing ratios in Victoria and California and addresses the following questions:

- What kinds of working conditions and relationships with management produce the ratio response?
- Are ratios a one-size-fits-all solution that is simply pulled out of thin air? Or does the determination of ratios result from sound analysis?
- What specific problems do ratios solve? Are they *the* answer to the nursing crisis and nursing shortages, or must they be viewed as part of a

broader strategy to solve the myriad problems—job satisfaction, burnout, recruitment, and retention—that nursing faces?

- Are ratios a cost-effective component of the patient-safety agenda?
- Are ratios, in fact, a key component of the integrity of the nursing profession?
- Finally, are the accounts of the history and implementation of nurse-staffing ratios relevant to other health-care workers and workers outside of health care who face ceaseless pressure to work longer hours and be more productive in the face of real and exaggerated global competition?

A Road Map of the Book

To answer these questions, section 1 of this book, which was written by Suzanne Gordon, recounts the struggle for ratios in California. Chapter 1 sets the historical and political context by explaining the impact of managed care—the cornerstone of U.S. health-care reform in the 1990s—on nursing practice and patient care in the most populous state in the United States. Chapter 1 also explains how nurses successfully campaigned for ratios by framing them as a patient-safety issue so they could mobilize the kind of public support necessary to overcome both hospital industry and political opposition to their proposed legislation.

Chapter 2 chronicles the lengthy process of administrative investigation and deliberation the California Department of Health Services followed to produce its final ratio regulations. Chapter 3 looks at how the hospital industry continued to mobilize against ratios; how the California Nurses Association responded to this renewed attack; and how subsequent political events and legal decisions finally thwarted Governor Schwarzenegger's opposition to the implementation of the ratio legislation. Chapter 4 examines the introduction of ratios at the hospital level. Here staff nurses, nurse managers, and directors of nursing assess the successes and failures of the ratio bill.

In section 2 on the Victoria experience, John Buchanan and Tanya Bretherton begin with two chapters detailing the working conditions and intensification of work in Victoria. These chapters, 5 and 6, also analyze the particular political context in which ratios emerged as a solution. Chapter 7 describes the campaign to gain staffing ratios and how the specific ratios were determined. Chapter 8 describes the implementation process and evaluates the impact of ratios on the nursing workload. Bedside nurses describe their responses to ratio requirements on their units. Nurse unit managers and directors of nursing explain that many nurse managers and directors of nursing have used ratios to establish better working relations with nursing staff and their union. Some have built on ratios to introduce innovations designed to both recruit and retain nursing staff. Chapter 8 summarizes the problems and concerns that ratios do not—and, in our view, cannot—resolve.

In the book's third and last section, in chapter 9 we evaluate the studies that explore the relationship of nursing and nurse staffing to patient outcomes. In it we also discuss studies that link workplace conditions to nurses' occupational illnesses and injuries. Although we believe that ratios are part of the solution to the nursing crisis and thus a way to improve patient care, in chapter 10 we carefully consider objections to them. Is there a scientific basis for linking nurse staffing to patient safety? What is really known about staffing levels and nurses' health? Are ratios too costly, and how can they be funded in different kinds of health-care systems? Do they cause hospital and emergency room closures? Do they deprofessionalize a group that has long sought greater professional legitimacy? Are they a one-size-fits-all solution? In this chapter, we also look at other proposed solutions to the nursing crisis.

In our concluding chapter we explain why we believe ratios are a necessary— but not sufficient—solution to the many difficulties nurses encounter as they try to deliver quality patient care in a complex, high-tech health-care environment in which often short-sighted considerations of cost, efficiency, and effectiveness dominate the decision-making process.

Although the issue of trade unions is particularly controversial in the United States, this book is largely a story of the action of nurses in labor unions. No matter what one's positions on trade unions, it's inarguable that they have been at the forefront of efforts to improve conditions for all of those who work for a living. In a previous era, people who worked in the traditional union territories of mining, construction, and manufacturing were the ones who championed advances such as the eight-hour day, the forty-hour week, and the now taken-for-granted weekends off and annual vacation. Today, partly reflecting the increasing importance of the service economy, union territory has shifted into sectors such as health and education. Standards set in these workplaces provide a benchmark for others. While issues of wages and allied conditions remain important, in today's world issues of quality of working life are increasingly viewed as central to people's experiences at work and in life outside it. In this context, the issue of work intensification is increasingly recognized as a growing problem. Lessons offered by nursing, therefore, are of central relevance to all with an interest in how work can be improved in an era in which so many people—many of them women—are now involved in producing services and not just products.

We believe that telling the story of ratios in Victoria and California will not only help nurses and patients elsewhere but also provide useful insights into the broader challenges of regulating and improving working conditions throughout the new global economy.

PART I

California: Managed Care, Hospital Restructuring, and the Ratio Response

1

Hospital Restructuring and the Erosion of Nursing Care in California and the United States

As a young recruit new to nursing, Summer Vanslager is both a statistic and a phenomenon. As a modern young woman she has an entire professional world open to her and could have decided to be a doctor, lawyer, or banker. Instead, she chose nursing because she wanted a career in which she could make a difference and be close to patients. Unlike her nursing foremothers, however, she is unwilling to put up with relentless self-sacrifice. During both her nursing school apprenticeship and her first year on the job, Vanslager found that the ratio of satisfaction to sacrifice was less than reassuring. In spite of this, Vanslager fell in love with oncology nursing and got a job on an oncology unit at Dominican Hospital in Santa Cruz, California, after graduation. By November 2004, she had been working for a year, which was enough time to convince her that unless something changed for the better, there was no way she would stay at the hospital working at the bedside for more than a couple of years.

When she was a student and learned from nurses on an oncology floor, she says, conditions were nothing short of "barbaric." "We were working with seven or eight patients. It was gruesome." Her patients had breast, lung, colon, or other cancers. They knew they could die. She knew they could die. They were getting heavy-duty chemotherapy. They were terrified. "You couldn't get any sense of who they were. There was no way to know the patients, let alone know what was the right equipment or medications and how to use it," she says. Had she entered the wrong profession, Vanslager wondered? Or was it just hospital work that was the problem?

The questions continued to mount when she graduated and went into the hospital workforce. Would she move on to less stressful work after a year or two or stay at the hospital bedside and thus contribute to ending California's—and the nation's—serious nursing shortage? Many newly graduated nurses shared Vanslager's dilemma. In fact, just as she was entering the workforce, several studies, including one conducted by Julie Sochalski, a University of Pennsylvania nursing workforce researcher, were quantifying the experiences of new graduates entering the hospital setting. Sochalski, for example, found that "raising particular concern is the increasing proportion of new RNs who are not working in nursing." More new male nurses than female nurses were leaving the profession, but "the proportion of female entrants who were not working in nursing also increased."[1]

At the time of this writing, new recruit Vanslager, going against the odds, had at least for the time being decided to remain at the bedside. Why? Because she believed that working conditions were changing for the better in California's acute care hospitals. In 1999, the California legislature passed AB 394, a statute introduced years earlier by Assemblymember Sheila Kuehl establishing minimum patient-to-nurse ratios in all acute care hospitals in the most populous state in the United States. After a complicated three-year process, the California Department of Health Services (CDHS) set minimum staffing ratios that would be phased in starting in January 2004. On medical/surgical floors and specialty units such as oncology (which account for the majority of patient capacity in any hospital), no nurse could be asked to care for more than six patients at any time, day or night. Other ratios applied to additional units. Moreover on January 1, 2005, the ratios would be even "richer." On medical/surgical and specialty floors, the ratio would be set at 1:5. By 2008, oncology units like Vanslager's would have a 1:4 ratio.

When Vanslager started work the ratios had just been implemented. "It was like a breath of fresh air," she said, as if just inhaling. "We could actually read charts. We could find out about our patients and deliver safe care."

She said her hospital abided by the ratios most of the time. In November 2004, they were planning to staff up to the 1:4 ratio that would have been implemented in January 2005. Then on November 12, 2004, just a few days after President George W. Bush was reelected, California governor Arnold Schwarzenegger announced that he was suspending the phase-in of the next stage of the ratios, which would have assured nurses like Vanslager that they would not be asked to take care of more than four patients at a time. He argued that the nurse-staffing ratios had created a health-care "emergency" and that the ratios were responsible for hospital and bed closures, staff cuts, and undue financial strain on California's hospitals.

Vanslager, like thousands of other nurses in California, remembers feeling stunned at this news. "I just wondered if he'd ever actually visited a hospital. If he knew what it's like to have so many patients and to try to take care of them," she recalled. The California Nurses Association, the union that led the battle for the staffing-ratio bill, immediately filed a suit against Schwarzenegger. The suit alleged that the administration had exceeded its authority, and the union demanded that the ratios be implemented as scheduled. Even though the public supported the bill, Vanslager worried about the outcome of this legal action. The governor had received campaign contributions from a state hospital industry that was a powerful force in California politics and adamantly opposed the implementation of the staffing-ratio bill.

In March 2005, however, Sacramento Superior Court Judge Judy Holzer Hersher issued a decision that rejected every claim the governor and the California Department of Health Services had made. The judge ruled that the phasing in of the ratios must continue. Later that year, the CNA, along with other unions representing public-sector workers, again battled the governor. Governor Schwarzenegger was pushing a statewide referendum, which, if passed, would limit public-sector unions' ability to use members' dues for political lobbying. When this referendum was soundly defeated in November 2005, the governor immediately stated that he would forego any further efforts to fight the implementation of the phasing in of the nurse-to-patient staffing ratios.

For nurses like Summer Vanslager, this was welcome news. "Thank God," she said. When I asked her what she would have done if the phase-in had not continued, she sighed. If things had not continued to change for the better in California hospitals, she said, she would have left hospital nursing. "Absolutely!" she asserted. "I would have gone into home care or hospice. I would not have been able to continue in such stressful work. I would have gone to work someplace where there is less physical labor and more time with patients."

We Can't Cut 'Em Fast Enough

Whether they are new nurses or more experienced and older ones, RNs who are involved in direct care throughout California have marched and rallied, stood in vigils in the cold and rain, and engaged in letter-writing campaigns and door-to-door political canvassing in support of ratios. During the mid to late 1990s nurses began to argue that they were working in an increasingly money-driven, rather than quality-oriented, health-care system in which managers were forced to focus more on the bottom line than on quality care. As Californians, moreover, they lived and worked in a state that has been hit by one of the most extreme forms of U.S.-style managed care.

After a decade of cost cutting and hospital restructuring in which nursing had been deskilled and deprofessionalized, organized nurses insisted that staffing ratios represented their attempt to assert professionalism. They did this through a legislated mechanism that they believed would give them greater control over their workload. As nurses involved in the fight for ratios in California and elsewhere in the United States emphasized to the public and policymakers, they believed that legislation was one of the only ways they could ensure patient safety and their own professional integrity. It was, moreover, a vehicle to protect their own health and well-being in the face of an epidemic of workplace injuries and stress-related illnesses. Indeed, they argued that patient safety and worker safety are interconnected. Nurses won't be there to take care of patients if they leave the bedside because of intolerable stress, stress-related illnesses, and increasing levels of occupational injury. They can't be attentive to patients' needs if chronic workplace stress leaves them so burned out that they are unable to muster empathy for their patients' pain and discomfort.

Many nurses in California believed that the only way they could gain a measure of professional control over their work was to make government an ally. They chose this path because they had tried everything else. They had tried appealing to their professional managers, the nurse middle-level and high-level managers who throughout the staffing-ratio debate declared themselves to be the guardians of nursing's professional integrity. Yet, when nurses begged hospital nurse managers for workload relief, they said they were told they were being alarmist, resisting change, and acting selfishly. Although managers argued that they were not cutting nursing care to the bone, in the twenty-first century many admitted that that's just what they did. As Jeanette Ives Erickson, senior vice president for patient-care services and chief nurse executive at Massachusetts General Hospital, said of the restructuring of hospital nursing in a recent U.S. public radio series on the nursing crisis, "We just couldn't cut 'em fast enough."[2]

In California, as floor nurses registered growing concerns about unit staffing, they say they agreed to work to implement patient acuity systems (sometimes referred to as patient acuity or dependency systems) that would computerize decisions about their workload and determine how many hours of nursing care patients would receive. As we shall see, hospitals did not abide by the data on acuity that their own systems generated. The legislative solution to eroding working conditions was, many bedside nurses argue, a last-ditch response to conditions that few contest were untenable and the existence of which even high-level executives have come to ruefully acknowledge.

The struggle for staffing ratios as a solution to the nursing crisis in California is one that engages some of the thorniest issues in U.S. or even global health care. When compared with the story behind and the state of ratios in Victoria, it becomes even more interesting—illustrating the differences between workplace transformation in Australia's highly unionized, public national health-care system and the privatized, market-driven system in the more politically polarized United States.

The key actors in this drama are the three nursing unions that fought for ratios; the California Healthcare Association, which fought against them; the Department of Health Services, which implemented (and then opposed) the law; and three California governors. Heading up this cast of characters is the California Nurses Association, an all-RN union that, until 1995, was part of the American Nurses Association. Because members of the collective bargaining arm of the CNA believed that the ANA was not acting assertively enough in the face of managed-care and health-care cost cutting, the unionized nurses split from the ANA in a bitter divorce whose reverberations are still felt today. Its twenty-four thousand members formed their own independent labor organization, which led the battle for ratios.

The other unions involved were the Service Employees International Union (a national union that was at that time affiliated with the AFL-CIO) that represented RNs and LVNs, many in public-sector hospitals. Finally, another union player was the United Nurses Association of California, which represents RNs in Southern California and which is affiliated with the American Federation of State County and Municipal Employees.

On the opposing side of the ratio dispute stood the California Hospital Association—later to be renamed the California Healthcare Association (CHA)—whose members include over four hundred, or over 85 percent, of the state's acute care hospitals. The CHA has been and still is opposed to ratios. In addition to the California Department of Health Services, which regulates the state's hospitals, critical players included California governors Republican Pete Wilson, who served from 1991 to 1999, Democrat Gray Davis, who was elected in 1998 and served one and a half terms from 1999 to 2003, and Republican Arnold Schwarzenegger, who replaced Davis in a special recall election in 2003 and was reelected in 2006.

The Reemergence of Ratios

Although the ratio legislation was enacted and signed into law in 1999, the story of California nurse-staffing ratios actually began with the passage of what came to be known as Title 22 in the 1976–77 state legislative session. This mandated a standard for a nursing presence on at least some units in acute care hospitals. It stated that "there shall be registered nurses, licensed vocational nurse and operating room technicians in the appropriate ratio to ensure that at all times a registered nurse is available to serve as the circulating nurse."[3] Although the appropriate ratio was not defined for the operating room, it was specified for intensive care units and intensive-care nurseries: "A ratio of one registered nurse to two or fewer intensive care patients shall be maintained" in intensive care, newborn nursing, and in ICUs "the nurse:patient ratio shall be

1:2 or fewer at all times. Vocational nurses may constitute up to 50% of the licensed nurses." Similarly, on perinatal units, the regulations mandated that "a ratio of one licensed nurse to eight or fewer infants shall be maintained for normal infants."[4]

Throughout the 1980s and early 1990s there was no movement to expand the use of ratios to include other acute care hospital units. With the advent of health-care cost cutting and hospital restructuring in the mid-1990s, nurses' work changed dramatically, and the idea of extending ratios to other hospital units surfaced.

After the election of President Bill Clinton and the failure of the Clinton health reform proposal, managed care produced a rash of hospital cost cutting and belt tightening that had an enormous impact on nursing.[5] Nursing care was restructured or reengineered, as hospitals replaced experienced and expensive registered nurses with what became known as "unlicensed assistive personnel" (UAP). Reports of staff cuts became common in the mainstream and industry media. Publications such as the weekly *Modern Healthcare* ran stories reporting that "from 1993 through January of 1996, 140 hospitals or systems laid off a total of 23,910 workers, or an average layoff of 171 workers per hospital." Their article "Jobs Go First," based on a survey of hospital administrators, revealed that more hospital executives said they would save money by cutting staff than by limiting capital improvements or research and development.[6]

California, which had the highest "penetration" in the nation of managed-care health plans, was the hardest hit of all the states. It thus had the dubious distinction of ranking fiftieth in the nation in terms of the nurse-population ratio.[7]

The hundreds of nurses laid off from California hospitals was not the only factor creating disaffection among the state's nurses. Work overload quickly became a major problem, not only because fewer nurses were taking care of the same number—or more—patients but also because patients themselves were becoming more intensely ill while in the hospital. This increase in patient acuity was a by-product of one of managed care's most significant cost-cutting strategies—reducing the length of hospital stay for patients.

Under the traditional fee-for-service coverage that managed-care plans aimed to replace, both doctors and hospitals profited by keeping patients in the hospital as long as possible. Because there was no incentive to limit lengths of stay, costs mushroomed.

The reduction of hospital stays accelerated in 1983, when, in an effort to rein in hospital expenses, the federal government instituted a hospital reimbursement system known as the prospective payment system (PPS) for Medicare, its program for older Americans. Under PPS, patients were categorized by what were called diagnostic related groups (DRGs), and no matter how long a patient stayed, the hospital received a flat fee based on the patient's diagnosis. Hospitals suddenly had an incentive to discharge patients sooner: if the DRG allocated payment for what was anticipated to be a three-day stay and the patient stayed only a day, the hospital pocketed the difference.

Many private health insurers quickly adopted the idea. Indeed, an influential early study by H. S. Luft that was published in 1978 in the *New England Journal of Medicine* concluded that virtually all the savings achieved by health maintenance organizations—the typical managed-care insurance plan—were due to lower rates of hospitalization.[8] Their lower cost was the main reason employers, who are the major purchasers of health insurance in the United States, welcomed HMOs so enthusiastically.

According to several studies, the incentives worked. The Princeton economist Uwe Reinhardt found that from 1980 to 1993 the number of days patients spent in the hospital was cut by more than 36 percent, leaving the United States with the shortest length of hospital stay in the industrialized world.[9]

As the leader of the managed-care revolution, California also led the nation in shortened length of hospital stay. In fact, California's record had become so pleasing to insurers and hospital administrators that they used it as a benchmark for physician practice elsewhere. One doctor interviewed in the mid-1990s reported that when he went to work at a small community hospital in New Jersey in 1996, he found a flyer warning that hospital management was now profiling physicians and benchmarking them on their discharge patterns. Doctors would soon learn whether their patients were staying in the hospital longer than patients cared for by other staff doctors and with those cared for by doctors in California. According to the announcement, "the last column tells us how many days would have been saved ("opportunities") if we were as efficient as the California hospitals."[10]

Alyson Kennedy, a fifty-five-year-old RN, also at Santa Cruz's Dominican Hospital, explains how shortened length of stay transformed nursing by comparing her patients on a medical/surgical floor in the 1980s with those she cared for in the 1990s:

> In the eighties, we had three nurses on a thirty-bed floor, with one charge nurse. That means that two nurses each had fifteen patients on the day shift, and ten patients on the p.m. shift—3:30 to 11:00 . . . that was the one I worked. In the eighties we had ten patients and we also had the same number in the nineties. The thing was those patients were very different. Back then, two or three of the patients you had were just spending the night before surgery. Many were staying longer after surgery. So there would be some patients who were just easier. You didn't have as many nursing interventions to deliver. The patients could walk and talk and take care of some of their own needs, like brushing their teeth or feeding themselves.

Nurses also had fewer intravenous medications to administer. "For pain control all you gave were IM [intramuscular] injections of Demerol and maybe an antiemetic [antinausea drug], and you did that every three to four hours. There weren't many IV therapies. They had IVs but you'd just hang up bags of fluids, not adding medications like antibiotics or pain medication," Kennedy said.

In the 1990s all that changed. The patients stopped coming into the hospital the night before an operation and started going home fairly quickly after surgery. Plus, there were many more intravenous therapies.

> We gave a lot more IV pain medications, like Demerol and morphine drips, which means there were more problems with people being overly sedated. Sometimes it was really overwhelming. You'd have ten rooms and maybe seven would be fresh post-ops, and you were just running the whole night and praying that nothing bad was going on in one of the rooms that you didn't know about. It seemed like the patients were getting sicker and sicker and sicker. There were no easy patients anymore. The easier ones were either outpatients or treated at home.

What is more, Kennedy said, the DRGs and administrative pressure to increase hospital "through-put" (a term that became common currency in the 1990s) meant that patients weren't just rushed out the door, they were also rushed off more expensive units like the ICUs to telemetry or medical/surgical units like Kennedy's: "You were getting patients who were monitored more closely on ICU, and you had to take care of them on a med/surg floor. But they were much, much sicker than the usual med/surg patient."

The increased patient load, Kennedy said, meant that there was too much work for one nurse to accomplish in her eight-hour shift. So more nurses were working overtime. According to Kennedy, hospitals would pressure nurses not to put in for overtime pay:

> When you're a new nurse, there's lot of pressure not to put in for overtime. At our hospital, before the union came in, we'd have meetings about overtime. My manager wanted to give me a written warning for overtime abuse. I remember I refused to sign it. I said, "It's not me; I'm a very efficient worker and a careful nurse. It's the system. You just can't have this many patients and expect nurses to get out on time. It's just not possible."

Which is why Kennedy feels that a flood of overtime work fueled the support for ratios:

> Not only are nurses doing their jobs, but we're punished for doing our job if you have to stay overtime. What do these people want? We're not machines here. We're doing the best we can. You're asking us to do something that's not humanly possible, to take care of all these patients. And yet somehow we're not supposed to put in for overtime or get breaks.

In fact, Kennedy became so discouraged by the situation that she quit nursing: "I just loved nursing. But I couldn't do it anymore." Eventually, it was the ratio bill, she said, that brought her back into the workforce.

Throughout the country nurses like Kennedy voiced their discontent by protesting and by leaving as she did. Diane Sosne, head of the SEIU's Nurse Alliance—the union's internal organization of RNs and LPNs—recalled the union's efforts: "After thousands of nurses rang the alarm bell in the early nineties on the dangers of short staffing on patient care and the nursing profession, the Service Employees International Union's Nurse Alliance conducted a national nurse survey of ten thousand SEIU nurses." The results were reported to the subcommittee on Health and the Environment of the House Energy and Commerce Committee in 1993, when the nurses testified on the erosion of hospital nursing care. Nurses described "the adverse effects of poor or inadequate staffing on patients and nursing staff."[11] The subcommittee decided that it needed an "independent assessment" of these problems and assigned the job to the Institute of Medicine (IOM), a unit of the National Academy of Sciences created to bring together "distinguished members of the appropriate professions who conduct examinations of policy matters pertaining to the health of the public." In 1994, the IOM assembled a sixteen-member committee of experts that included nursing academics, nursing administrators, a professor of law, a professor of economics, a health-care consultant, and a hospital administrator—but not one staff nurse or representative of a staff nurses' union or organization. Their mandate was "to determine whether and to what extent there is a need for an increase in the number of nurses in hospitals and nursing homes to promote the quality of patient care and to reduce the incidence among nurses of work-related injuries and stress."[12]

The same month, nurses from across the United States marched on Washington to protest cuts in nursing staff in acute care hospitals. A nursing magazine called *Revolution*, edited by critical-care nurse Laura Gasparis Vonfrolio, organized the march. Nurses from California were among the twenty-five thousand RNs, including frontline nurses, academics, and students, who proceeded along Pennsylvania Avenue to the Capitol. Along with nurses from the SEIU and other unions, the president of the CNA, Kit Costello, spoke on a dais positioned directly in front of the Capitol building. The following year nurses rallied again in Washington, and once again they warned that restructuring of nursing staff was hurting patient care, reducing nurses' job satisfaction, and increasing their burnout. Nurses predicted that layoffs and the hospitals' failure to fill nursing positions created by attrition would create a serious shortage by the end of the twentieth century.

Industry groups, such as the California Healthcare Association, insisted that nurses were being alarmist. Nursing executives and middle-level managers argued that reports of patient harm were exaggerated and anecdotal, and that there was no scientific evidence to back up the staff nurses' claims. Staff nurses, they insisted, were afraid of change.[13] Nursing executives also insisted that ratios would deprofessionalize nursing, taking staffing decisions out of the nurses' control and allowing government bureaucrats to dictate to nurses.

Although the hospital industry claimed that nurses' concerns could not be scientifically verified, the process of verification was, in fact, already beginning. One of the first researchers to look at the problems that hospital restructuring had created was the Boston College professor Judith Shindul-Rothschild. In both 1989 and 1994, Shindul-Rothschild surveyed Massachusetts nurses (928 and 856 in each year, respectively) about their working conditions. The nurses represented a geographical cross-section of hospitals of all kinds in Massachusetts. In 1989 only two nurses reported difficulty providing safe patient care due to inadequate RN staffing. In 1994 that figure sharply rose to 49 percent of all respondents, and nurses reported marked deterioration in patient care as numbers of RNs decreased and unlicensed personnel increased. In 1989 no nurses reported patient deaths. In 1994 nurses reported fifteen patient deaths due to inadequate staffing levels. For example, in an intensive care unit an alarm sounded on a patient's ventilator, signaling that the patient was going into cardiac arrest. The nurse was too busy with other patients to respond, and the patient died. In another case, a patient was accidentally disconnected from a ventilator, and the nurse was so busy she was unable to observe this fact. Six patients committed suicide. A teenager killed himself in a psychiatric unit at night. Another young man hung himself on a general medical floor. Yet another patient in a community hospital hung himself in a jacket restraint and was discovered by nurses too late to be saved.[14]

The Campaign Begins

To deal with the eroding care researchers were beginning to document, the California Nurses Association proposed its first staffing-ratio bill. The CNA launched a political campaign to lobby legislators. To win broad public support the organization also paid for radio, television, and print ads that ran in California newspapers and the *New York Times*. One dramatic advertisement featured the up-close image of a hand on a patient call button. "It's 3 a.m. WHO WILL COME WHEN YOU NEED HELP?" the headline asked. The ad copy asserted that "hospitals and HMOs are cutting care to make record profits. Patients are paying the price. Just ask any registered nurse who provides direct care." The ads asked members of the public to write letters to a

"Patient Watch" program "if your care or the care of your loved one suffered because of short staffing."[15]

People did indeed send in heart-wrenching accounts of tragedies or trials that had occurred because of a lack of expert nursing care. "Our family has suffered from the death of our daughter because of short staff and/or inadequate care in a local hospital. At about 3 a.m., Tuesday, June 7, she vomited and aspirated the vomit, causing cardiac arrest and then seizures. She then went into a coma and was in the coma until she died," a parent wrote.

Another parent, the mother of a premature baby, sent the following story. "I can't count the number of times I saved my son's life and the life of the child in a neighboring room. The nursing was five (patients) to one (nurse); at least that is what they told us. We had things happen (like) being told to pay for a babysitter to watch our son if we wanted to leave. We would go for eight hours without seeing a nurse."

What was interesting was that many patients and family members did not attribute their problems to the failings of individual nurses but to the system as a whole. "Nurses do a terrific job, but more nurses are needed to nurse the patients in the hospitals, not just to hook up patients and take the vitals," a San Francisco resident wrote.[16]

In spite of this barrage of complaints from both patients and nurses, the Republican-controlled state legislature and Republican governor Pete Wilson refused to consider the staffing bill. Instead, a compromise was reached. The state of California would promulgate regulations requiring that all California hospitals implement what were known as "patient classification systems" (PCSs). The regulations that were finally implemented in January 1997 were the product of negotiation and discussion among state nursing associations and the California Hospital Association.

According to the California Code of Regulations, Title 22, "Licensing and Certification of Health Facilities and Referral Agencies," all licensed and certified general acute care hospitals in California had to purchase and utilize some sort of PCS. As stipulated in the regulations, "The hospital shall implement a patient classification system . . . determining nursing care needs of individual patients that reflects the assessment made by a registered nurses . . . of patient requirements."

PCS systems were to create a "method to predict nursing care requirements of individual patients." Systems were to establish a "method by which the amount of nursing care needed for each category of patients is validated for each unit and each shift, and each level of licensed and unlicensed staff." Hospitals had to "validate the reliability of the patient classification system for each unit and each shift," and administrators had to develop a written staffing plan based on the needs determined by the PCS.

These plans had to include:

- Staffing plans, as determined by the PCS for each unit, that documented on a day-to-day, shift-by-shift basis the variance between required and actual staffing patterns.
- An annual review by a committee of nurses of the reliability of the PCS. The members of the committee were to be appointed by the nursing administrator, and half of the committee had to include nurses giving direct patient care. Any adjustments needed in the PCS to "assure accuracy in measuring care needs" had to be made "within thirty days."
- A process, developed and documented by the hospital, by which "all interested staff may provide input about the patient classification system, the system's required revisions, and the overall staffing plan."[17]

Title 22 created an in-hospital "process" that allowed interested staff to comment on hospital staffing plans. Nurses did, in fact, express many concerns about the reliability and accuracy of these systems. Throughout 1997 and 1998, nurses in California argued to their administrators, the media, legislators, and the public that hospitals were not abiding by their own acuity-measurement systems. Interested nurses, they contended, had difficulty expressing their concerns about these systems because they weren't "transparent and easily accessible." As Deborah Burger, 2007 CNA president and a nurse in Santa Rosa, explained, Title 22 did not mandate a standardized patient acuity system in California hospitals. She said that there are more than six hundred patient acuity systems in hospitals in the state. Because these tools are proprietary, nurses weren't—and still aren't—clear about how the data they input about patients and their needs is translated into a determination of how many nursing hours per patient day a particular patient needs. Even when nurses were able to fathom the complex computer algorithms, they argued, hospitals weren't staffing according to the numbers that patient acuity systems generated.

These concerns are reflected in more objective discussions of the use of patient acuity systems to determine nurse staffing. In 2005, for example, James Buchan, professor in the Department of Management and Social Science at Queen Margaret University College in Edinburgh, conducted a review of staffing ratios in Australia and California for the Royal College of Nursing in the United Kingdom. On the subject of patient acuity systems, Buchan wrote:

> Various locally developed and proprietary systems are being used. Some are generic, and have scope for widespread application, others have been specifically developed to be applied within one specialty, or area of practice, such as ICU or midwifery.
>
> The challenge with using "off the shelf" or bespoke systems of workload assessment and staffing determination is that their application can all too easily become a numbers game, an end in itself rather than a decision support

mechanism. They can also be time intensive to use, can be "data hungry," and can fall into disrepute if their recommended staffing levels are not then implemented by the organization.

The other major point to note when selecting a system is that there is no single "right" answer to the question, what is the best staffing level for this ward? Research has demonstrated that different systems applied in the same care environment will give different staffing "answers."[18]

In other words, patient acuity systems, which are often said to be the sharp instrument that is needed to replace the "blunt instrument" of staffing ratios, may be equally dull.

That is precisely what nurses in California argued. Kelly DiGiacomo was one of them. The forty-seven-year-old mother of two, who was later to play a surprising role in the ratio saga, has been a nurse since 1995. She entered the workforce just at the height of restructuring and has always worked at a Kaiser Permanente hospital in labor and delivery, newborn nurseries, pediatrics, and now telemetry. Her first job at Kaiser was at the Morse Avenue Hospital in Sacramento. Her voice was filled with exhaustion just at the thought of her initiation to hospital RN work. "They were constantly threatening us with layoffs and downsizing," she recalled. In fact, she was so fearful about losing her job in labor and delivery that she soon took a job in a pediatric clinic. "A lot of nurses were so nervous about all the layoffs that they either left the hospital, like me, or left nursing. I think," she added parenthetically, "that that made the nursing shortage even worse."

"The work," she continued, "was just very, very heavy. Back then you could be canceled anytime. They could call you two hours before your shift, if they were kind enough to do that, and let you know they didn't need you. There were no ratios, and things were just crazy. I remember one time on the postpartum unit when I had fifteen moms and babies. It was so unsafe. You just felt like you were just running, throwing pills at your patients. You dreaded what to do if they asked you a question."

That particular night, DiGiacomo recalled, she came home from work, threw herself on the couch in her uniform and fell asleep. The next day, when she woke up bleary eyed, she was surprised to find herself still fully clothed. "Many times I thought about leaving nursing," she recalled. "I was torn between my love of the profession and the craft of nursing and my love of people and of my patients. But these extreme working conditions were just too much."

They precluded not only patient safety but a life outside work, time to refuel and also to fulfill other caregiving responsibilities. She had a twelve-year-old daughter and a sixteen-year-old son and a husband who was being treated for leukemia and who couldn't work. She said, "I was the sole breadwinner. I couldn't quit. I just kept thinking, how many nurses out there are like me? We have families, young children, and maybe a family member who's really sick, and we're taking care of these really sick people under these incredible conditions."

Although hospitals dismissed the complaints of nurses like DiGiacomo, they were confirmed in 1998, when the California Department of Health Services surveyed over 160 of California's acute care hospitals. The CDHS found that 61 percent of facilities were out of compliance with Title 22 patient classification systems, and 87 percent were deficient "in the specific sections that require the facility to establish a PCS and to staff based on patient needs."[19]

Once again, nurses believed that legislatively mandated ratios were the only way they could be assured that they wouldn't be asked to care for too many patients. RNs recognized, moreover, that ratios were hardly a revolutionary solution to work overload and that they were common in other sectors. For years, for example, firefighters have had regulatory limits on how many firefighters must be on a fire truck. In many states, by regulation, family day-care providers can't take care of more than a certain number of infants and a preset number of toddlers, and federal regulations stipulate that one flight attendant is required for every fifty seats on a commercial aircraft. CNA nurses wanted similar limits on the number of patients they cared for. On medical/surgical and specialty units (the vast majority in a hospital) they proposed a ratio of one nurse to three patients, with other ratios proposed for other units.

In support of the argument for ratios, the Institute for Health and Socio-Economic Policy (IHSP), a CNA-sponsored nonprofit research and policy group, conducted a study analyzing 18.2 million California discharge records as well as other government and hospital data. It found an 8.8 percent increase in the average number of patients cared for by each full-time RN and a 7.2 decrease in the number of full-time RNs employed during the period from 1994 to 1997. Between 1995 and 1998, the number of patients per staffed bed had increased by 7.7 percent, and this increase took place in the state with the second lowest ratio of RNs to patients in the United States.[20]

As the IHSP published its results, more national data on the nursing crisis were published. Shindul-Rothschild, in collaboration with the *American Journal of Nursing*, applied her Massachusetts survey to RNs across the entire country. In November 1996, the *AJN* published a report of responses from over seventy-five hundred of those RNs. Sixty percent said patient length of stay had decreased; 73 percent reported they had less time to teach, talk to, or comfort patients or families. More disturbing, 69 percent said they had less time to provide basic nursing care. Sixty percent of nurses said that they had fewer RN colleagues providing direct patient care to work with, and 66 percent said that patients were sicker and they had to care for more of those sicker patients.[21]

In 1996, the IOM also released its findings, *Nursing Staff in Hospitals and Nursing Homes: Is It Adequate?* The report was both satisfying and infuriating to many nurses giving direct care. The study validated nurses' concerns in exhaustive detail. It stated unequivocally that managed care and hospital restructuring were focused on reducing operating costs and that both had transformed work processes and roles and jobs. It stated that "staff reductions or changes in the labor mix are at times implemented without attention to the organizational changes that might facilitate the possibility of better patient outcomes with fewer, more appropriately trained and used staff."[22] The report documented that poorly trained nursing assistants were replacing RNs. One study of particular relevance was conducted in California and found that most hospitals were using these ancillary personnel. Researchers found that 99 percent of California hospitals reported fewer than 120 hours of on-the-job training for newly hired ancillary personnel. "Only 20 percent of the hospitals required a high school diploma. The majority of hospitals (59 percent) provided fewer than 20 hours of classroom instruction and 88 percent provided 40 or fewer hours of instruction time."[23] This evidence confirmed that the use of nursing assistants who lacked proper training could add to—rather than reduce—nurses' workloads.

The report also confirmed that hospitalized patients were more acutely ill and documented the increasing hazards in the nursing workplace: "Whereas the injury and illness rate in private industry as a whole has been stable or declining slightly since 1980, the rates for hospitals and nursing homes during the same period have increased by about 52 percent and 62 percent, respectively."[24] The report also confirmed that there was increased stress and violence in the hospital workplace.

Nonetheless, the IOM argued that there was not enough research documenting the relationship of size of nursing staff to quality of care and that there was "a serious paucity of research on the definitive effects of structural measures, such as specific staffing ratios, on the quality of patient care in terms of outcomes when controlling for all other likely explanatory or confounding variables."[25] The IOM did not, therefore, recommend staffing ratios as a remedy for the many problems its own committee catalogued in such extensive detail. Instead, it suggested a series of voluntary measures. Although they did not explain how such nurses could cope with the eroding conditions they documented, the committee recommended that hospitals should employ more advanced-practice nurses. They should document "evidence that ancillary nursing personnel are competent and that such personnel are tested and certified by an appropriate entity for this competence." They recommended further training for nursing assistants. The report also advocated the inclusion of RNs in restructuring and redesign schemes, as well as the monitoring and evaluation of effects of organizational redesign on patient outcomes, patient satisfaction, and nurses themselves.

Because the committee thought there was no conclusive scientific evidence connecting nurse staffing to patient outcomes, it recommended that the

National Institute of Nursing Research and other agencies conduct and fund research in this area. Finally, the report recommended "that an inter-disciplinary public-private partnership be organized to develop performance and outcome measures that are sensitive to nursing interventions and care, with uniform definitions measurable in a uniform manner across all hospitals."[26]

For nurses who were begging for immediate relief this report was a grave disappointment. Diane Sosne of the SEIU Nurse Alliance said:

> Despite a decade of the health-care industry's cost-cutting measures, which frequently cut nurse staffing to bare bones and caused patient care to suffer, and despite testimony after testimony documenting nurses' concern regarding the patient's safety, the IOM report fell woefully short on conclusively linking the importance of adequate nurse staffing necessary for delivery of quality patient care. The report failed to exercise leadership on what every registered nurse in the country knew—that safe staffing levels are the difference between life and death.
>
> Nurses were warning that poor staffing conditions and deteriorating patient care were demoralizing nurses to the point where many would vote with their feet. The IOM report missed the opportunity to call national attention to the issue and no action was taken. The result, conditions continued to deteriorate and thousands of nurses continued to leave our hospitals.

The Study Is Political

Interestingly, even as the IOM report was released, more studies were confirming nurses' concerns. Two of these were from the American Hospital Association itself. One was the publicly released report *Eye on the Patient* prepared by the American Hospital Association and the Boston-based privately funded research group the Picker Institute. It was based on a survey of thirty-seven thousand patients and thirty-one focus groups held in twelve states. The report revealed widespread concern about the quality of care—or the lack of it—in the nation's hospitals. Of even more concern was "Reality Check: Public Perceptions of Health Care and Hospitals," a confidential report sent out by the president of the American Hospital Association, Dick Davidson, to the association's more than five thousand member hospitals.

Summarizing the comments of focus group participants, "Reality Check" stated:

> The key indicator that people referred to as a measure of the quality of their hospital care was the nurse. They hold a strong belief that skilled nurses are being systematically replaced by poorly trained and poorly paid aides. Their perspective on the "thinness" of hospital nurse staffing was reflected in a universally

mentioned experience: "If I hadn't stayed in the hospital room with my mother (or child or spouse) they never would have gotten the correct medication or care on time." People believe that the profit motive is behind the reduction in nursing care. They are angry at the reversal in health care priorities that they believe this represents.[27]

In "Reality Check," Davidson was warning member hospitals that they were "at risk of losing public support in maintaining their place at the table of health care decision making. As they lose the image of being 'on the side' of the patient, they lose the public legitimacy to exercise the authority that their expertise would otherwise entitle them."[28] The message seemed obvious: continue with policies that fail to ensure adequate nursing care and government will have to intervene.

This is precisely what many nurses in California were hoping legislators would do. A number of critical changes took place in the research and political arenas in 1997 and 1998. On the research front, several key studies appeared that validated nurses' contention that there was indeed a connection between nurse staffing and patient outcomes. At least three major studies affirmed a connection between adequate nurse staffing and fewer medication errors, fewer decubitous ulcers (bedsores), and more patient satisfaction.[29] Blegan and Vaughn found that when there were more registered nurses in the nursing-staff mix there were fewer medication errors. Kovner and Gergen documented a relationship between the number of full-time-equivalent registered nurses on duty per patient day and urinary tract infections, pneumonia, blood clots, and serious respiratory problems after surgery.[30]

On the political front, Democrats had taken control of the California legislature. Armed with more evidence and more public complaints about poor patient care, the ratio bill was reintroduced and finally passed in 1998. The Republican governor, Pete Wilson, however, quickly vetoed it. But in 1999 Gray Davis, a Democrat, won the governor's race. Nurses in the CNA and other unions had backed his candidacy in great part because he had promised to sign their bill.

When Davis took office, Assemblymember Sheila Kuehl once again introduced the bill. Given the hospital industry opposition, nurses knew its passage wasn't assured. So once again, they began to organize to do education and outreach not only to unionized nurses but also to nonunion nurses and the public. RNs brought petitions to their workplaces asking their unit mangers and administrators to support the bill. Many of these nurses recognized that management support would be unlikely, but they believed that this was a way to get more staff nurses involved in the campaign. The CNA also took campaign materials to California nursing schools and asked students and working nurses to write letters and make phone calls to state senators and assemblymembers.

This produced nearly ten thousand letters, some of them five or ten pages long. Nurses also wrote letters to the editor and op-ed pieces and conducted press conferences at the local level. They spoke at hearings, church groups, and community and consumer organizations and appeared on TV and radio.

The bill passed the California Assembly. Nonetheless, nurses were worried it might be defeated in the senate. The day of the senate vote, twenty-four hundred RNs gathered at the state capitol building in Sacramento. Eight hundred miles to the south, in Los Angeles, hundreds of nurses from fifty hospitals, many of which were not unionized, joined a rally in support of the bill. This clear demonstration that the staffing issue was of concern to all California nurses, the CNA believes, convinced a number of senators who'd been ambivalent about supporting the bill to vote for it.

The nurses' final campaign was waged to make sure Gray Davis signed the bill into law. Although he had told the CNA and other unions that he would support the legislation, he faced an intense lobbying campaign from the hospital and HMO industry, which urged him to veto the bill when it was finally passed. In a series of letters to the governor, hospital and health-care administrators outlined their objections.

Kenneth K. Westbrook, senior vice president of operations for Tenet, the second largest for-profit hospital chain in the United States, insisted that this was a "one-size fits all" solution to a problem that was, in fact, "complex and diverse." Ratios ignored the critical nursing shortage; hospitals already had difficulty filling vacancies and the ratios would be an unfunded mandate that would add an undue burden on hospitals and "lead to unintended consequences for our patients."[31]

The California Association of Catholic Hospitals took the position that hospitals should be the ones to make staffing decisions and that their decisions should be based on the assessment of patient-care needs, "not on numbers." They complained that whatever ratios might be mandated couldn't be met because of the nursing shortage, and they urged the governor to focus on increasing the number of students who graduate from nursing schools.[32] The Association of California Healthcare Districts pleaded that rural facilities "operating on slim financial margins would be irreparably hurt."[33] The Association of California Nurse Leaders echoed the one-size-fits-all argument and added that the solution to nursing's problems was graduating more students from nursing schools. Like the American Nurses Association, they favored the creation of "nurse sensitive patient outcome indicators and further scientific research to improve patient care."[34]

In a three-page letter to the governor, the California Healthcare Association outlined similar concerns and added more. The CHA began by warning that "ratios could have unintended consequences for patients. For example, hospitals may need to limit admissions in order to meet ratios, depending on the specific ratios adopted. Absent new revenue, laboratory, pharmacy, and other hospital services may have to be cut back to fund more nursing positions. These changes also will have adverse consequences."

Ratios would put inflationary pressures on nursing salaries and benefits. But since nurses' wages had stagnated over the past twelve years, higher salaries might have actually eased the shortage. The CHA also expressed concern about the nurse shortage, warning that hospitals might have to compete for nurses through bidding wars that would pit rural and inner-city hospitals against each other. Then the association, which adamantly opposes nurses' unionization, insisted that "ratios" should not be determined through the political process but should be collectively bargained.

The association suggested that nurses' unions were trying to create a "controlled economy." Ratios would place California at the edge of a slippery slope from which there could only be a precipitous fall. If signed, "other unionized hospital employee groups will certainly sponsor the same job benefits for their membership . . . and will continuously lobby the state for tighter ratios to benefit their membership."

Finally, the CHA insisted that nurse staffing wasn't really a serious issue since the Joint Commission on Accreditation of Healthcare Organizations (JCHAO)—a nonprofit organization largely financed by the hospital industry itself that accredits U.S. hospitals—hadn't "flagged nurse staffing levels as a general problem" and the Institute of Medicine in its 1996 report presented little evidence of patient harm. If such august bodies insisted there was no problem, how could there be? Nurses were just trading on anecdotes and horror stories, the CHA insisted, and ratios would not enhance patient outcomes.[35]

Faced with such arguments, it seemed that Governor Davis might waffle. In order to convince the governor that the unions and their supporters were in fact willing to compromise on a number of critical issues, the bill's sponsor, Assemblymember Kuehl, said she would agree to offer a bill the following year that would delay implementation of the ratios from 2001 to 2002. This would give the state more time to determine the appropriate ratios. Given that assurance and the intense lobbying by the public and the state's RNs, Davis signed the bill.

AB 394 Gets Signed

In November 1999, with AB 394, California became the first government in the world to guarantee nurses and patients a minimum staffing ratio. The legislature and people of California recognized that the care nurses deliver is, in fact, a matter of life and death.

The preamble to the legislation unequivocally stated that the Legislature

finds and declares all of the following:
(a) Health care services are becoming complex and it is increasingly difficult for patients to access integrated services.
(b) Quality of patient care is jeopardized because of staffing changes implemented in response to managed care.
(c) To ensure the adequate protection of patients in acute care settings, it is essential that qualified registered nurses and other licensed nurses be accessible and available to meet the needs of patients.
(d) The basic principles of staffing in the acute care setting should be based on the patients' care needs, the severity of condition, services needed, and the complexity surrounding those services.[36]

As a superior court judge in California would rule in 2005, in passing the bill the legislature declared that the accessibility and availability of nurses is essential "to ensure the adequate protection of patients in acute care settings."[37]

This was emphasized in Governor Davis's statement that accompanied the bill when he finally signed it into law. "Registered nurses," he wrote "are a critical component in guaranteeing patient safety and the highest quality health care. Over the past several years many hospitals, in response to managed care reimbursement contracts, have cut costs by reducing their licensed nursing staff. In some cases, the ratio of licensed nurses to patients has resulted in an erosion of care."[38]

AB 394 mandated that the Department of Health Services work to create "regulations that establish minimum, specific, and numerical licensed nurse-to-patient ratios by licensed nurse classification by hospital unit." The bill explicitly stated that the ratios were to be a minimum that established a baseline for each unit. These minimums were not to replace the existing patient classification systems. Hospitals were required to assign additional staff in accordance with the documented patient classification system for determining nursing care requirements. In its insistence on this, the bill was deliberately not a one-size-fits-all piece of legislation.[39]

To answer another hospital-industry concern, the bill authorized the CDHS to give waivers of the minimum staffing requirements to rural hospitals to increase operational efficiency, but only if the waivers were proved not to "jeopardize the health, safety and well-being of the patients affected."[40] The bill also granted some leeway to the University of California teaching hospitals.

To protect patients, the statute also prohibited "nurses from being assigned to a unit unless that nurse has received orientation and demonstrated the ability to 'provide competent care' to patients." Under the statute, hospitals could not replace licensed nurses with unlicensed personnel and ask them to perform clinical activities such as medication administration, IV therapy, tube feedings, inserting catheters or nasogastric tubes, doing endotracheal suctioning, assessing a patient's condition, or educating patients and families. Even if a registered nurse was ostensibly supervising the nursing assistant in performing these duties, that would violate the statute. Finally, AB 394 required that the department "review these regulations five years after adoption and . . . report to the Legislature regarding any proposed changes."[41]

Because the Davis administration took the hospital industry's concerns about the nursing shortage to heart, in January 2002, the governor announced a Nurse Workforce Initiative that allocated $60 million to address the nursing shortage. The initiative funded "five regional workforce collaboratives to train 2,400 new licensed nurses" and included money to expand training and preceptor programs in hospitals, community colleges, and the state university system. It also funded a statewide media recruitment campaign. The California state budgets in 2001–2002 and 2002–2003 also included "$4 million for 1,000 additional student nurse training programs at community colleges across the state."[42] The bill assigned the job of determining appropriate ratios to the Department of Health Services.

As soon as the governor signed AB 394 into law, nurses in California breathed a very long collective sigh of relief. "Oh my gosh," said Kelly Di-Giacomo, "I felt like there was finally hope. Someone recognized this is just crazy. People finally realized what we need to take care of patients. We were validated and vindicated." This sense of hope also buoyed nurses all over the United States—and across the globe—as they confronted the serious problem of work overload. One of those nurses was Belinda Morieson, secretary of the Victorian Branch of the Australian Nursing Federation, who was in the middle of her own fight to protect nurses and patients from work overload.

As early as 2000, before the final ratios had even been stipulated, nurses who had been inactive began to reenter the workforce, and nurses from other states started moving to California. According to Board of Registered Nurses (BRN) statistics, in 1999, the number of RNs with active California licenses was 735 per 100,000 population. In 2000, the figure edged up to about 738; by 2001, it was 745; by 2002, it had jumped to 765 and, by 2003, to more than 788. In 1994, 1995, and 1996, during the period of layoffs and restructuring, the BRN "endorsed"—that is, issued California licenses to nurses from out of state—3,115, 3,398, and 3,656 out-of-state nurses in the respective years. In 1996–97, as the nurses were waging their ratio campaign, that number increased to 4,560. By 2000–2001, it took a great leap forward to 7,845.[43]

Nurses in California hoped that as the legislation was implemented and the Department of Health Services began its search for the appropriate staffing ratios, their workloads would decrease and patient safety enhanced. And indeed, some more progressive hospitals, like those in the Kaiser system, as we'll see later, began to initiate their own process of investigation that would result in a 1:4 ratio on medical/surgical units at least two years before the state-determined ratios were put into effect.

2

Not Out of Thin Air

Critics of staffing ratios often claim that there is no scientific evidence suggesting that there is a perfect number of nurses to match a perfect number of patients on any given hospital unit. This is certainly a legitimate concern that we will discuss in chapter ten. After considering many critics' comments, however, one gets the impression that they believe the numbers the California Department of Health Services—or unions in favor of ratios—proposed were arbitrarily plucked out of thin air. In fact, the Department of Health Services embarked on a long process of investigation and discussion to determine the ratios that eventually became part of the regulatory process. Similarly, union ratio proposals were carefully researched.

The CDHS reviewed the literature on nurse staffing and patient outcomes, heard the testimony of experts and interested parties, and conducted studies to reveal the realities of staffing in the state's hospitals. It sought the recommendations of professional medical organizations and looked into working conditions and staffing solutions in other states and in other countries including Australia. The department collected information about nurse staffing from the Office of Statewide Health Planning and Development (OSHPD) and solicited input from professional nurses on its own staff. As it considered final ratio numbers, between 1999 and 2003, the department received over thirty-eight hundred phone calls, e-mail messages, and postcards from working nurses. CDHS staff participated in town hall meetings (many of them organized by the CNA) and attended rallies where nurses talked about their on-the-job experiences.

During this period a number of studies (discussed in more detail in chapter nine) were published that significantly influenced the debate and discussion. Researchers including Linda Aiken and her colleagues at the University of

Pennsylvania School of Nursing and several others were documenting impressive links between nurse staffing and patient deaths and preventable complications.[1] This research also charted a continuing nursing crisis with escalating levels of job dissatisfaction and burnout and problems with nurses' health. More and more nurses were saying they planned to leave the profession, and hard-won new recruits were moving through a revolving door in and out of hospital work or, like Summer Vanslager, considering doing so. In addition to documenting heavy patient loads, researchers were also beginning to study another disturbing trend: nurses were working longer and longer hours.[2] Even physicians were reporting that they were increasingly concerned about poor staffing, with "64% rating nurse staffing levels at their hospitals as 'fair' or 'poor.'"[3]

As it studied the evidence, the CDHS considered four proposals from the organizations that had taken the lead in fighting for or against staffing ratios: the California Healthcare Association, the Service Employees International Union, the United Nurses Association of California, and the California Nurses Association.

The California Healthcare Association based its proposal on meetings held with the Association of California Nurse Leaders. The ACNL, an organization of hospital nursing administrators is, like its national counterpart the American Organization of Nurse Executives, closely associated with the American Hospital Association (AHA). The nurse executives and the CHA assembled a statewide taskforce to identify the ratios they considered to be "clinically appropriate for all major patient care units." They investigated hospital units' ratios, talked with designers of patient acuity systems and solicited input from chief executive officers and chief nursing officers from all California hospitals.

The CHA's ratios were based on several assumptions that they had reiterated in their campaign against the ratios. They argued that there were no sound studies defining or determining RN-to-patient ratios and continued to insist that the implementation of any ratios be delayed until such studies materialized. They repeated their concerns that hospitals couldn't afford ratios and that government mandates would deprive patients of individualized care. It would not, the association insisted, be financially viable for hospitals to hire staff to meet the ratios and at the same time abide by another set of new mandates requiring that hospitals make their buildings earthquake safe and implement the mandates of the Health Insurance Portability and Accountability Act (HIPPA). Once again, they insisted there were not enough nurses to meet the ratios—no matter what those ratios might be. The CHA proposed 1:10 ratios on medical/surgical units as well as ratios for other units (see table 1).

The Service Employees International Union also presented a proposal. To calculate its ratios, the SEIU created committees of RNs and LVNs in various hospital units. In a series of conference calls, the committees decided to base their ratios on the premise that "hospital staffing is a team effort." SEIU nurses urged the CDHS to consider all categories of hospital workers, not just RNs and ancillary nursing staff when determining ratios, which, they argued, should include "those things which every nurse on every shift must do, what every nurse will always do for at least some patients, and what every nurse will often do for some patients." They recommended the ratios that could be filled by registered nurses or licensed vocational nurses. The CDHS deemed their approach "democratic, creative, and instructive."

The proposal made by the United Nurses Association of California was based on anecdotal reports from their nurse members.[4]

The California Nurses Association submitted the most extensive of the union proposals. To produce its 122-page document, nurses researched various studies and methodologies that had been used to try to determine ratios. These included staffing by outcomes, by diagnosis related groups, and by acuity. The

Table 1. Comparison of Ratios Proposed by the California Healthcare Association, the Service Employees International Union, the United Nurses Association of California, and the California Nurses Association

	CHA (RNs only)	SEIU (RNs and LVNs)	UNAC (RNs only)	CNA (RNs only)
Critical Care Unit	1:2	1:2	1:2	1:2
Burn Unit	1:2	1:2	1:2	1:2
Neonatal ICU	1:2	1:2	1:2	1:2
Labor and Delivery	1:3	1:2	1:2	1:1
Antepartum	——	1:3	——	——
Postpartum	1:4 couplets	1:3 couplets	1:3 couplets	1:5
Well Baby Nursery	1:8	1:6	1:6	1:5
Postanesthesia Service	1:3	1:2 Adults 1:1 Peds	1:2	1:2
Emergency Department (ED)	1:6	1:3	1:3	1:3
ED Critical Care	——	1:2	1:2	——
ED Trauma	——	1:1	——	——
Operating Room	1:1	1:1 plus 1 LVN and 1 Tech	1:1	1:1
Pediatric Unit	1:6	1:3	1:3	1:3
Step-down Care Unit	1:6	1:3	1:3	1:3
Specialty Care Unit	——	——	1:3	1:3
Telemetry Unit	1:10	1:3	1:3	1:3
Oncology Unit	1:10	——	1:4	——
General Medical/ Surgical Unit	1:10	1:4	1:4	1:3
Subacute/Transitional Care Unit	1:12	1:5	1:5	1:4
Behavioral/ Psychiatric Unit	1:12	1:2/1:3/1:5 (by acuity)	1:5	1:4

CNA was critical of each of these methods because they believed they did not adequately capture nurses' contributions to patient care and patient outcomes. The union was particularly concerned about patient classification systems because the "lack of PCS uniformity statewide has in part led to the considered distrust which many nurses evidence concerning individual hospital PCSs. Some nurses suspect that the individual hospital PCSs serve as a kind of internal public relations program to justify inadequate staffing to a reduced nursing workforce in order to meet budgetary rather than patient care goals."[5] The CNA therefore decided to create a different model.

Vicki Bermudez, the Regulatory Policy Specialist for the California Nurses Association who acted as the petitioner for the union in its court case against Governor Schwarzenegger's suspension of the ratios in 2005, explains the complex process. The union used data from a study conducted by the Institute of Health and Socio-Economic Policy and published as "California and the Demand for Safe Nurse to Patient Staffing Ratio" (March 2001). IHSP evaluated 21.7 million patient-discharge records from 1993 to 1998, which had been collected by the California Office of Statewide Health Planning and Development. Using the 3M Corporation's "All Patient Refined DRG Severity Sub-Class System," OSHPD assigns every patient discharge a "severity of illness" rating. This ranks each discharge on a 1 (minor acuity) to 4 (extreme acuity) scale. Because the OSHPD patient-discharge data does not reveal the unit in which a patient received care in the hospital, the CNA wished to create a process that would identify where patients with a particular diagnosis related group would stay in the hospital. So they tried to develop a tool that would determine the average acuity of patients by hospital unit.

To do this, the CNA asked twenty-five experienced nurses from twenty-two hospitals across the state to come together to evaluate 490 DRGs and indicate where patients with these diagnoses would be placed in their hospital setting. They were instructed not to identify where they believed the patients should be placed but rather where patients would actually be placed in their hospital. The 490 DRGs included, "respiratory system diagnosis with ventilator support," "diabetes over the age of 35 years," and "subtotal mastectomy for malignancy without complications." Among others, the units included the intensive care unit, medical/surgical unit, direct-observation unit, and postpartum unit. The nurses then analyzed the nurse placement of the DRGs and determined the average acuity of these units by using the DRG acuity data from the OSHPD discharge data analysis.

Because California had regulated nurse-to-patient ratios in the intensive care units since 1975 (a minimum of 1:2 at all times), these ICU staffing ratios were used as the benchmark for staffing ratios for the other hospital units. In effect, if the average DRG acuity in the intensive care unit was found to be 4 (extreme) and the average medical/surgical unit acuity was found to be 2 (moderate), then it would be reasonable to conclude that patients in the ICU were twice as acute as patients in the medical/surgical unit. Using such a relationship of acuity to ratios, the ICU unit with an average acuity of 4 would represent a minimum of 1:2 at all times (the already undisputed regulation for staffing in the ICU). A unit with an average acuity of 3 would represent a minimum of 1:3 at all times and a unit with an average acuity of 2 would represent a minimum of 1:4 at all times.

The CNA did not contend that these acuity examples actually reflected the findings of discharge data analysis. They were simply trying to illuminate the relationship between California's longstanding ICU staffing ratios and the proportional ratio that would be proposed for other units based on acuity differences of patients in each hospital unit. The IHSP study asserted a linear relationship between patient acuity and the intensity of nursing-care needs. In effect, they contended that higher-acuity patients required more nursing care and lower-acuity patients required less nursing care.

After considering the proposals submitted by the CHA and the three unions, the CDHS decided that the proposals reflected "the interests of the submitting organizations and their best recommendations but do not present an adequately supported, documented basis for their specific proposed ratios." To reach what it considered a "more objective consensus of workable, reasonable standards that would improve nurse staffing levels and quality of care to patients," the CDHS decided to do its own study to "determine how acute care hospitals were currently staffing their units with licensed nurses."[6] It asked researchers at the University of California at Davis to help with this research and to work with the department to develop an on-site hospital survey.

Determining the Workload in California Hospitals

Researchers first analyzed data that the Office of Statewide Health Planning and Development had collected. Could this data be used to calculate staffing minimums? Not really, they decided. It contained too many methodological pitfalls. OSPHD data calculated how many "productive hours per patient day" (PHPD) nurses put in. But how was the word *productive* defined? Many of these so-called productive hours were spent away from the bedside. Nurses might be attending a professional education seminar in the hospital, acting as managers, or doing quality reviews. Productive hours might not consider when a nurse was on a break and thus not involved in patient care. This meant that "the PHPD are likely to overestimate the actual amount of bedside care, and the magnitude of the discrepancy may vary from hospital to hospital."[7] Moreover, nurses' workloads increase when they admit or discharge a patient. The PHPD did not capture that work. This is particularly important in the contemporary hospital environment. More than 40 percent of hospitalized patients spend only about twenty-four hours in the hospital, which means that a nurse's workload increases not just because they're working with more patients but because more patients are admitted and discharged during a shift.[8]

Other variables add even more complexity to the definition of nursing productivity. Is every patient the same? No. That means every productive patient hour is different. And is every hour that a nurse puts in the same? Not, the CDHS concluded correctly, if that nurse is being "floated" out of her usual unit: "An RN assigned to the labor and delivery unit who is floated to the medical/surgical unit may not be as productive as the regular medical/surgical staff."[9] Although the report doesn't explicitly say why this is so, it is because the labor and delivery nurse is not as knowledgeable about medical/surgical patients as a medical/surgical nurse is and thus may be less efficient.

Then there was the term *patient day*. That was assumed to be the usual twenty-four-hour allotment. But, "for any given hospital, this may or may not be true." Because of the way hospitals calculate their daily census, they get a snapshot of the sum of patients who are in the facility at a particular moment in the day, say midnight. If a hospital admits patients right after midnight and discharges them the next day just before midnight, that hospital will appear to have fewer patients than a hospital that admits patients in the late afternoon. Thus, depending on how hospitals calculate their censuses, they appear to have more or fewer nurses per patients.

"A hospital census is a dynamic," explained Thomas Smith, senior vice president, Patient Care Services and Chief Nursing Officer of the Cambridge Health Alliance in Massachusetts, "so what most hospitals do is pick a time of the day when they calculate their nursing hours per patient day. Usually it's midnight."

He elaborated that unfortunately "the midnight census tends to understate the nursing workload. For example, you could start the day with thirty patients, ten might then go home, followed by the admission of another twelve. So the midnight census is not reflective of that variation." Smith cited the example of a busy thirty-five-bed cardiovascular unit whose patients have very short stays. "Eighteen to twenty patients would go home," Smith pointed out. "As soon as they left there'd be another eighteen to twenty. It was a ostensibly a thirty-five-bed unit, but really nurses might be taking care of forty or even seventy-five patients in a day."

That's why, he said, frontline nurses often complain that their administrators are not taking into account all the activity that's going on with patients over the course of a day. Some administrators, he added, might contend that activity level doesn't matter. Their attitude is "There's a patient in that bed, and they came and went. What's the big deal? So stop worrying about it." It is, he said, a very big deal for the nurse who's taking care of this revolving cast of new patients whose conditions and responses have to be factored into any plan of care—no matter how rapidly executed.

The CDHS understood this and chose to deal with the limitations of the OPHD data by trying to get a "clearer picture of nurse staffing in California acute care hospitals."[10] To do this, the UC Davis researchers sorted California's 495 acute care hospitals into six categories: (1) academic medical centers; (2) those owned by the HMO Kaiser Permanente, which has twenty-nine acute care hospitals in California and employs almost 25,000 RNs, not all of whom work in acute care facilities; (3) small and rural hospitals; and (4) other public, (5) private, and (6) state hospitals. The researchers then visited ten academic medical centers, ten Kaiser hospitals, twenty small and rural hospitals, ten other public hospitals, thirty other private hospitals, and ten state hospitals. They distributed a nurse-staffing questionnaire to individual units. It asked about nurses' education, length of employment, and years of practice. Researchers also collected shift-specific data for the seven days before the date of their study visit, which could be conducted on a weekday, a weekend, or a holiday.[11]

The researchers found that in labor and delivery, postpartum, medical/surgical, and oncology a small fraction of hospitals—5 percent—had 0.55, 2.00, 3.17, 2.44, and 2.50 patients per nurse while 95 percent had 2.00, 8.67, 8.00, 8.5, and 7.50 patients per nurse. For example, mean patients per RN on medical/surgical units ranged from 2.70 to 11.10.[12] Even on critical care units, which by well-established law could not exceed two patients per nurse, nurse-to-patient ratios were often violated: patient-to-nurse ratios ranged from as low as 0.50 to as high as 4.80 patients per nurse. Another study done by the California Nursing Outcome Coalition Database Project (CalNOC) had analyzed data from fifty-two acute care hospitals between April 1998 and June 2000 and found "wide variation across units within the same type of cohort."[13]

Based on their assessments, literature reviews, consultations with various interested parties, analyses of staffing ratios in Victoria, Australia, and what they insisted was their real world picture of nurse staffing, the CDHS made the recommendations that were to be implemented in all California acute care hospitals. It is important to note that, as in Australia, either licensed vocational nurses or registered nurses could theoretically fill the ratios. Regulations clarified that LVNs could constitute up to 50 percent of licensed nurses on units so long as they did not exceed their scope of practice. LVNs cannot give intravenous medications and administer blood products. Although they cannot do complex patient assessments or develop plans, they can provide information that RNs use in producing these.[14] LVNs could not be used when the hospital's PCS found that a patient needed care from an RN.[15] The regulations stipulated that "a hospital cannot reduce overall staffing by assigning licensed nurses to duties customarily and appropriately performed by unlicensed staff."[16] In other words, a hospital could not get more work out of an RN or LVN by assigning that person transport, housekeeping, or secretarial duties.

The recommendation would not allow hospitals to average the number of patients and nurses during a single shift. As the report by the CDHS stated bluntly, "If CDHS were to permit averaging (as an alternative approach) there would effectively be no limit on the number of patients who could be assigned to one nurse at any given time." For example, the report postulated that a twenty-four-bed unit could be staffed with six nurses on day shift, four nurses on evening shift, and two nurses on the night shift. The unit would thus succeed in employing on average one nurse to six patients over the twenty-four-hour period. They point out that "the actual care provided, however, would be 1:4 on day shift, 1:6 on evening shift, and 1:12 on night shift. While facilities always have the option of increasing staffing above the minimum required levels . . . the regulations are written to prevent, at any time, the assignment of fewer nurses to care for patients than the minimum level specified in these regulations."[17]

Thus, as their "Statement of Reasons" (the document the CDHS wrote to explain the rationale for their ratio proposal) went on to explain, "the ratios are the same minimum standard for every shift." They are to operate at all times, that is, when nurses are on breaks and "represent the leanest staffing the Department believes is compatible with safe and quality patient care in the acute care setting." They also represented, the CDHS said, "the maximum number of patients assigned to any one nurse at any one time."[18]

The Ratio Report

What were those maximums to be? On labor and delivery units, the ratio would be 1:2 or fewer at all times—a standard that had been recommended by the American College of Obstetricians and Gynecologists, the American Academy of Pediatrics, and the Association of Women's Health, Obstetric and Neonatal Nurses. This was, in fact, a standard of care for 95 percent of hospital shifts in the state. On postpartum units, the ratio would be 1:4 mother-baby couplets, again a standard closely conforming to that recommended by the same organizations. According to the CDHS, 90 to 95 percent of shifts were at 1:8 total patients, while 75 percent were at 1:6. This meant that 5 to 10 percent of shifts were worse than 1:8, while 15 percent were better than 1:8 but not as good as 1:6.[19] In the postanesthesia recovery unit where fragile patients recover after surgery, the ratio was to be a minimum of one nurse to two patients or fewer at all times. This "would increase staffing at the leanest 10–25% of hospitals" and would follow recommendations of the California Society of Anesthesiologists.[20]

In the busy hospital emergency departments (ED) of the most populous state in the nation, the ratio was to be 1:4 or fewer at all times and for critical-care ER patients 1:2 or fewer, as on all critical-care units. Because triage and radio nurses play a central role in the ED, where they man radios and talk to emergency medical personnel and then triage patients when they enter the unit, they would have to be registered nurses and could not be counted in the ratios. These nurses could, however, assist their colleagues if there were no patients waiting to be assessed and assigned to the proper physician or service and if they didn't have to respond to radio calls. The California Chapter of the American College of Emergency Physicians stated that these were the minimum acceptable ratios.[21]

Because patients in step-down units are more unstable than those on regular floors but not fragile enough to be in the ICU, so that they are "literally just a step away from needing intensive care," the ratio there was to be 1:4—a ratio that the CDHS mandated be changed to 1:3 in 2008. "This is clinically appropriate," the department explained, "because of increased patient acuity and the required level of care in step-down units. Enriched staffing is needed to address this increased patient fragility and complexity of care and treatment."[22] If patients are so fragile, why was the department waiting to enrich staffing until 2008? Because it honored the industry's concerns that hospitals would be unable to meet mandated ratios due to the state's nursing shortage. By waiting until 2008, the state would have more time to produce the type of nurse who was now in short supply because the job requires "advanced education, training and certification."[23]

Ratios were also to be richer on telemetry units. These are units that care for stable cardiac patients or patients whom doctors and nurses suspect may have a heart condition or disease, all of whom need constant monitoring for potential or actual cardiac problems. Fifty percent of hospital shifts on telemetry units, the report stated, were currently staffing at 1:4 while 75 percent of shifts were at 1:5.6. According to the "Statement of Reasons," "When the ratio shifts to 1:4 it will enrich staffing for more than 50 percent of shifts on telemetry units statewide. This is necessary because the expanded use of telemetry reflects the prevalence of heart diseases in the United States."[24]

Finally, the recommendations addressed the medical/surgical floor and the specialty unit—the heart of nursing care in the hospital and of the debate about ratios. The majority of patients in a hospital are either on a medical/surgical or specialty floor. Medical units care for patients with every imaginable ailment from diabetes to dementia to congestive heart failure or cellulitis.

Surgical units deal with patients monitored after surgery. Specialty units include such specialties as oncology or neurology. As of January 1, 2004, the ratio was to be set at one nurse for six patients for med/surg and 1:5 for specialty units. On January 1, 2005, ratios would go to 1:5 for med/surg and 1:4 for specialty units.

> According to OSHPD's data, 75% of California's hospital shifts are already staffed at a level of 1:5.6 or richer for medical/surgical units. The CDHS's on-site study of hospitals statewide confirmed staffing in those unit types at 1:6 for 75% of all medical/surgical and mixed unit shifts. The CDHS decided to set the starting point for the minimum ratios at this level, to improve staffing on those shifts in the leanest 25th percentile.[25]

All these ratios were considered to be the minimum baseline for nursing care. They were represented to apply to the slowest, lowest-intensity shifts with the least acute patients, for example, evening and night shifts. Higher-acuity patients and shifts like the day shift, where there was a greater intensity of work and more tests, procedures, admissions, and discharges, were supposed to trigger extra staffing for which the levels would be determined by using patient acuity systems.

Although neither the unions nor the hospital industry got precisely what they wanted, these are the ratios that were to be put into place starting January 1, 2004.

For a series of dry documents, the collection of reports and recommendations that lay out in intricate detail the debate about which ratios were appropriate in California hospitals makes fascinating reading and raises equally fascinating questions. An analysis of the multiple studies of the realities of staffing in California hospitals makes it clear why so many nurses had become discouraged about their working conditions and suspicious about hospital management's willingness or ability to address their concerns. Time and time again, studies commissioned by the state verified that staffing was short on many hospital units. Even on those critical-care units that had been supposedly regulated for more than twenty years, violations of the 1:2 legally mandated ratio seemed to routinely occur. Researchers found that on other units, sometimes staffing was "rich" while in the same hospital and on the same or a different unit it might be quite "lean." In other words, a nurse could not predict whether she would come to work and find herself taking care of eleven increasingly ill patients or three. Neither could the researchers.

It also seemed that some hospitals were abiding by the patient acuity systems and that their staffing was just what the ratios recommended. This suggested that some hospitals—or was it some units in some hospitals?—were bad apples and that ratios were needed to bring them up to standard. But which hospitals were they? And were they staffing appropriately on all units? The answers were: Who knows? and Apparently not. Nurses didn't know and—more important—patients couldn't predict from moment to moment or shift to shift whether they would be safe in a particular hospital or on a particular floor.

The hospital industry insisted that the ratio bill wasn't needed. The industry's solution was to strengthen patient acuity systems. How was the state to do that when the industry itself either refused to abide by or simply ignored PCS data?

The voluminous reports on staffing in California's hospitals make the CHA's ratio proposals even more disturbing. The industry's proposals would not have simply continued the status quo about which many California nurses and patients complained but would have actually made the situation worse. The CDHS data revealed that many hospitals and many shifts in different hospitals were already staffed according to the ratios that the state eventually recommended. For them the ratios would not interfere with care delivery, so why would ratios force them to close beds, lay off staff, or curtail services? What the industry proposed—ratios of 1:10 and 1:12—would, however, have significantly set back patient care in a state already suffering from a series of setbacks. Had those ratios been enacted, California hospitals would have walked into the trap AHA president Dick Davidson warned about in his 1996 confidential memo. By further eroding a standard of care that was already contested, the hospital industry would have forfeited any claim for a place at the decision-making table or that it was protecting the public. Yet the hospital industry seemed ready and willing to take that risk.

The testimony and literature reviewed and cited raises serious issues not only about the hospital industry's claims to legitimacy and leadership but also about some California nurse administrators' claims to be leaders of the nursing profession as a whole. In its statement of reasons for every ratio determined, the CDHS cites standards articulated by a variety of professional organizations—the California Medical Association, the American Academy of Pediatrics, the Association of Women's Health, Obstetrical, and Neonatal Nurses, the American Association of Critical Care Nurses, the Emergency Nurses' Association California State Council, and many more—that agree that the ratio delineated is, in fact, the best practice and best standard of care. How, for example, could the California Association of Nurse Leaders ignore this impressive body of research and commentary? As we will see when we examine the studies that correlate nurse staffing and patient outcomes, this mystery deepens even further when one considers the quantity of data establishing a connection between nursing care and patient deaths and preventable complications.

3

The Hospital Industry Response

In the satiric movie about the tobacco industry, *Thank You for Smoking*, the son of the well-paid tobacco industry lobbyist asks his father what he considers to be the best thing about the American form of government. Without blinking an eye, the morally challenged character Nick Naylor replies, "The endless appeals process." In response to the ratio bill, the California Hospital Association began to mobilize that relentless process to stall the implementation of ratios in the state.

In fall 2003, as soon as the Department of Health Services announced its ratios, the California Healthcare Association ran a series of seven seminars around the state. Participants in the seminars were nurse administrators and managers and the presenters were nurse executives and lawyers who worked with the hospital association. They included Patricia McFarland, executive director of the California Association of Nurse Leaders; Dorel Harms, vice president for professional services of the CHA; and William L. Abalona and Gregory W. McClune, lawyers employed by the CHA. According to the association, the goal of the seminars was to "analyze California's staffing ratio regulations; examine policy implications as they relate to staffing regulations; identify two strategies for implementing staffing ratios; explore strategies for best practices as they relate to implementation of nurse staff ratios."[1] The CHA distributed PowerPoint slides and handouts, which were provided to us by a nurse who attended one of the seminars.

Seminar leaders began by explaining the legislation and highlighting the consequences of noncompliance. Among other things, if hospitals failed to abide by the law, the CDHS could suspend or revoke a hospital license. Noncompliant hospitals could lose a trauma center designation, be accused of negligence, and would become vulnerable to civil suits. If a patient filed such a suit, the hospital could be liable for payment of punitive damages.

Much of the presentation, however, seems to have been devoted to showing nurse managers how they could undermine the ratios' credibility with the public. Managers were informed about the process of obtaining "a voluntary suspension of license or licensed beds" and responding to any nurses who filed forms alleging that the hospital was not in compliance with staffing ratios.

Presenters discussed how administrators could justify downsizing, that is, staff layoffs, by closing beds temporarily or placing beds in "suspense" of closing them over the long term. Forms requesting that a hospital be allowed a reprieve from the ratios, "program flexibility requests," were given to participants. Administrators were told how to report a "health care emergency" that resulted in an inability to meet staffing ratios. They received copies of sample news releases explaining why a facility had closed a unit. These materials specifically blame unit closures on the new staffing law. Sample letters to employees and medical staff were supplied. These letters again blamed unit closures on the staffing bill.

The PowerPoint presentation made no mention of any potential benefits from the law. For example, no mention was made of the efforts of Kaiser's highest echelon nurse administrators who implemented ratios in their hospitals even before the CDHS announced its ratio requirements. Nor was there any discussion of positive developments in Australia.

Although the CHA might argue that it was legitimately trying to help administrators prepare for a worst-case scenario, these presentations were given in the fall 2003. The ratios were not, however, implemented until three months later, in January 2004. One CNA member who attended a seminar at Washington Hospital in Fremont reported that the presenters were openly hostile to the ratios. Their comments, she said, included the following:

- "When ratios were written, common sense walked out of the door."
- "Ratios were signed into law because there was a Democratic governor."
- "When ratios were passed, we moved away from policy and moved into politics."

Did You Really Mean "At All Times?"

As soon as the ratios were implemented, the CHA filed a lawsuit in California Superior Court to contest the ratio bill. In its suit, the CHA contended that the regulations were contrary to the purpose of the authorizing statute, that the entire set of nurse-staffing regulations, section 70217, was "arbitrary and capricious and not supported by the administrative record," and that

CDHS actions were procedurally unfair. The heart of its suit, however, was a challenge to the CDHS's interpretation of AB 394 because the regulations "repeatedly state that the specified ratios apply 'at all times,' " that is, when nurses are not on their units because they are on breaks.[2]

Nurses in California are, by law, allowed two fifteen-minute rest breaks and one half-hour meal break for every eight-hour shift. If they work twelve hours, they are to have the same two fifteen-minute rest breaks and two half-hour meal breaks. Nurses are not supposed to work longer than four hours without a break. When they are off the unit, someone else has to take over the burden of the care of their patients. The hospital association wanted nurses who had a full supplement of patients to add another to their caseload. This would mean that for fifteen minutes or half an hour, a nurse would be taking care of more than the number of patients ratios stipulated. From a hospital's point of view, the demand that ratios apply "at all times" added to their onerous burden. Hospitals would have to abide by ratios while nurses were caring for patients on their units. If a nurse took a break, the hospital would have to add enough staff to make sure that there was coverage for that nurse's patients and that other nurses, shouldering their own patient loads, would not have to add another nurse's patient complement to their own. To do this would obviously require more outlay of funds by the hospital.

While hospitals considered the "at all times" rule to be an unacceptable burden, many nurses felt that being asked to add more patients to their load was also unacceptable. Looked at superficially, shouldering any more patients for only fifteen minutes or a half an hour might not seem like much. The problem is that, for a certain period each day, it returned nurses to a situation they believed was unsafe for both themselves and their patients. A nurse wouldn't be asked to fill in for just a short fifteen minutes, she could be asked to substitute for perhaps two or three or even more nurses who went off on break. Thus, she could be spending several hours a day caring for patients far in excess of the ratios.

Even if that nurse had to cover only one other RN's patients for an hour, that extra load would be unsafe, staff nurses argued. Sick and vulnerable patients don't schedule their crises or needs around their nurse's break and lunch times. A nurse taking care of six patients on her own as well as those of a nurse who was at lunch or on break could discover that several of those patients had serious and urgent needs while she was juggling eight or ten other patients. It could thus be 1997 or 1999 all over again—not 2004, when legislation was supposed to protect patients and their nurses from such unsafe conditions.

In spite of nurses' protests, the CHA claimed that, during the rule-making process the Department of Health Services had commented, "Nurses do not need replacement for breaks."[3] The association also argued that "assist" and "relieve" had one and the same meaning. To defend this position, the CHA of-fered a truly novel interpretation of the words *assist* and *relieve*. The common definition of one nurse offering *assistance* to another requires the presence of two nurses—the one who's assisted and the one who is doing the assisting. When a nurse goes off for a coffee break or for lunch, the nurse who takes over her patient load is commonly considered to be *relieving* rather than assisting the nurse who is no longer physically present. The association disagreed.

According to the CHA, it would be fully within the letter of the statute and mandate for a nurse assigned a particular patient load to be assisted by a nurse (with the same patient load) even though the nurse assisting was not present and available to do the assisting because she was, in fact, off the unit on a break. Or, as the CHA argued, the "regulation does not require physical pres-ence as a prerequisite for an assignment for the purposes of the nurse-to-patient ratios."[4] Even the fact that this "assistance" could last up to half an hour was not enough to transform "assisting" into "relieving."

On May 24, 2004, the California Superior Court denied the plaintiffs' case, dismissing all its claims. Rejecting the CHA's request to scuttle the entire bill, the court stated that it could not rule on the wisdom of a particular piece of legislation and refused to comment on the CHA's contention that the regula-tion was contrary to public policy. As to the CHA's other contentions, the court declared them to be "without merit."[5] The CHA, the court stated, could not challenge the at-all-times provision because of "DHS's response to one comment during the rulemaking process . . . California Healthcare Asso-ciation's reliance on this response is misplaced."[6] Moreover, the court stated that "assist" and "relieve" did not mean the same thing: "The 'assigned' nurse must remain responsible for the provision of direct patient care. To do this, the assigned nurse must be present on the unit. If the assigned nurse is not present, another nurse would not be 'assisting' but instead would be taking over and assuming the assigned nurse's responsibilities."[7] The court catego-rized the CHA contention that there was "no data or analysis" regarding how many nurses would be required to take care of patients as "really an attack on the ratios themselves" and found there was "adequate support in the record for DHS' actions in adopting ratios."[8] CDHS furthermore provided "suffi-cient notice of the proposed regulation," and the court refused to declare the ratio bill invalid.

Finally, and perhaps most important, the court ruled that applying the ratios to break periods "is not new and is consistent with the plain language of the regulation. Any other interpretation would make the nurse-to-patient ratios meaningless."[9]

In another move against the ratios, in February 2004, assemblymembers Robert Pacheco and Tom Harmon introduced AB 2963, which was sponsored by the California Healthcare Association. The bill would have required the Department of Health Services to evaluate the ratios on medical/surgical units that went into effect in 2004 by January 1, 2005. This provision would have overridden the more reasonable and rational requirement that ratios be evaluated five years after their implementation. The bill would also have delayed implementation of those medical/surgical ratios pending an evaluation establishing that hospitals could recruit enough nurses. Implementation of the ratios would also depend on proof that CDHS's estimates of fiscal impacts on hospitals were accurate; that 1:6 ratios hadn't prevented hospitals from hiring and retaining staff; and that there were measurable improvements in patient care that justified additional costs to hospitals.[10] The legislature did not pass the bill.

At this point nurses believed that legal and legislative challenges to ratios had been soundly defeated at the ballot box, in the courts, and through the ongoing political process. Little did they know that even bigger challenges lay ahead. Those came in the form of the election of Arnold Schwarzenegger as governor of California and the reelection of George W. Bush as president.

Enter the "Terminator"

On October 7, 2003, movie star and bodybuilder Arnold Schwarzenegger, of *Terminator* fame, leaped into a brand-new role. He ran, as a Republican, for governor of California and beat 134 other candidates in a special election that ousted Democrat Gray Davis two years before his term of office was officially over. The push for a special election had been financed by a right-wing opponent of the Democratic governor and took advantage of the fact that voters disapproved, among other things, of Davis's handling of the state's energy policy. Schwarzenegger had accepted campaign contributions from the state's hospital and insurance industry, and nurses worried about the impact he would have on state health-care policy. In 2003, they got a preview of coming attractions when he vetoed a bill that, like similar regulations in Victoria, would have mandated lift teams and lift equipment in California hospitals. Such regulations would have helped protect nurses, many of whom were aging, from the risks in lifting patients who, due to the obesity epidemic in the United States, were increasingly heavy.

Most nurses did not dream, however, that the new governor would attack the widely popular nursing ratios. But that's precisely what he did. Just a day after George W. Bush was reelected for his second term as president, Governor Schwarzenegger announced an emergency action. The Department of Health Services, at his behest, was issuing an emergency regulation suspending the ratio phase-in until 2008. The department would also "clarify when licensed nurses shall be counted toward ratios" and changed the record-keeping requirements for emergency rooms. This new emergency regulation gave emergency rooms permission to deviate from ratios when they were "saturated" with patients, rather than only during a health-care emergency. This provision essentially allowed hospitals to violate ER ratios at almost any time, since the number of patients an ER receives can never be predicted and ERs are constantly "saturated."

This new CDHS emergency regulation echoed all the arguments the CHA had mobilized to oppose the ratios. The emergency regulation stated that the nursing shortage prevented hospitals from hiring enough nurses to comply with AB 394. It insisted that hospitals didn't have enough money to hire the nurses because of "pressures of managed care, inadequate Medi-Cal reimbursement rates, an ever-increasing uninsured population receiving health care through emergency departments, and unfunded mandates (including seismic retrofit)."[11]

The CDHS contended that, in some cases, the ratios were responsible for the closure of two hospitals, as well as for the closure or decrease in services at hospital emergency rooms and patient-care units. Thus, it declared that the ratios were causing a health-care emergency, which was why an emergency regulation was "necessary for the immediate preservation of the public health and safety."[12]

As soon as the governor announced the Emergency Regulation terminating staff ratio phase-in the CNA went into action. The nurses' association immediately filed a suit in California Superior Court arguing that the department had exceeded its authority. The suit contended that the CDHS claims were inaccurate and violated the intent of the legislature and, thus, the will of the people of California. The legal proceedings, which went on for more than a year, consumed millions of taxpayer, union, and hospital dollars. The initiation of the second phase of the ratios was delayed by months. Kelly DiGiacomo said nurses felt like they'd "received a punch in the stomach." Perhaps the longest-lasting, albeit not surprising, result of the emergency regulation was to create an emergency not for the nurses and their ratios but for the governor himself.

Once Schwarzenegger announced the termination of the ratio phase-in, nurses initiated a statewide—even nationwide—campaign to put public and political pressure on the governor to rescind the emergency order.

Arnold Schwarzenegger proved to be a particularly vulnerable target for political protest. He was known for his swagger and boasting, his alleged groping of women, his misogynist comments, and his crass bravado. Indeed, he seemed to repeatedly play right into the hands of California's angry nurses who, it appeared, were better organized than he was. In December 2004, for instance, the governor spoke to an audience of about ten thousand participants at a women's conference in Long Beach. Nurses were outside picketing, and he stopped his speech to inform his audience to "pay no attention to those voices over there. They are special interests. Special interests don't like me in Sacramento because I kick their butt."[13]

Many Californians were shocked by his comments. However, the governor wasn't cowed by this public outrage. In fact, in his January State of the State speech, he lumped nurses in with a broader group of "special interests" that he chose to attack that included teachers, police officers, and firefighters. The CNA was emboldened by these attacks and struck back with more protests and ads against the governor. One ad, which ran in California newspapers as well as the *New York Times*, pictured the governor glowering at an audience and shaking his fist. The headline read "California nurses take 'special interest' in their patients. Is that what he meant?" and went on to criticize the governor for what the nurses contended was his own pandering to the special interests of hospitals and insurance companies, from whom, nurses insisted, he had received part of the $26.6 million in campaign contributions he'd raised in his first year of office.

When Schwarzenegger appeared at an event, which would always be covered by the press and photographers, nurses were always in the crowd outside the barricades. They even followed him to what were supposed to be more discrete fund-raising dinners at supporters' homes and flew a light plane over his events, towing a banner declaring, "California is not for sale."

It was at one of these protests that Kelly DiGiacomo was catapulted into the national—even international—media spotlight. Governor Schwarzenegger was making an appearance at a movie premiere of *Be Cool* with its stars John Travolta and Uma Thurman in Sacramento. As celebrities paraded into a downtown theater, nurses picketed outside. The CNA was able to get one ticket for one nurse, and DiGiacomo, all five-foot-two of her, entered the movie theater. She was dressed in her nurse's uniform; she didn't have a purse and was not carrying anything other than her ticket, ID, and a cell phone. She took a seat near the front of the theater. As she kept an eye out for the governor, she made a couple of calls.

Suddenly, two burly security officers approached her and asked her to move to the back of the theater. She refused. They asked for her ticket and ID, which she gave them. They looked at her, gave them back, and again asked her to move. Once more she refused. They left and she sat back down. Then a highway patrolman, six foot four, by her estimate, came to ask her if she'd like to speak with the governor. Pretending that she would have that opportunity, he escorted her out of the theater into an adjoining room. "For an hour," she said, "they interrogated me like I was a terrorist or a criminal. Over and over they asked for my name, date of birth, Social Security number, who I was with, why I was there. I kept asking if I could leave, and they wouldn't let me.

They kept me away from the governor until the movie premiere started and the governor had left the stage."

Finally, they let DiGiacomo go and she rejoined the nurses' picketing outside the theater. Quickly, however, the news that Schwarzenegger, the bulky bodybuilder, had appeared to be scared of a tiny California nurse made headlines. In one story, he was dubbed "the Paranoid Governor." The *Los Angeles Times*, the *New York Times*, and national radio and television stations interviewed DiGiacomo. Media in Australia, New Zealand, and even China reported on the story. "The reactions," she recalled, "ranged from hysterical laughter—that a nurse could be so threatening to the governor—to outrage. People equated it with Rosa Parks being asked to move to the back of the bus." Nor did the attention quickly evaporate. "I thought I'd have my fifteen minutes of fame and it would last a few days." But no, she said, it dragged on.

The Court Rules against Schwarzenegger

The California Superior Court gave the governor another defeat when it ruled against the CDHS emergency regulation in March 2005. The Superior Court decision is worthy of close attention. In ruling against the Department of Health Services and its emergency regulation, the court reviewed the history of staffing ratios, the failures of the patient acuity systems, and the hospital association's arguments against AB 394. This historical outline highlighted how carefully thought out the rule-making process was and how cautiously—some nurses might say overcautiously—the CDHS approached the determination and implementation of ratios.

Here were the facts as the court outlined them:

Ratios did not supplant patient acuity systems but rather established a minimum-staffing baseline, which the patient acuity systems should, when necessary, supersede. Waivers for rural hospitals were available, and teaching hospitals were given special consideration. To deal with the concern about the nursing shortage, a multistage phase-in was created so that hospitals could find additional nurses and schools could produce new recruits to add to the existing professional stream. To make sure this happened, the Davis administration allocated funds for recruitment and education. The court underlined—not once, but many times—that AB 394 was considered to be such a fundamental patient-safety measure that it ultimately precluded concern about hospital finances: "Concerns of 'operational efficiency' were intended to be subordinate to the health and safety of the patients." General acute care hospitals were not given "the authority to base ratios on such considerations."[14] Further:

> The Court finds that the statutory language unambiguously establishes that the purpose of the proposed minimum staffing ratios is to enhance the *quality* of care, i.e., to protect the health and safety of patients in acute care hospitals in California. It was not designed to remedy the nursing shortage nor to address the business and fiscal constraints faced by hospitals.[15]

In the emergency regulation, the CDHS argued that by suspending the phase in of the 1:5 ratios, it had full authority to initiate further delays in implementing ratios. The court flatly rejected that argument. Considerations of nursing shortages and hospital finances, it reiterated, were outside the CDHS's rule-making authority. To bring those considerations into the regulatory process was proof that the agency was indeed, as the CNA contended, exceeding its authority.

The court also found that the CDHS was not consistent in its positions. This finding seemed to confirm the CNA's contention that legislation was the only alternative available to hospital nurses who wanted some assurance that their workloads would be controlled. As Vicki Bermudez argued to the court, the CDHS had proved to be a fickle guarantor of patient safety and nurses' health and welfare. The CDHS had inconsistently argued both for and against ratios. It urged the legislature not to pass the bill and encouraged Governor Davis to veto it. Then it turned around and forcefully explained and defended its rule-making process and the ratios it had established. Finally, in this latest campaign, it opposed the very regulatory process it had earlier created and supported.

The court also addressed the contention that AB 394 had produced unintended consequences for patients and the people of California. Legislators, the court ruled, always understood this risk and determined that—minus workload control—the risk to patient safety was even worse. The legislation, the court said, was not intended to protect all of the citizens or residents of California but just a segment of them—patients in acute care hospitals. Because the legislation and ratios accomplished this goal, the court could not simply "ignore this language in interpreting the meaning of the statute."

The decision attacked another CDHS assumption—that it had the discretionary authority to halt the ratio phase-in of 1:5 because this decrease in workload represented "discretionary enrichments" of staff.[16]

Not so, the court insisted. The ratios were not presented as an "enrichment" strategy but as a minimum baseline. PCS systems were the discretionary devices designed to "enrich" staffing and assure individualized patient care. But on their own, the court reminded its bickering parties, these systems were not working as intended, a fact the CDHS itself had established in its earlier "Statement of Reasons." Thus, the CDHS could not reasonably argue that in delaying the phase-in of the ratios it was merely delaying an enrichment device, the proverbial fat rather than the muscle. According to the court, it was cutting muscle. "Nothing in AB 394 gave the

DHS the discretion to 'enrich' the ratios beyond the minimum necessary to ensure the adequate protection of patients in acute care settings. Rather, as DHS properly determined, any 'enrichment' to the minimum staffing ratios was intended to be implemented in accordance with the Patient Classification System."[17]

It would thus be "illogical to interpret AB 394 as requiring the DHS to adopt minimum staffing ratios, while simultaneously giving DHS the unbridled discretion not to implement those ratios."[18]

Throughout its ruling, the court reiterated that because of the paramount concern for patient safety, shortages and economic impacts were outside the rule-making process. To invoke the Emergency Regulation with the express intent of addressing problems of possible hospital closings or reduction of services due to financial strains caused by the ratios or difficulties finding nurses to fill the ratios was "inconsistent with the fundamental purposes of the statute to ensure that nurses be accessible and available to meet the needs of 'patients in acute care settings.' "[19]

Finally, the court turned its attention to the issue of whether "the Emergency Regulation was reasonably necessary to achieve the purposes of the statute."[20] Here the court's ruling was even more scathing. The court declared unequivocally that the "evidence" the CDHS marshaled to substantiate its claim that the ratio bill was responsible for facility closures and shutdowns was specious at best and fallacious at worst.

When it announced its emergency regulation, the CDHS cited articles in several newspapers that, the department contended, blamed hospital and unit closures on the ratio bill. In fact, the court retorted, those articles established no such link. Quite the contrary. The *Pasadena Star* covered the shutdown of Santa Teresita Hospital in Duarte "but made clear that the hospital's 'financial woes' preceded the state-mandated increase in the ratio of nurses." As the article put it, "Santa Teresita's finances have been teetering on the brink of crisis for the past three years." An article in the *Los Angeles Business Journal* mentioned hospitals that had closed or downgraded psychiatric units, but the article explicitly stated that the ratios on these units would not be affected by the emergency regulation.

The Court pointed out that according to articles in the *New York Times* and the *Los Angeles Times*, allegations that ERs, like the one at Robert F. Kennedy Medical Center in Hawthorne, California, were shutting down because of the ratio bill were equally unfounded. As we will discuss at greater length in chapter nine, emergency rooms were not experiencing difficulties because of the staffing bill but because of the U.S. health-care system's failure to provide health insurance to vast segments of the U.S. population. This produced ERs full to the brim with nonpaying customers, people reliant on charity care. Similarly, state-mandated earthquake retrofitting was partially responsible for the crisis in ERs. An article in the *San Jose Mercury News* reported that ERs in

Santa Clara County were having problems accommodating patients and attributed some of these problems to the staffing bill. The article hastened to point out that those patients treated in ERs were getting "higher quality care." According to the reporter, it was "too early to tell" if the new ratios are "too much of a strain on hospitals trying to meet the mandate."

Hemet Valley Medical Center was also laying off staff, allegedly because of the ratio bill. But, in fact, an article in the *Riverside Press Enterprise* documented that the facility had been in dire financial straits since 1998 and that it had laid off seventy employees the year before AB 394 went into effect.

"None of the 'evidence' establishes any basis to postpone the minimum 1:5 ratio for medical/surgical units," the court declared.[21]

The final legal blow to the CDHS emergency regulation was the court's finding that there was really no emergency in California hospitals and thus no rationale for an emergency regulation. "An emergency regulation requires a finding that it 'is necessary for the immediate preservation of the public peace, health and safety or general welfare,'" the court restated the law. Courts "generally give deference," it went on to elaborate, to an agency's judgment. But not always. Particularly if there is no "evidentiary support" justifying the declaration of such an emergency.[22]

In this case, the CDHS insisted that it had received "reports" of compromised patient care (which were in fact nothing that the department hadn't heard before). Yet the department still went full speed ahead with the rulemaking process, established the ratios, and created a timetable for their implementation.[23] CDHS then argued that it had not anticipated the magnitude of these "reports." Yet, on the subject of hospital closings, the department itself admitted that it couldn't be certain that "reports" of hospital closures were in fact true and that "it does not have data to support or refute these and other claims that have been made about problems caused or exacerbated by the current nurse-to-patient ratios."

"The Court finds that it was an abuse of discretion for the DHS to determine that deferring the 1:5 ratio for Medical/Surgical Units was necessary for the immediate preservation of public health and safety."[24] The court also ruled against the other changes to the bill that the CDHS proposed—altering emergency room ratios and the at-all-times rule.[25]

When the court issued its ruling on March 5, 2005, many nurses in California celebrated as did nurses and other people elsewhere in the United States. In November 2005, many hospital nurses were even more jubilant. On November 8, 2005, California voters resoundingly defeated a series of proposals placed on a referendum ballot initiated by Governor Schwarzenegger in a special election viewed as a crucial test of his personal popularity and probusiness agenda. The special election presented a series of referendum questions that, if passed, would have lengthened the probationary period before a teacher in the public schools could get tenure and would have required public-employee unions to get written consent from members before spending dues money for political purposes. Many observers believed that this latter measure specifically targeted the California Nurses Association, which had lobbied so hard against the governor on this issue. Had it passed, the restriction on funds would have limited the ability of nurses' unions to raise money to lobby for measures such as the ratio bill.

In this high-profile struggle involving teachers, firefighters, police officers, and many other public employees, media commentators widely credited the California Nurses Association with finding the first chink in the governor's armor—and sparking the grassroots countercampaign against the referendum. The nurses' union organized a coalition of teachers, firefighters, public employees, and other citizen groups to oppose the ballot initiative. The coalition enlisted the support of two famous actors, Annette Bening and Warren Beatty. In the company of the actors, nurses held a four-city tour in Southern California to counter the governor's message. The association ran an ad campaign contrasting the critical role nurses play in the health-care system with the governor's efforts to raise money from corporate sources. A traveling billboard—rolled out on the back of a flatbed truck—showed a calm but authoritative-looking nurse with a stethoscope around her neck next to a photograph of the governor who, once again, was grimacing angrily with his fist up in the air. The headline over the nurses' photo read "She heals." Over Schwarzenegger the headline was "He wheels and deals." Underneath was a caption: "Dedicated to patient health, not corporate wealth."

As the campaign wore on, opinion surveys showed that RNs were more popular than the governor and that picking a fight with them was not a winning strategy. The voters of California rejected all of the governor's ballot propositions. Immediately after the election, he announced that he was abandoning his adversarial stance toward public employees, teachers, firefighters, and nurses. In fact, angering the right wing of the Republic Party, he hired a Democrat to be his new chief of staff. More important, almost as soon as the referendum was defeated, the governor's lawyers quietly dropped their appeal of the Superior Court ruling that supported the staffing ratios. The governor said he would no longer oppose implementation of the safe nurse-to-patient staffing ratios. Kelly DiGiacomo said, with an undisguised note of triumph:

> When Schwarzenegger announced that he'd given up fighting us on the ratios, we felt vindicated. It was nurses in California who were the ones who took him on. We made him change his policies. More than that we made him change his style. The public didn't like what he was doing to nurses. If he was reelected that's only because he made these concessions. Otherwise he came very, very close to not even being able to run again.

4

Ratios Redux

In 2005, Nancy Donaldson of the California Nursing Outcomes Coalition (CalNOC) Data Base Project, Linda Burnes Bolton, chief nursing officer of Cedars-Sinai Medical Center in Los Angeles, and four other researchers—three from Cedars-Sinai and one from Kaiser Permanente—published the first analysis of the California staffing ratios in the journal *Policy, Politics, and Nursing Practice*. The research compared the first six months of 2002 with the first six months of 2004 when the 1:6 ratios went into effect. The researchers reported that most medical/surgical units were already meeting the mandated staffing even before ratios went into effect but added that hospitals had, nonetheless, significantly increased their staffing after ratios. As they staffed for ratios, most hospitals had not, as some feared, replaced RNs with LVNs. Hospitals were, however, cutting ancillary staff.

The heart of the article was what it claimed to be its most serious finding: patient care had not improved because of ratios. Using the ANA's nurse-sensitive indicators, the researchers focused on incidents of falls and bedsores. Here, they said, they found no statistically significant improvement in either problem after ratios were implemented.[1] The clear inference to be drawn from this study, according to the authors, was that ratios were not useful because they did not improve patient care.

There are, however, a number of methodological and political problems with this particular study, some of which were highlighted in an editorial written by David Keepnews, the journal's editor. Keepnews pointed out that "an honest reading would caution against anyone concluding that staffing ratios have no impact on patient outcomes." Keepnews noted the contradiction between the assertion that hospitals were staffing to ratios before ratios were mandated and that staffing had increased significantly after ratios.

"Were many hospitals, in fact, already meeting yet-to-be-required staffing levels—and, if so, what would explain their 'staffing up' following implementation of the requirements?" he asked. Were hospitals adding nurses to relieve, rather than assist, nurses for meal, rest, and bathroom breaks? Keepnews cautioned that the first six months of 2004 may not have been an appropriate time frame for a study: judging the efficacy of ratios only a few months after they'd been implemented was probably premature. Finally, he suggested that the questions the researchers addressed were far too narrow. Unaddressed issues, for example, were how the ratios affected "recruitment and retention of nurses, nursing overtime worked, patient experiences of care, and the impact (positive or negative) on hospital finances and services."[2]

Other researchers have had similar concerns. Sean Clarke at the University of Pennsylvania School of Nursing finds the study intriguing but worries that it is too early to judge the impact of the ratios on the basis of those results alone. "I have faith in the staffing trends the authors identified," he says. "It's clear that RN positions increased to meet ratios, while overall, non-RN positions decreased. But this only demonstrates that hospitals moved to comply with regulations but may have cut back on the types of personnel the legislation doesn't cover." Indeed, Clarke found it interesting that hospitals apparently did not, as some had feared, use the "licensed nurse" provision in the ratios to replace RNs with LVNs but instead hired more RNs (who are more expensive but have a broader scope of practice).

Several researchers share Keepnews's concerns that the research design was not sophisticated enough to offer conclusive evidence about the impact of ratios. Donaldson and colleagues performed a simple before-and-after comparison of the rates of a small handful of complications of care averaged over short periods of time. More patient outcomes that could be influenced by a complex change such as ratio implementation need to be studied for longer periods of time before conclusions can be drawn.

Joanne Spetz, an economist who teaches at the University of California, San Francisco School of Nursing, has studied nursing labor markets and the nursing workforce since the early 1990s. Spetz believes that the jury is still out on the ratios and that, at the time of our interview in the fall of 2007, there was no published research that provides evidence that ratios are working—or not working—to improve either recruitment and retention into nursing or patient care. She argues that the CalNOC study is both premature and that the two problems measured are actually not useful in judging nursing's impact on patient care.

Spetz explained that nurses are not the only personnel that have an impact on pressure ulcer prevention through maintenance of the patient's skin integrity: "It's not entirely clear whether you need an RN to perform all of those functions versus having able-bodied nurse personnel turning the patient. You also need to have the right kind of bedding and mattress." Spetz is concerned that Donaldson's data point to other factors that may have a negative impact on bedsores. "There is some evidence in the Donaldson data that RN hiring has caused displacement of some unlicensed personnel. If some of those unlicensed personnel were involved in things that have to do with preventing pressure ulcers then having more RNs isn't going to have an impact on pressure ulcers," she said.

Spetz was equally uncertain about the validity of using patient falls as a measure to judge the efficacy of ratios. Once again the question is how much influence do licensed nurses versus unlicensed personnel have on patient falls. "My read of the literature is that you might do better to have an unlicensed person to serve as a bedsitter," she said. "You want to have an RN do the initial assessment to identify patients who need the intervention, but in the end it's not clear that substituting RNs for aides or LVNs is going to reduce your fall rate."

She expects to see more positive outcomes of the ratios appear when researchers look at the problem of failure to rescue. Spetz surmises, "Having a nurse who has the kind of clinical knowledge and critical-thinking skills that a registered nurse has makes it possible for the nurse to say, 'I don't like the way this patient is looking. I'm worried this patient is going to go south.' The signs of a very early complication are quite subtle." Unfortunately, the CalNOC study does not include failure to rescue.

The time frames (2002 and 2004) of the study may not have been well chosen either. Researchers at the University of California, Davis, documented that in 2002 the majority of hospitals in California were staffing their units at 1:6, before the ratios were determined and implemented. If most hospitals were staffing at these 1:6 ratios, one would not expect to see much of a difference when that specific ratio was mandated in all hospitals. Surely, the most appropriate time to do an assessment of the results of ratios would be when the ratios significantly changed to 1:5. This is presumably why the legislature stipulated that ratios should be evaluated five years after implementation, not after five months.

To fully evaluate the impact of ratios on patient safety a research design would have to involve data from several years both before and after implementation. It would also have to use statistical techniques that evaluate changes over time through the period when patients might have been affected, with an eye to whether there is improvement, decline, or stability in the measures.

The potential biases of the participants and the data used also raise concerns. CalNOC uses data that hospitals voluntarily report. Spetz wonders whether this fact creates a kind of selection bias:

I anticipate that the hospitals that choose to report to CalNOC, or the National Data Base of Nursing Quality Indicators (NDNQI), or any other quality programs, are the hospitals that care about quality. If they already care about quality and are doing something about it in these dimensions, there's also the question about how much more improvement could they get. It was a limited sample, and we don't know if the results for these outcomes . . . might not be seen statewide.

CalNOC itself is closely allied to the Association of California Nurse Leaders, which fought the ratios and continues to oppose them. Moreover, four of the researchers—including the chief nursing officer—are from Cedars-Sinai Medical Center. During the study period, the hospital nursing department was involved in a bitter dispute with the California Nurses Association over a union election that would have granted collective bargaining representation to Cedars-Sinai nurses. Although the union won the election, the nursing administration appealed its findings all the way to the National Labor Relations Board in Washington, D.C. The NLRB eventually overturned the election and said a new election would have to be held. The election was never held. The relationship between some of the researchers and the union that was the main proponent of the ratios was not mentioned in the article.

Working Nurses Talk about the Importance of Ratios

Because the CalNOC study seems to raise more questions than it answers, I talked to individual nurses and managers regarding their views of the 1:5 ratios that, in March 2005, were finally phased in. Most of the nurses I interviewed all argued that ratios—while not the final solution to their problems—have changed things for the better for them and have made their hospitals safer for patients. For the first time in over a decade, nurses know they can come to work certain that they will not be asked to take care of an impossible number of patients.

Kathy Sackman, president of the United Nurses of California (UNAC), which represents RNs at thirteen Kaiser hospitals in Southern California as well as nurses in other hospitals, says that most hospitals are staffing according to the ratios at least 80 to 85 percent of the time. Kaiser, Sackman reports, has been particularly assiduous in working with unions not only to staff to ratios but also to staff above them—at 1:4. When the ratio bill was passed, Kaiser's nurse unions, with the exception of the CNA, began to organize working groups to analyze medical/surgical units at all the facilities. The groups, Sackman says, "looked at current positions, vacancies, and how many additional staff would be needed, as well as the cost for each. This took about a year and a half, and Kaiser recruited two thousand nurses to bring the ratios up to where they needed to be."

Depending on the hospital, Sackman says, most units staff to the 1:4 ratios most of the time. Some Kaiser hospitals, she adds, have trouble with recruitment, because hospitals are in a downtown area where they are in competition with surrounding facilities that are also trying to recruit nurses. Examples she cites are Kaiser Sunset and West LA, both in or near downtown Los Angeles.

Non-Kaiser hospitals, such as most unionized Tenet facilities, where UNAC represents nurses, are also staffing to ratios, Sackman says. In the facilities where it represents nurses, UNAC is trying to get language on ratios included in their labor contracts. "In our last negotiation with Tenet we got contract language to maintain state ratios. This gives us an option to go through the grievance procedure if nurses say their unit never staffs to ratios. We can demand documentation like schedules and vacancy rates and find out why they're not. We can take the issue through the grievance procedure." Sackman explains that without this the union's only option is to lodge a complaint with the Department of Health Services. "They want to be helpful, but they are overwhelmed and not staffed up the way they need to be."

"Basically the facilities are staffing according to ratios," said CNA president Deborah Burger.

> In fact, we now have ratio language in a number of contracts with, for example, Catholic Healthcare West and the UC [University of California] system. We put ratio language into the contract just in case some crazy people decide to take it upon themselves to change the law with a stroke of a pen. At least our patients are protected in the contract. This kind of contract language sets a precedent so that even the private hospitals that aren't under a CNA contract feel obligated to staff according to ratios because this is now the community standard. When you're out in the community talking about how safe your hospital is, and when patients have a choice about what hospital they'll go to, they'll choose the one that has more nurses.

Burger believes that the ratios have allowed nurses not only to provide safe basic nursing care but also to "claim back things that they had to give away or could not do because they didn't have the time, the physical or emotional energy. Nurses can now talk to a patient a little longer than you would have before the ratios to do some really good psychosocial interventions. Some of those things are necessary, but when you're short staffed, you do the things that are a priority."

Although Burger does not work in in-patient care, she nonetheless works for Kaiser in Santa Rosa, where she notes that the impact of ratios spills over into her clinic work with high-risk diabetics. "My patients have a lot of what we call comorbidities—hypertension, renal insufficiency, problems with ulcerating wounds, and many other issues," she said. Before the ratios, when she met with patients who'd just gotten out of the hospital, she'd often discover that they didn't know much about how to take their insulin or what signs or symptoms to look for if they took too much or too little medication. They didn't know how to care for the wounds that are one of the most prevalent risks of diabetes, the ulcers on a foot or leg that, if not properly treated, can lead to an amputation. Nor did they understand how their blood sugar affected their healing. This was because nurses on the hospital unit didn't have time to educate them.

With ratios in place, she said, "patient education is much improved and patients know when to contact a doctor or nurse when they notice an early sign or symptom of infection or of a medication reaction. When I see patients who had been hospitalized, they have received more patient education and better teaching about their chronic conditions. Nurses now have time to provide this in the hospital."

People don't usually ask clinic or home-care nurses about the impact of ratios because they consider them to be peripheral to their application. Yet as care has eroded in hospitals, clinic and home-care nurses notice and have to deal with the fallout. Home-care and clinic nurses find that patients have complications that could have been prevented with proper education—problems with wounds or infections. The patients don't know how to take their medications and thus experience preventable side effects or complications due to the interaction of different medications. They don't know how to adjust their diets and exercise patterns and provide basic self-care, much less cope with complex treatment regimens.

Burger believes more workforce researchers should make the connection between adequacy of hospital nursing and the work of home-care nurses. As an example of a researcher who does understand this link, Burger points to the work of Linda Aiken at the University of Pennsylvania School of Nursing. As discussed in part 3, Aiken has documented the link between nurse staffing and preventable complications and patient mortality "Aiken's work makes the connection," Burger said, "but a lot of people don't."

Most staff nurses, of course, do connect the dots. "When we went from one to ten or more patients on the telemetry unit to one to five it was a total transformation," said Kelly DiGiacomo. "After the ratios it was totally different. You felt safe. You felt patients were safe."

For Alyson Kennedy, who is in her mid-fifties, the ratios are critical to helping return to and remain in the workforce. For her, the issue is the wear and tear of nursing's hard physical work. Lifting and turning patients takes its toll on nurses who, in this predominantly women's profession, have more musculoskeletal injuries than many men in traditionally male professions. It is ironic that today a longshoreman, whom some might see as the quintessential male physical laborer, no longer touches crates and bales but pushes a button on a lifting device that does the work for him.

In the state of Victoria, one of the strategies the government used to both save money and attract older nurses back into the workforce was to mandate lift teams and lift equipment in all public hospitals (as mentioned, Governor Schwarzenegger vetoed precisely this kind of legislation in California in 2005). Aging nurses like Kennedy have to lift patients who weigh two hundred or even three hundred pounds or more without the help of the devices medical equipment manufacturers have produced for safe lifting. Even though getting help from another nurse or two doesn't guarantee that a nurse or all the nurses will not get injured, it certainly makes it less likely. But if nurses have eight or ten or twelve patients, they're running too fast and hard to help one another if a patient falls, needs to be turned, or needs help to get to the bathroom. Each extra patient added to the workload is an invitation to injury.

"It makes a huge difference in the wear and tear on your body the fewer patients you have to take care of," Kennedy explained. "I feel like I could easily do another ten years. I actually did leave, for a brief period, five years ago. I went to beauty school and became an esthetician, and I missed nursing so much that I really wanted to come back." The ratios convinced Kennedy to do just that. "I wouldn't have returned to nursing if I knew I was going to take care of ten patients. No way. Ratios and the fact that I was offered half-time convinced me to return to the hospital. Now I can see myself working into my sixties."

How older nurses fare in the workplace is one key to easing today's nursing shortage. The average age of the nurse in the United States is forty-seven. Hundreds of thousands of nurses are over fifty. They could retire in five years, or they could last another ten or fifteen years. Making adjustments in their workloads, as Kennedy attests, is particularly important if older nurses are to retire later rather than earlier.

For nurses outside of California, who don't have ratios, either because there is no state legislation or because they have no union contract regulating workload, sheer physical exhaustion is a critical variable in their decision to leave nursing. Sarah Jeffers (not her real name), a nurse who recently retired to Las Vegas, recounts a typical story. The sixty-two-year-old nurse had worked in the same Ohio hospital for thirty-four of her thirty-nine years in nursing. In her last two years working on an orthopedic floor, her patient load jumped from three to four patients, then to five or sometimes even six patients. Most were elderly men and women admitted for hip or total joint replacements. It took almost two hours to prepare each of them for surgery. But Jeffers also cared for patients who'd just come out of surgery. If they didn't get pain medication, they wouldn't be able to do their rehabilitation exercises. Without frequent monitoring of vital signs, they could develop a wound or a urinary tract infection. If they weren't carefully shifted in bed, they could develop the kind of excruciating bedsore that could cost between $4,000 and $70,000 to heal. At her age, she couldn't tolerate the heavy patient load coupled with the long hours.

"I wasn't ready to retire," Jeffers said with regret. "I would have worked for another two or three years. I loved my job. I loved going to work. But I couldn't work those long hours with such heavy patient loads."

Improvements in workload will affect more than the retention of nurses like Kennedy or Jeffers, who have been in the hospital workforce for twenty to thirty years. They will also determine the longevity of newer, but older, recruits into nursing. Peter I. Buerhaus, a nursing workforce researcher who has produced major studies on the nursing workforce, has documented that as hospitals and the profession attempt to deal with the nursing shortage by recruiting new candidates to the profession, many of them, according to Buerhaus, are women and men age fifty to sixty-four.[3] For them, workload—and work hours, which are also escalating—will be a key variable in retention.

A Management View of Ratios

It is not surprising that so many staff nurses favor ratios. What is more surprising is that a number of nurse managers and executives also do. A 2004 report written by Joanne Spetz, who is hardly a cheerleader for ratios, said that "some hospital nurse executives quietly expressed support for the ratios." This is in spite of the fact that their industry association—the CHA—has aggressively opposed the mandated ratios.[4]

One of the not-so-quiet nurse executives who has voiced support for AB 394 is Marilyn Chow, vice president of patient-care services for the national office for Kaiser Permanente. As Kaiser's chief nursing officer for the entire nation, Chow oversees a great many nurses in a great many places. As perhaps the largest employer of nurses in the state of California (about 20 percent of nurses in California work at various Kaiser facilities, not all of whom at its twenty-nine acute care hospitals), Kaiser took the lead on the ratio issue, implementing 1:4 ratios of licensed nurses on their medical/surgical units in 2002, before the DHS even announced its final ratio decision.

Chow's attitudes toward and actions implementing ratios stem from two intertwined factors. One is her understanding of escalating patient acuity. The other is her desire to make Kaiser, as she puts it, the employer of choice for nurses as well as a national clinical model.

Unlike many of her colleagues, Chow does not question the legitimacy of ratios. Nor does she believe they are, as many managers depict them, some dark and dangerous revolutionary experiment. "I know there's a lot of controversy about ratios across the country," Chow acknowledged. "When I thought about the issue of ratios, I thought back to when the ICU ratios of 1:1 or 1:2 went into effect in California and in other parts of the country in the 1970s. Who were the ICU patients then, and where are those patients now?" Chow asked.

"Many people would say and agree that the med/surg unit patient [of today] is as sick if not sicker than the ICU patients of the 1970s. So we've got regulations that address that, and, in addition, we have a patient classification system, which is another check. If a patient needs more care they should get it," she answered. Because patients on medical/surgical floors today are as sick as those on ICUs in the 1970s, Chow thinks that implementing ratios on those floors, as Kaiser has done, is a very "reasonable" move.

Chow also favors ratios because she sees it as part of Kaiser's strategy to make the system "a great place to work and national clinical model." She explained that when she became the chief nurse at Kaiser in California in 2000 she examined several issues about the nursing workforce. The first, she said, was "How do we get the workforce we need? That's the whole on-boarding process of recruitment and retention." The second aspect she looked at was learning: "In our exit interviews we learned that people considered career development issues as well as supervisor issues. So we created different educational opportunities to help with career development."

The third was leadership—Did nurses who left Kaiser have problems with managers? It turns out that some did. So Chow focused on developing better leadership programs. The fourth area was practice and the work environment. Here, she said, ratios were one way to enhance nursing practice and nurses' working conditions. The fifth issue was research—getting evidence for practice. And the sixth was quality and safety for patients and workers. She concluded that "ratios fit in with what we were doing to become an organization of choice and national clinical model. They didn't exist in a vacuum."

One influence on the early introduction of ratios was meetings Kaiser held with what it calls its labor partners under its labor-management partnership. Several unions represent Kaiser nurses, including the Service Employees International Union (SEIU) and the United Nurses Association of California/UNAC (part of AFSCME). Kaiser met with these groups and understood that they favored ratios. Chow also ascertained that the DHS/UC Davis research would probably produce ratios of 1:6 or 1:5. So in 2001 the company began the slow process of implementing 1:4 ratios of licensed nurses on its medical/surgical units. The CNA, which represents nurses at Kaiser in northern California, is, however, critical of the labor partnership approach and chose not to be a member of the partnership. The union has criticized Kaiser's early implementation of ratios, arguing that it was simply a ploy to replace RNs with LVNs. Whatever the motivation, Kaiser and Chow have been supportive of the ratio process, which is certainly more than one can say of other health-care companies and nurse executives.

Chow said that Kaiser's data indicates that the ratios have helped in recruiting and retaining nurses. She said, "We've looked at retention and recruitment, and over the past five years we have decreased our turnover and vacancy rate from double digits to single digits." As of fall 2006, Kaiser's vacancy rate was 6 percent. Many hospital vacancy rates are in the double digits.

Although Chow believes that ratios are necessary, she, like many of her colleagues, is concerned that in implementing ratios, hospitals will deprive nurses of ancillary support:

> When I hear my other colleagues who aren't supportive of ratios, I understand that perspective. There are just a finite amount of dollars, and you have to choose where you're going to spend them. When I heard some nurses talk about it, on the one hand, they like having ratios. On the other hand, if it means [having] ratios at the expense of having an aide or less support staff, they'd rather have support staff. That's where the jury is out from the perspective of front-line staff. At the end of the day, what I care about is if nurses have the feeling they have the supports they need to deliver safe, quality care. Even with ratios, sometimes nurses still say it isn't a good use of their time to do these daily activities that they could use an aide [to do].

Although Chow agrees with her Australian counterparts that government-mandated ratios could give nurse executives leverage in their budget discussions with other hospital executives, she emphasizes that they need to be developed in a flexible way and that their efficacy and cost need to be constantly reevaluated. Technological advances, she points out, can dramatically affect nursing, and patient care and ratios must take into account the dynamic nature of health-care delivery. Finally, Chow worries that ratios could bust hospital budgets if other health-care workers followed the nurses' example and demanded workload regulation. "If you get everyone coming with their minimum ratios, what do you do then?" she wondered. "The people who are running hospitals as well as staff need flexibility and that's where the challenge of ratios comes in."

Another chief nursing officer, Karin J. Bernsten, who directed nursing services at a one-hundred-and-ten-bed hospital in 2005 and is currently director of quality risk and care management at another hospital in San Diego, is also supportive of ratios. The author of two books on patient safety, Bernsten says that

> appropriate ratios are important for patient safety in a market in which there are so many growing responsibilities for nursing staff. Patients are more complex; acuity today is much higher as inpatient procedures and complexity increase. Regimens of medication have increased substantially over the last two decades; today your average patient can be on anything from nine to eighteen different medications. It takes a high skill level to coordinate that care.

Plus, she says, nurses are using sophisticated monitoring equipment, dealing with patients on ventilators, and manipulating such equipment as wound vacs, which apply suction to heal and dry wounds.

"Appropriate ratios are critical to make sure from a safety standpoint that each patient is getting the optimal care," Bernsten says, adding that she believes the 1:5 or 1:4 California ratios are appropriate.

Bernsten acknowledged that the ratios made her job more challenging. "You had to extensively plan to make sure you had coverage available. With good planning it made you focus more on making sure there was a balance of licensed nurses to the appropriate ratios." It also, she said, "protected the nursing budget. You can't slash the budget because you have the ratios. Sometimes you have to shift from nonskilled ratios; you may have to have fewer unit clerks in order to meet the ratios. But you are providing higher skill."

Bernsten emphasized the fact that ratios allow nurse executives to move the patient not only more safely but sometimes more swiftly through the system:

> If you coordinate that efficiency correctly, this can help you, for example, decrease the patient's length of stay because you're managing that care more appropriately. If instead of a nurse handling eight patients, that nurse is handling four or five, they can actually help with making sure, say, the testing is done on time. They can actually move the patient through the system more safely in a way that takes less time. The longer the patient stays in the hospital, studies show that patients are at risk for infections, falls, or medication errors.

Even some chief nursing officers who are critical of ratios acknowledge that the ratios have had a positive impact. Judith McCurdy is the CNO at Arrowhead Regional Medical Center. This is a 373-bed hospital in San Bernardino County, near Los Angeles. The hospital employs eight hundred nurses who are represented by the California Nurses Association. McCurdy said she feels she has a good relationship with the nurses' union. McCurdy's hospital depends on public financing from Medi-Cal and Medicare, whose reimbursement rates have gone down, not up. She criticizes ratios because they represent an unfunded mandate for which, at least in her case, no funds are likely to be made available. She would be more supportive of ratios if she had the flexibility to apply the 1:5 or 1:4 ratio over a twenty-four-hour period rather than for each shift. "If they would say this is what you have to have in a twenty-four-hour period, I would have one less nurse on nights and one more nurse on days," she explained. "Or I would adjust that, depending. Ideally, what I would have is an extra nurse who comes in and works from 4:00 in the afternoon to 8:30 at night. Because that's when I have my admissions and discharges."

Nonetheless, McCurdy understands that ratios were needed because patient acuity systems just weren't working. "The good news is," she said, "it forced hospitals to have to provide enough resources for nursing, because some were really running skimpy and nursing service often didn't have enough clout to increase the staffing." McCurdy candidly admits that "the system we had before, the acuity-based system, in some ways could be gamed, played so you really didn't have to provide staffing." In some hospitals, medical/surgical floors with patients with very intense nursing needs were "running a 1:8 ratio. That's really skimpy, even if the nurse worked with one certified nursing assistant. One CNA is not enough."

Several middle-level managers I spoke with also expressed support for ratios. Kelly DiGiacomo is one of them. Since her brush with Arnold Schwarzenegger's security forces, DiGiacomo has, in fact, become a manager at Kaiser. When asked how the ratios affect her job and why she supports them, she took a deep breath and released a rush of reasons:

> I'm a manager now and no longer in the union, but I'm still a patient advocate and a nurse advocate. I know that patients are going to be safe. I know that my nurses aren't going to be so danged exhausted and frustrated every day that they want to quit. I know that I can retain my nurses. I know that if my nurses are happy and can practice safely, then the patients are going to be happy and get good care, and that all equates to Kaiser being the employer of choice and being the choice for health care for patients.

DiGiacomo believes that many managers support ratios, whether silently or not. "All the managers," she said, "they're still nurses, and many, many managers were really rooting for us and wished they could have been out there protesting too. I never had a manager treat me badly because of my protesting for the ratios."

Another manager at a Kaiser hospital said that she thinks, with some reservations, that ratios have, for the most part, helped nurses and patients. Judith Forrest°, who at fifty-five was an older nurse, had been assistant manager in the telemetry unit for a year and a half when I spoke with her. Ratios help "prevent burnout because [nurses are] not so overwhelmed with patients," she said. "It gives them time to reflect on the care they are giving patients. That's a positive aspect." When Forrest worked as a staff nurse, she wasn't able to spend time to talk with the patients and find out who they were and to incorporate their concerns into her care. "I probably felt frustrated about it," she admitted. "You knew the patients would want to talk to you about something. You didn't have the time to sit with them and talk to them as much as you would have liked." She acknowledged that "nurses today now have the opportunity to take that time. Whether they take it or not is up to the individual nurse."

Forrest is, however, concerned that ratios could "stunt the growth" of some nurses. She believes they could prevent nurses from taking advantage of opportunities to learn more. Her ward, for example, is made up of two units. If there's an interesting procedure being performed on one unit that a nurse could learn from by observing, but she's on the other unit, the ratios would keep her from going over to the other unit to watch. She also thinks that nurses get complacent when they have too few patients—three or fewer. This happens, she says, because Kaiser has a policy of "no cancellations." If the patient census is down, nurses can't be told not to come to work, which means they might actually have fewer than five patients. "It's kind of coddling them," she said of the situation. When I asked whether this "no cancellation" policy has anything to do with ratios or is, instead, another matter—which could be happening with or without the ratio bill—she responded, "Oh yes, you're right, I hadn't thought of that" and agreed that ratios were not responsible for this "coddling" of nurses.

Forrest grudgingly conceded that ratios helped her as a manager, because if nurses are less burned out, they are less frustrated, and if they are less frustrated they give her fewer problems. There is, she hastened to add, a flip side—newer nurses. "There are," she explained, "some nurses who haven't practiced very long. They think five patients is the max, and if they have five patients they're so overwhelmed they can't possibly do anything else and how dare we expect them to take care of five patients. On the other hand, it's a very good thing, because older nurses are very glad they have only five patients instead of seven."

Forrest does believe that ratios have helped put nursing on the public and medical map. "I think that it's about time that the public and doctors understand what nurses do and how valuable they are to the practice of medicine. It's making the medical field stand up and pay attention to nurses," she said. The heated debate about staffing and nurse-to-patient ratios has encouraged researchers to study the impact of nursing on patient care and to demonstrate that nurses aren't there only to "fluff your pillow or wipe your butt." And for Forrest, "It's about time."

Deborah Burger believes that ratios help managers do their jobs more effectively. "Before the ratios," she said, "nurse managers were constantly being harassed and harangued to keep in budget, to keep the staffing down to the most minimal level so they could continue to make profits." Managers, she added, were sandwiched between administrators at the top, who wanted to nurses to do more with less, and nurses at the bottom, who were begging for more staffing. They also suffered from the same process of work intensification as the nurses they supervised, as they were being assigned more nurses to oversee. Although managers may need ratios as much as staff nurses do, Burger believes that ratios at least allow them a bit of relief. She said, "Now they can say, 'Wait a minute. There's the ratio law, and this is the number of patients we have; this is the number of nurses I have to provide.'"

Joanne Spetz's 2004 report confirms this view:

One chief nursing officer said she was looking forward to the ratios in medical/surgical units changing to 1 nurse per 5 patients in 2005 because she would be able to demand funding to staff at a level she has always wanted. Nurses seem to be gaining more power and greater decision-making authority as a result of the minimum ratios.

In the past, when a unit manager believed the admission of more patients to the unit would overtax the nursing staff, the manager may have been unable to enforce a closure of the unit to new admissions. Physicians usually had control over whether more patients were admitted to a unit. Under the minimum ratios, a unit manager must refuse new patients until more staff is available on the unit, and physicians have no recourse. In order to support higher patient loads, unit managers can demand higher budgets to hire more staff, and the medical staff of a hospital must support higher personnel budgets to secure greater capacity.[5]

Some evidence on the success of ratios comes from statistical analysis of the number of nurses who are migrating to California from other states. According to Spetz the "number of new RN licenses issued by the California board has risen substantially in the past two years, but it remains unknown how many of these licenses are held by foreign-educated nurses and travelers from other states."[6] Data from the Board of Registration of Nursing document that between 1994 and 1999, the number of endorsements slowly climbed from 3,115 to 4,880. From 1999 to 2006, it leaped to 10,472.[7] In June 1999, there were 246,068 RNs with active licenses in California. By 2006, there were 309,918.[8] In 1997, the Board of Registration of Nursing had predicted that by 2006 there would be 257,716 active RN licensees. In fact, in 2006 there were 52,202 more than that. Some of these nurses are recruited from foreign countries; others come from out of state. When I was in Mississippi after the ratios had passed, nursing academics there complained that they were losing many of their new graduates to California because of the ratio law. Needless to say, the California Nurses Association, not surprisingly, attributes this to the passage of the ratio bill and the improvement of working conditions in the state. Although the CNA argues that the number of out-of-state nurses obtaining a license in California has increased by 47,186, the California Hospital Association counters that "42,820 nurses left California during that period of time. Thus, California had a net increase of only 4,369 out of state nurses during the past five years." What the CHA fails to mention is that this net increase is almost the precise number of nurses researchers estimate would be needed to fill the ratios.[9] Moreover, the hospital association does not consider how many more nurses would have left the state—and how many fewer would have entered it—without AB 394 and the implementation of ratios. With a few notable exceptions, most of the nurses interviewed for this book said that their hospitals had been complying with the ratios DHS had established. Both quality of care and quality of work life had improved.

Linda Aiken, Sean Clarke, and their colleagues at the University of Pennsylvania School of Nursing received funding from the National Institutes of Health to examine staffing influences on patient and nurse outcomes in California and Pennsylvania. The group has also received funding from the Robert Wood Johnson Foundation to extend the work to New Jersey. The researchers view ratio legislation as a complicated policy intervention that merits detailed study by as many groups as possible and using as many data sources as possible. "To our knowledge," said Clarke and Aiken, "we're the only group not affiliated with either labor or management who have asked nurses on the ground experiencing these changes for their impressions and observations about staffing and its consequences through surveys. We're also going to use data sources that other groups are using to get as clear a picture as possible of impacts." Research results of Clarke and Aiken's study of the impact of ratios are discussed in chapter 9.

Problems with the Application of the Law

Although many nurses are supportive of AB 394, many are critical of the enforcement process. Nurses themselves must report violations of the law to the Department of Health Services. If the department decides that the violation is serious enough to jeopardize patients, investigators are required to arrive at the institution within two working days. If it is deemed not to be a threat to patient safety, the DHS has up to seventy working days to investigate. The law does not give the DHS the power to fine or financially penalize hospitals found to be in violation of the ratios. Hospitals must create an action plan to address the violations.

"Although DHS enforcement of the ratios is relatively weak, other mechanisms exist to ensure that hospitals adhere to the ratios," Joanne Spetz wrote in her 2004 article assessing the ratios just as they were being implemented. "Medicare and Medi-Cal [the state Medicaid program] require that hospitals comply with all laws and regulations. These programs can audit hospitals retroactively by examining payroll and staffing records. Moreover, these programs can deny payment retroactively if a hospital is found to be out of compliance."

As the CHA warned its members in its early seminars on the ratio bill, anyone who sues a hospital for medical malpractice can subpoena staffing records. "In addition, staffing records can be subpoenaed in medical malpractice cases. If a hospital is not in compliance with all laws," Spetz writes, "lawyers can make a case for negligence on the part of the hospital, and California's $250,000 cap on malpractice awards might not apply."[10] In a suit for damages related to a medical error or injury, a hospital could be at fault not because it failed to follow ratios but because it was violating a de facto standard of practice that, because of the ratio bill, was now communitywide.

Because the Department of Health Services is severely underfunded, Deborah Burger said ratio enforcement depends on nurses' willingness to file unsafe staffing complaints, which the department can then investigate. Nurses do report violations of the ratios. They seem to be more concerned about violations of the intent of the entire law than with violations of only the ratio.

It is important to stress that violations of AB 394 include more than violations of the mandated staffing ratios. The law clearly stipulates that the ratios are minimums, not maximums, and that staffing of units is not to be based on ratios alone but on ratios plus data generated by patient acuity systems. "If a patient classification system indicates that more nurses than the minimum are needed for a shift, the hospital must staff more richly as suggested by the patient classification system," Spetz wrote.

It is often here that the rubber meets, or in many cases doesn't meet, the road. Spetz has hinted at some of the reasons for this: "The patient classification system requirement has been criticized because it does not provide guidance about the types of patient classification systems that are acceptable, nor are there strong enforcement mechanisms."[11]

According to a health facilities evaluator nurse who works for the Department of Health Services in licensing and certification, the mechanisms available to monitor and determine whether there are violations in the law are woefully inadequate. The evaluator said, "All of the hospitals are violating the law, cutting corners. Most nurses don't report the violations. When they do, we have little funding. We don't have a special program or taskforce, and most of the staff are not capable of handling all the stuff we receive when there is a complaint." The evaluator explained that when a complaint is made to the DHS, "hospitals will send boxes and boxes of paperwork—schedules, acuity-classification data—and there is not enough staff to even go through the vast quantities of paperwork the complaints generate."

The evaluator believed that there need to be significant financial penalties to hospitals if the law is to be taken seriously. "They should be at least $10,000," the evaluator said, insisting that more nurses should complain about staffing violations. Although this evaluator argued that "all the hospitals are violating the law and cutting corners," the evaluator also said that things were better with ratios than they had been. In ICUs, hospitals may now assign a nurse two patients instead of one—but not three, as previously—and on medical/surgical floors, they may assign six or seven instead of five—but not eight or ten, as they had been getting before.

Many of the nurses I talked with concurred that their hospitals were cutting corners—primarily by failing to comply with the portion of the law stipulating that these bare minimums be exceeded when patients were sicker.

Nurses insisted that managers and administrators were reluctant, if not downright recalcitrant, to provide patients with more nursing care. CNA president Burger outlined the problem:

> In California there are over six hundred acuity-system tools. Many of them are designed to take budgetary constraints into consideration. Most of them are proprietary, which means that the nurse puts in the data and then the program spits out how much staffing you need. We went to staffing ratios in the first place because people felt that administrators were manipulating the acuity system either in the black box or when a nurse would put in the information. Most nurses know how many nurses, how many aides and LVNs they need to provide care for patients. But managers, they feel, are manipulating the acuity systems.

Chief nursing officer Judith McCurdy explains how these systems can be, as she puts it, "gamed." To determine patient acuity and thus calculate how many nurses are needed per shift, managers "apply a certain amount of time or hours to do a task. So let's say it's a bath. Let's say you assign ten minutes for a bath. In the olden days that might have been enough because patients could participate in some of their care. Today patients are sicker. It could take fifteen minutes to do a bath. Then patients are assigned a level of care—one to five. Each one of these patients requires so many hours of care."

The problem, McCurdy explained, is that the determination of how many hours of care a patient receives is driven by how many tasks the nurse has to do for each patient and how much time is allotted for each task. As a manager, she said, all you have to do is reduce the amount of time for each task and you've reduced the hours of nursing care a patient receives. This is in spite of the fact that your acuity-based system says that a patient is a level 1, that is, someone who needs the highest level of care. "These systems didn't recognize that patients in the hospital are sicker and sicker because we are discharging them sooner," she said.

Hospitals, McCurdy explained, could game these systems before the ratios, which was why nurses pushed for ratios. And they can clearly game them with ratios in place. "Nursing," McCurdy reminded us, "is the largest expense in the hospital. The only way to make money is to cut nursing labor costs." This is especially true for for-profit hospitals that "have to have so much return on their investment."

What McCurdy describes as a preratio problem is, according to nurses like Summer Vanslager, also a post-ratio problem. Vanslager says that Dominican Hospital, in Santa Cruz, has for the most part stuck to the ratios. In her experience, when a patient's condition—and the nurses caring for that patient—begs for more nursing care, managers won't comply with that aspect of the law. "We really started pushing them. We'd say, 'Look these patients, they are really heavy. We're having to check on them every hour and do certain procedures with them.' When you have so many patients with all these procedures you can't possibly pay attention to other patients."

In addition, Vanslager pointed out, you can't work safely if a patient is experiencing out-of-control pain or another emergency. All of this results in nurses who have—even with ratios—fourteen hours worth of work on their plate and seven hours to do it in. Which is why, she said, nurses are putting in a lot of overtime because they can't get to all their work—particularly the charting that has to be put off until the end of shift. She said:

> Our managers are very reluctant to give us more nurses. When we get a new supervisor responsible for doing the staffing, they'll say, "Oh it looks like you guys have got a heavy load." Then the longer they work with us, they start to find it very easy to call people off and call up certified nursing assistants [CNAs] to come in for the night. "We don't need you to work," they say to the nurse. They'll give you the bare minimum of nurses at the beginning of a shift regardless of how many people are in the ER or how many people we expect to admit. They're not taking into account that it takes time to admit a patient and that different patients have different needs. For example, the patient who's coming up from the ER may need blood, which requires a certain amount of monitoring.

How acuity is determined and what acuity systems include in—or exclude from—their calculations is one of the major things that Barbara Williams, a member of the CNA executive committee, contends with on a daily basis. A clinical nurse specialist in adult psychiatry at Dominican Hospital, Williams is also cochair of the hospital's professional practice committee and has been on all its negotiation teams since the early 1990s. She explained that multiple factors intensify the work of the nurse.

One of those factors is technology. Today hospitals are introducing a variety of computerized systems into the process of patient care. These include electronic health records (EHR), electronic medication administration records (eMAR), and computerized physician order entry (CPOE) systems. Nurses must use these computerized systems at the bedside—scanning barcodes for medications that are administered to hopefully avoid medication errors and charting on the computer as they are giving care to the patient.

Williams insisted that technology, while it may make patient care safer, can also make it more arduous. "In our hospitals, they are actually putting the whole patient chart online," she explained. Rather than leaving a patient's room and writing data into a chart or entering it into a computer at the nurses' station, the nurse brings the computer to the patient's room and enters information while she is caring for the patient. Williams explained:

> If you had a perfect system, computers could make things simpler. In fact, they make things more complex. Many of the systems aren't very good. The one we

have, Cerner, is basically a spreadsheet, so it's not clinical-staff friendly. During its initial phase-in, it had a lot of problems—pages you had to go through, buttons you had to click. All this created a lot more work. People were missing dialogue boxes. If you're trying to communicate something that's not in those boxes, you may communicate the right things but they may end up in the wrong section of the chart so people can't find the information they need. What the technology does is force the nurse to take care of the technology, and taking care of the patient becomes secondary.

Williams believes that computerized systems are not designed from a clinical point of view. Moreover, the fact that nurses need to constantly monitor for and adjust to the problems of the technology is not factored into computerized calculations about the nursing workload.

Experts in the problems and promise of information technology confirm the legitimacy of nurses' complaints. Ross Koppel is a medical sociologist at the Center for Clinical Epidemiology and Biostatistics in the School of Medicine at the University of Pennsylvania and a principal investigator of hospital workplace culture and medication errors. He has studied the impact of computer technology on work organization, patient care, and error. Hospitals now consider computerized charting, medication ordering, and entry systems to be a silver bullet to solving many hospital problems and improving patient safety, he explained. Although these systems offer many benefits, they all too often obscure or ignore critical information that physicians and nurses need to treat patients. "Some nurses and doctors find the data entry and retrieval process with these systems to be onerous, rather than time saving," he explained, adding:

> Clumsy and inefficient computer interfaces will continue to distract from patient care and require extra time for each patient. You have to move the mouse around to the next field or you have to find the next field on a form that's unnecessarily filled with empty fields [boxes]. The time and effort needed to make these interfaces truly efficient for health-care providers has not been taken, which means the technology can increase the nursing workload.

Michael Cohen, director of the Institute for Safe Medication Practices, agrees. As Cohen and his staff have investigated medication errors, they find that bar-coding systems can't claim 100 percent accuracy. These systems simply don't work with all packaging and all medications. Nurses are thus forced to take extra time to work around or work through the many glitches they create. As more and more hospitals computerize, dealing with computer glitches has become part of the new nursing workload.

In their fight against nursing ratios, hospital executives insisted that strong acuity systems would make ratios unnecessary. AB 394 took the ratio concept and the acuity concept and married them. The problem is that hospital executives seem to have forgotten that the state has mandated that acuity trumps ratios, which are, by law, supposed to determine the minimum—not maximum—amount of care patients are to receive. In this way they try to turn a floor into a ceiling. "Since these are minimum standards, there's no hospital in the world that's going to say, 'OK, we're going to meet the ratio at night, and we're adding to the day shift.' Not going to happen," Judith McCurdy stated emphatically. Like many other hospital managers, she insisted that the ratios represent the legislation's last word on the subject of staffing. By conveniently forgetting or ignoring the acuity mandate, she, like other hospital executives, can continue to contend that these ratios are inflexible:

> It's so inflexible, we can't flex that. If they would say there's a twenty-four-hour minimum, then great, that would be ideal, then I could flex those nurses to match the work flow. You have all your tests and procedures, admissions and discharges, patient education, family interventions . . . your doctor rounding, everything—all done during the day. I could have a change of ten patients within a four-hour window—ten in and ten out. But the day is not when I can have the most resources.

She can't, by law, she insists, add another nurse on days and take a nurse off nights when things are, in her view, slower. "No hospital is going to say you staff to ratios and in addition we'll give you these extra people," she insisted. "I know hospitals don't have enough money to do that." Given this inflexibility, and the determination to define the law as one of its parts rather than the sum of its parts, it is not surprising that nurses believe that hospitals are picking which parts of AB 394 they will comply with and which parts they feel free to violate.

Another enforcement problem nurses worry about is hospital efforts to cut back on ancillary staff and save money by forcing nurses to leave work if the hospital census is down. Ingela Dahlgren, a member of the Service Employees International Union and a critical care nurse at Northridge Hospital Medical Center in the San Fernando Valley area of Los Angeles, explained the predicament: "The ratios have provided us with a tool. We can now say to management, 'No, you cannot give me more patients. It's against the ratios. I need to have five patients on med/surg, on telemetry; if you do, you are not compliant with ratios.' "

The problem in her hospital is that management, while generally complying with the nursing ratios, is trying to save money by laying off ancillary personnel. Because there are no ratios for aides or secretaries, Dahlgren said, her union is constantly fending off the hospital's attempts to lay off critical workers who help nurses do their job effectively. In her case, the hospital has laid off unit secretaries and a category of worker called a "patient care associate."

These are higher-level nursing assistants who have more training than the standard certified nursing assistant and who help with lab draws and doing electrocardiograms (EKGs). "We have no lab staff, no phlebotomists," Dahlgren said. "They were let go. Nurses could do a blood draw or an EKG. The problem is we have so many things to do and oversee, we just don't have time." Nurses, Dahlgren said, are also perfectly capable of answering the phone. But how can they do that and care for their patients? she asked. Yet, the hospital, constantly complaining about the bottom line, would like them to care for patients *and* do the work of ancillary staff.

Nurses always argue that the hospital needs a full complement of staff—not just RNs or LVNs. In enacting AB 394, legislators clearly did not intend to decrease—but rather increase—the level of care. Dahlgren insisted that administrators now use the law to threaten nurses. When nurses complain about the loss of ancillary staff or want more nursing care for patients, their administrators will use the law against them. "Well, we have had to staff the hospital fully with RNs, so to balance the budget we have to let go PCAs and secretaries," they respond.

So, she wondered, who will go next? Will they lay off respiratory therapists and then insist "nurses can do that as well? Pretty soon, if we don't fight it, I'll be all alone on the units and will mop the floors, go down and pick up my food and get my patients in the ER, or stop by the OR and see if they have something for me, and go on with my day."

The Paradoxical Role of Ratios in Hospital Public Relations

Outside California, few nursing managers and administrators, whatever their private feelings, will publicly support nurse-staffing ratios as either one of the solutions to the nursing shortage or as a mechanism to promote greater patient safety. They will insist that there is simply no proof, no scientifically documented perfect number of nurses that assures quality patient care on any particular unit. Interestingly, some of the same managers who publicly oppose staffing ratios seem to have also embraced the concept in their advertising and public relations materials that boast of the nursing care in their hospitals and that are used to recruit and retain nurses. When I have spoken at a number of teaching hospitals in the United States, chief nurse executives have proudly confided that their hospitals staff at 1:5 or 1:6. Why, I've asked? "Well, because that's the ratio Linda Aiken identifies in her study," one responded. "We know that's the ratio that means safe patient care," another said. When I have spoken on radio shows promoting my book *Nursing against the Odds*, nurses have called up to tell me that their hospitals are different. One nurse from

Vanderbilt Medical Center in Nashville, Tennessee, called in to a talk show I was on to inform me that I'd gotten it all wrong—at least when it comes to her hospital. Then she proudly told me why Vanderbilt was different: It has 1:4 ratios on med/surg.

I have also spotted hospital advertisements that put support for ratios in black and white in the pages of newspapers or nursing journals. An advertisement seeking applications for nursing jobs at the University Medical Center in Tucson, Arizona, announced that UMC was, at the time, the only "Magnet hospital" in Arizona. Magnet hospitals go through a process of credentializing from the American Nurses Credentialing Center and are supposed to be magnets for nurses, because among other things, they give nurses a greater voice in patient care and have strong nursing leadership. The advertisement boasts the Magnet logo of the American Nurses Credentialing Center at the top right-hand corner and the letters UMC at the top left. Right under the hospital logo is the following assertion. "1:4 is our way of life. You can believe it."

The ad goes on to say, "We maintain a nationally recognized nursing environment with low RN-to-patient ratios and a genuine commitment to professional and personal development."

One to four. You can believe it. Is that it—the perfect number?

PART II

Australia: Nurses and Work Intensification in Public Hospitals in Victoria—Context, Response, and Legacies

5

Working Life for Nurses in the Late 1990s in Australia: A Snapshot

In 2000, Rachael Duncan, a neurosurgical nurse, was working part-time and studying for a master's degree at the University of Melbourne School of Nursing. At work, she was routinely assigned six very sick patients on an ordinary section of the floor and four in its "high dependency" area. "You left work feeling like a wet rag," she recalled.

> There was a very poor skill mix on the floor. A lot of casual [temporary] nurses were making up the numbers. Nursing is always hard work, but you never got ahead, you were always chasing everything. It was very demoralizing. You never felt like you'd done your job. Everyone was stressed—the nurses, the doctors, even the cleaners. Your ability to be civil was pushed to the limit. I copped agro [got complaints] from other nurses all the time, so it was harder to be civil around stressed-out family members of patients who were very sick.

Duncan finally got a break, but thanks only to her maternity leave. With some trepidation, she returned to work after the birth of her child. New staffing ratios in the state of Victoria had recently been implemented and were now firmly in place. On units like Duncan's, the rule was five nurses to twenty patients.

On her first days on the job, Duncan thought she might be experiencing a temporary illusion. "I remember when I came back for those first five shifts. I would leave feeling I'd done my job well. I enjoyed it. I was actually energized when I left work instead of exhausted. Well, maybe I just struck a quiet day, I thought. But no, things had changed." Nurses were taking care of four patients on the regular unit and two in the high-dependency area. "I remain busy," she said. "There are always things to do. But what has changed is that there are other hands and heads to help you. There are just more skilled people around and more permanent staff instead of casual nurses to help you when you need it."

Now when a patient's condition suddenly changes and Duncan has to drop everything to deal with the emergency, there is far more coverage of her other patients. Duncan cited one instance in which she was taking care of four patients, including one who had just undergone brain surgery. Everyone thought he was getting better. Then, unexpectedly, the patient developed a pulmonary embolism. Duncan immediately went into overdrive. She "bagged" the patient (manually helped the patient breathe by moving air in and out of his lungs), then administered anticoagulants and did about a dozen other things that precluded her checking on her three other patients. "We got the patient stabilized. I took him up to the ICU and came back down and wrote up my notes. By the time it was all over, it took about two hours."

Before the ratios, Duncan said, she would have resumed her full patient load, knowing that other patients' medications were missed, their vital signs not taken, or their dressings not changed because there were not enough colleagues to cover for her. In this case, when she checked on her other patients, she found that everything had been done and she even had time to decompress. She said, "You're so knackered after a critical incident like that. You've just had this huge rush of adrenaline as it's unfolding and you need to calm down so you can really focus on your other patients. You need to return to your work slowly. I couldn't do that in the past. Now I can because I don't just have extra hands to help me, I have hands that know what to do."

An Overview of Overwork

Rachael Duncan's experiences are typical of many nurses working in public hospitals in Victoria, Australia's second-largest state. Indeed, her earlier experience was part of a ubiquitous situation before ratios. In order to better understand the issue of workforce planning and the impact of overwork, in the late 1990s, the New South Wales, Queensland, and Victoria nursing unions all commissioned independent researchers to conduct surveys of their members. In 1999, the Australian Nursing Federation–Victoria commissioned John Buchanan, Jill Considine, and colleagues at the University of Sydney to survey its more than twenty thousand public-sector members.[1] Our survey's data represents the most comprehensive snapshot of the working life of nurses in Victoria prior to the introduction of ratios.

Management often dismissed nurses' complaints about overwork. Politicians often claimed that the labor shortage could be managed with better recruitment and retention strategies. They argued that unions were not accurate when they said that work intensification was endemic to the system. The problem was that some employers simply "behaved badly." Our research built on the work of researchers in the United Kingdom, Continental Europe, and Australia that emphasized the validity and credibility of employee perceptions of stress, workload, and changes in work pressures.

This body of research differs from other data used to inform decisions about the efficiency of the health-care system. Government statistical indicators and state-commissioned research in this field typically focus on issues of supply and demand. This includes aggregate changes in the skill profile of the workforce, incoming graduate numbers, and patient evaluations of the standard of health care provided. Other large-scale workplace industrial relations surveys in Britain (the Workplace Industrial Relations Survey, or WIRS) and Australia (the Australian Workplace Industrial Relations Survey, or AWIRS) instead largely rely on employee observations for their insights. Although there is certainly disagreement about this approach, Mark Beatson, a UK-based labor market economist, and others argue that quality of employment is best measured through subjective (employee) assessments of job satisfaction.[2] Influenced by this methodology, unions had data collected on the scale of work intensification for nurses across the respective state sectors. This approach allowed the unions to both observe and understand the impacts of overwork, as well as the long-term implications for patient safety and care. It also provided some insight into the processes that had contributed to workplace change.

The Victoria public hospital survey sought nurse feedback on a wide range of working arrangement concerns, including shift work, access to and frequency of breaks, overtime, overlap time for staff to hand over duties, orientation, in-service education, and workload, as well as their perception of the adequacy of current nurse-patient ratios. The study was based on a random sample of four thousand members and achieved a 43 percent response rate.

The survey found a workplace culture that both accepted and actively encouraged work intensification, particularly through the use of overtime. Alarmingly, almost half of all nurses (46%) said that working overtime was an accepted part of workplace practice and that most expected to "have to do it" as part of their normal duties. Only 29 percent of nurses said they worked overtime by choice. Just over one quarter of nurses (26%) said management required them to work overtime. Nurses themselves clearly linked overtime to understaffing. More than two-thirds of all respondents indicated that they would like their employer to employ another person rather than expecting staff to work overtime. When asked about their preferences for overtime hours, more than 50 percent of nurses said they would prefer not to work any at all. Most disturbingly, only 18 percent of the nurses were always paid for their overtime hours, while 31 percent were never paid for it.

Under the Victoria public-sector nursing enterprise agreement, the main contract between the government and its nurses in the public sector, nurses are formally entitled to reimbursement for overtime worked. Custom and practice, however, can affect whether this legal entitlement is enforced. For instance, administrative protocols at some hospitals may require senior management authorization for overtime payments. This means that a designated period of notice (e.g., twenty-four hours) is required before a claim for overtime can be approved. In many cases, the need to work overtime may not become apparent until the last few hours of a shift, if managers have difficulty finding staff for a nurse who calls in sick. Because of concerns about patient care, nurses will stay and work additional hours at the end of a shift even though they know they won't be able to claim payment for the overtime worked. In other cases, the staffing budget may not provide enough money to cover all overtime claims, so the unit (both manager and nursing staff) may agree to a custom of "time off in lieu" (or TOIL) of overtime worked. Because understaffing inevitably makes it difficult to locate replacement staff, nurses are often unable to take accrued "time off in lieu" or additional leave days because they simply cannot be "spared."

Overtime practices were not the only problematic aspect of nurses' working life in 1999. More than eight out of ten nurses were not, at the time, taking regular full meal breaks. Of these, over 70 percent never received payment for their additional work time. In addition, shifts between workers were not well synchronized, so that nurses could not complete just one handover for all their patients to one incoming nurse. Multiple handovers were part of the working arrangements for 44 percent of members, and, of these, 77 percent said that more than one handover per shift caused an increase in workload.

To estimate the magnitude of nurses' voluntary contribution to the healthcare system, the questionnaire asked nurses to record the number of hours provided as unpaid overtime in the week of the survey. Using the week of the survey as an observation period, 4,304 nurses (almost 32 percent) had worked unpaid overtime in that week. These nurses put in a staggering total of 7,319.5 unpaid hours of overtime.

Why did nurses contribute so much unpaid labor to the system? According to our interviews, nurses adapted and accommodated to excessive work because of concerns about patient safety. Mary Snell*, a senior nurse working in a major public hospital in the outer suburbs, described it in the following way, "You have an obligation; it runs deeper than just the job. . . . People who don't work in the industry wouldn't understand it." Or as Sue Brock*, a part-time registered nurse working in an eldercare facility, said, "We can't just walk off the job. We have live-in residents here. If they can't get someone to staff a shift, well, you can't just walk away."

Nurses' Views of Staffing Problems

One of the most important findings of our initial research for the Victorian Branch of the ANF was that nurses made a direct link between their rising workloads and staff shortages. The study asked nurses about their current workload, if they favored ratios, and if they believed ratios would really ease the burden of their workload. More than half of all the nurses surveyed (51%) reported that they were currently required to work to nurse-to-patient ratios on day shifts that they believed were inappropriate. More than half of the survey respondents (56%) attributed excessive workloads to inadequate nurse-to-patient ratios.

Nurses, the study reported, did not believe there was a "quick fix"—for example, hiring more novice nurses or staff from temporary agencies—to relieve their burdens. Thirty-eight percent said that adding high proportions of recent graduates and inexperienced staff to the mix would cause additional workplace problems, as they would have to mentor novice nurses to "cover their backs." Additionally, of those nurses actually working in areas with high quotas of agency staff, 87 percent said temporary nurses were a significant concern, with over one-third of these respondents reporting that temporary agency staff's lack of familiarity with the work environment made them less efficient. Indeed, over half of those concerned argued that temporary agency staff's unfamiliarity with the working environment, lack of loyalty to a particular workplace, and inappropriate qualifications for particular areas increased the workload for regular staff.

Calculating the Personal Costs of Overwork

Both surveys of and interviews with nurses showed a workforce stressed to the point of exhaustion. It is well documented that high levels of persistent workplace stress is a pernicious health hazard. The United States National Institute for Occupational Safety and Health states that "problems at work are more strongly associated with health complaints than any other life stressor—more so even than financial problems or family problems."[3]

Stressful work (as opposed to challenging work, which may stretch a worker's capabilities) can have a range of detrimental health consequences including hypertension, stroke, heart disease, depression, and many other illnesses. Plus, work-related stress is guaranteed to aggravate chronic and preexisting illnesses.[4]

Stress at work, of course, affects all workers. Nurses, however, experience a range of pressures that other workers do not necessarily encounter. Because their work puts them into daily contact with the sick, dying, suffering, and vulnerable, nurses are at an even higher risk for—and indeed suffer from more—stress-related illnesses. Plus their concern for patients and patient safety means that nurses will often act as a personal buffer between quality patient care and workload pressures to uphold their duty of care. Our research found an overwhelming majority of the survey respondents (87%) felt a high level of work-related stress.

Of those who had recently been stressed, over half said that the major source of stress was inadequate nurse-to-patient ratios, while a third said that low staff morale was the greatest source of stress. Nurses' workload problems didn't only have a negative impact on the individual nurse but also on their families and the community. More than one in three of the nurses who had partners or children were not satisfied with their ability to spend time with them. Half of those surveyed said they were dissatisfied with their ability to spend time pursuing social and community interests.[5]

Responses also illuminated the detrimental professional implications of overwork. We see it in what we call the "dormant entitlement" effect. Put in lay terms, this occurs when, because of a hostile workplace or overwork, nurses do not make use of benefits to which they are contractually or legally entitled. Overtime pay was only one of the entitlements that nurses sacrificed. Other hard-won benefits that had long sustained professional and career development in the industry were under threat—for example, professional education. Without the ability to learn about new medications, procedures, treatments, and advances in nursing interventions, it is very difficult, if not impossible, for nurses to deliver the highest quality patient care. That's why nurses had fought for and won paid study leave—so that they could enhance their skills and knowledge in a dynamic, constantly changing high-tech healthcare system.

Because of union-negotiated contracts, paid study leave was available to almost 70 percent of members at the time of the survey. Yet less than half of respondents (47%) had recently applied for it. Among those who had applied for study leave, the amount of time granted away from work was minimal. Sixty-three percent indicated that the leave amounted to only one or two days in a year. Of those who had applied for study leave, a third had their applications rejected. The reasons for the rejection varied. Managers told 37 percent of staff that other nurses had already taken study leave, and 28 percent were told that no replacement staff were available. Sixty percent of nurses had been told by their managers that budgetary restraints meant they could not have study leave. Some nurses were denied leave because managers insisted that the subject the nurse would be studying was not relevant to her clinical area or that the nurse had not been in the workplace long enough to qualify for leave.[6]

If nurses cannot leave their units to learn about new therapies, advances, and research, then in-house unit-based education becomes critical. Yet, when we asked about in-house education, nurses' answers were equally disturbing. The length of time devoted to, and conditions surrounding, patient handover play an important role in determining whether nurses have paid work time available to devote to training and development activities. As Lisa Fitzpatrick, secretary of the Victorian Branch of the Australian Nurses Federation explains, in Victoria, nurses' work is scheduled not by using a twenty-four-hour day but rather a twenty-six-hour day. That means that between the completion of the a.m. and the beginning of the p.m. shift, a two-hour overlap period occurs when one group of nurses is leaving work and another is arriving. The bulk of the overlap between morning and afternoon shift—the "double" handover or shift overlap—is a scheduling technique used to ensure that nurses remain for a period of time after their "rostered" hours and formal "rounds" have been completed. This time is not used for frontline patient care but is devoted to tasks such as restock and check of rescus trolleys (what are known in the United States as "crash carts," which contain equipment to resuscitate patients if they have a cardiac arrest), checking medicines and oxygen cylinders, ordering medicines, or attending training and education seminars. During the cost cutting of the 1990s, however, the traditional educational uses of the double handover were largely eliminated.

Results of our survey showed that 82 percent of members thought that in-service education should be conducted during the period of overlap in staffing. This activity, however, had been withdrawn for more than a quarter of all respondents. Furthermore, although 62 percent of members thought specific clinical teaching should be done during periods of shift overlap, 31 percent said it was no longer available. About 30 percent of nurses indicated that teaching, in-service education, and professional development tasks had simply been abandoned.[7]

Because of reductions in shift handover periods, other vital work activities like handover itself and time with patients were affected. Almost 40 percent of nurses said they had no time for team building. Thirty-four percent said they couldn't debrief with their colleagues, and almost 20 percent said there were no more or fewer ward meetings. More alarming was that almost 25 percent did not have time to do maintenance and safety checks and 18 and 17 percent respectively said they couldn't communicate with patients or patient's families because of a reduction in handover periods. Faced with the choice of providing basic patient care or engaging with colleagues or engaging in emotional work with patients, nurses in Victoria were putting essential patient-care duties first.[8] At the end of the 1990s nurses were increasingly convinced that personal and professional development came last, if at all. On many units it had simply become impossible to build teams, get much needed social support, or debrief with colleagues. The result was a significant decline in workplace morale.

When asked, nurses gave particularly poignant accounts of the personal and professional implications of an overworked health-care system. Karen de Silva*, a nurse unit manager, who worked in the system in Victoria for more than fifteen years and who was at the time of our interview with her working in a large coordinating public-hospital facility in the outer suburbs, described what had become a common phenomenon: "I can only call it the bad old days. We had become task oriented, habitual. I don't believe we were doing what we had been trained to do."

Patrice Arnold*, a registered nurse in a public acute facility, described the working environment in hospitals of the late 1990s:

> It was not happy; no one enjoyed it. We didn't really get to spend time together as nurses, as colleagues. Many, many times I would go home and not be able to think about going back in for the next shift. I felt really sorry for the young ones, these kids coming straight out of uni [graduating from a nursing school in a university. You could tell how hard those first few months were for them. We lost a lot of them because they simply couldn't cope. . . . I remember the look on the face of one girl straight out of uni; you could see by the look on her face she thought, "What have I done? This is not what I thought nursing was about."

As one nurse unit manager told us, the nurse's role had become so habitual that it was undermining the integrity and unique contribution of nurses: "I think you could argue that it had gotten so bad in some places that anyone could do what we were doing." Gerry Redman*, an orthopedics nurse based in Sydney, New South Wales, in 2002, talked about his experiences in the decline in quality of nursing, simply because of the pressures of too many patients, too few staff:

> Quality care? In the last years there is no quality. We do clinical stuff we need to do, but there is no quality. We had a woman last week who was incontinent of faeces, and her daughter told us, but it took us twenty minutes to get there because we had all these post-op people and obs [observations] and spewing and bleeding and god knows what. Twenty minutes she had to wait before we could get her out of her own faeces![9]

By the mid-1990s, nurses, hospital administrators, and policymakers with the State of Victoria all agreed that the quality of working life for frontline workers in the health sector had significantly declined. These groups diverged, however, on what they thought were the reasons for this decline and what should be done to remedy it. Health-sector management believed the issues could be handled within the organizational structures already in place. Among organized nurses, especially those in Victoria, the problems were regarded as more deep-seated.

6

How Did It Come to This?
The Factors Driving the
Intensification of Nursing Work

When they contemplated the nursing shortage in Victoria, health-care policymakers and administrators commonly highlighted the effect of forces from the "demand" and "supply" sides of the issue. They pointed to the new demographics of an aging population, an aging nursing workforce, and the changing lifestyle preferences among young professionals. Many nurses and their unions, however, argued that additional forces were creating the shortage of nurses. The most important was the government's increasing preoccupation with cost control and the adoption of modern management methods with the aim of injecting greater financial discipline into the organization of hospital services.

Official Accounts of the Nursing Problem: Labor Shortages from Supply and Demand Imbalances

When policymakers discussed the crisis in nursing they used the concept of a generic "nurse shortage"—bolstered by statistical evidence of persistent unfilled vacancies. This offered policymakers an expedient way to explain a range of problems affecting the Australian health-care system as a whole and the Victoria health-care system in particular. For example, throughout 1998–99 the Productivity Commission (a national independent economic research body funded by the federal government) used public-hospital surveys to gauge the adequacy of labor supply given current health-care needs. The report found that by the late 1990s, for every one thousand people, Australia only had 4.1 active nurses.[1] The Commission dubbed this an "alarming" ratio in government-service terms, because it would be grossly inadequate to respond to the anticipated increase in health demands arising from an aging population. When a Commonwealth Senate inquiry into nursing released *The Patient Profession: Time for Action* report, it identified critical shortages in almost all areas of the health-care service throughout Australia. Psychiatric, mental health, and eldercare services faced particularly acute shortages. Other sources corroborated this data.[2]

By the late 1990s the Victoria health system faced a number of demands that were qualitatively and quantitatively different from those that nurses had faced even a decade earlier. The system throughout Australia, as in the rest of the industrialized world, faced the challenge of serving a very different demographic profile of patients. Most notable is the significant pressure to be placed on the health system by the large baby-boomer cohort entering retirement in the 1990s. A report commissioned by the Victoria government charted the changes that occurred between 1971 and 2001. Average life expectancy of men in Victoria was 68 years in 1971 and 77.5 years in 2001. For women, average life expectancy increased from 75 years to almost 83 years over the same period.[3] All of this meant that people would live longer, without necessarily being healthier, and that they would need higher levels of nursing care.

The demographics of the nursing workforce were also changing. Between 1986 and 1996 there was a distinct shift in the age of Australia's nurses. In ten years, the proportion of nurses under the age of twenty-five decreased by 13.4 percent, while the proportion of nurses over the age of forty-five increased by 11.1 percent.[4] Since the typical nurse was an older woman working part-time, health-policy stakeholders and people involved in direct patient care were also concerned about what would happen as more and more nurses prepared to retire. To make matters worse, the average age of students taking up undergraduate nursing degrees in the 1990s had increased to 24.5 years, reflecting large increases in the numbers of mature age students.[5] In the long term this meant an aging graduate population. In other words, an older cohort of inexperienced nurses would enter the workforce at precisely the time when many older nurses would be retiring.

Broadening the Definition of the Problem: New Funding Models and Allied Management Strategies

While demographic forces were clearly shaping the situation, they were not the sole factors determining the nursing crisis. Studies by and of nurses, which focused on their views and experiences, added a significant new dimension to understanding the nursing problem. By viewing staffing issues and the delivery of health care through the prism of nurses' experiences, these studies unveiled a complex network of factors driving the health crisis.

Mary Chiarella, until recently the chief nurse in New South Wales (the key senior policy advisor to the state government on issues that have an impact on nursing), explained that in the early 1990s, as Australian federal and state governments began to worry about containing costs and increasing productivity in their national health system, "the need for 'productivity savings' became the call. Nurses and other health care professionals were asked to do 'more with less,' 'work smarter, not harder,' and comply with other similar euphemisms."[6] Hospitals began to develop spending-cut targets. To cite only one example, in 1991–92 one New South Wales hospital was told it had to cut $7 million (Australian), with $3.5 million coming from cuts in nursing jobs. "By 1994, the 'productivity savings' had been so effective," Chiarella writes, "that there was a declared shortage of specialist nurses." Without job prospects, nurses were looking for work outside hospitals and even in other fields. Over six years, the New South Wales nursing workforce lost one thousand positions.[7]

The link between new funding priorities and the labor-management strategies associated with the recasting of nursing work has several permutations. The shift to a cost-control approach to managing illness, injury, and disease has been thoroughgoing and is now all-pervasive. This approach shortens patients' length of time in the system (particularly as inpatients). This is also known as "patient throughput," which in turn increases patient acuity. As patients get sicker, however, more nurses are not assigned to meet their increased requirements for care. Nurse managers—whose burdens also increase—provide less support, and there is often fewer ancillary staff to do cleaning, transport, provide security, social work, or dietary services. Moreover, new technologies—such as those that collect and report data—are also added to units, all of which changes both the job of the nurse unit manager and staff nurse.

These changes in the objective conditions of work have major implications for the subjective experience of work. In particular, they are diminishing some of the intrinsic, less tangible rewards—time to support patients and build supportive teams of nurses—associated with nursing work. In combination all of this creates more stressful and less rewarding work that now lacks the intrinsic rewards that used to attract and retain nurses. Nurses and exnurses often expressed frustration that they were constantly exhorted to "cope" with these developments, as identified in a detailed qualitative study of eighty-seven NSW nurses and exnurses on why they were leaving the profession in the late 1990s and early 2000s.[8] Even among nurses who remained in the system, significant numbers were seriously contemplating leaving.[9]

A significant and growing literature has corroborated nurses' insights about these interconnected developments. Throughout the 1990s researchers documented the emergence of public management as a dominant force in many countries throughout the Western world.[10] These dynamics were experienced most intensely in Victoria where the public-management model took a particularly virulent form. The small-government new-managerialist approach was vigorously pursued after 1992 following the election of the Liberal government headed by Premier Jeff Kennett. The radical reshaping of health care in the state went through two distinct phases. Phase one overtly pushed nurses out of the system through mass layoffs. Phase two covertly squeezed nurses from the bedside through the imposition of unsustainable workloads and deteriorating working conditions.

Phase One: Pushing Nurses Out of the System

Within two years of being elected in 1992, the neoliberal and Reagan-inspired Kennett government slashed permanent employment in the public sector. About 16 percent of the health workforce lost their jobs outright.[11] Kennett's "2050 plan" targeted almost forty Victoria public hospitals for restructuring and consolidation into seven administrative networks. The goal was to introduce "competitive neutrality" to the public-hospital operating environment, which was to be accomplished through either outright hospital closure, reducing hospital budgets, or full or partial privatization of a large number of metropolitan and regional-care facilities.

The Kennett government argued there was an oversupply of nurses, so it eliminated two thousand nursing positions. The government offered these nurses huge buyouts (so-called redundancy pay). Belinda Morieson, then secretary of the Victorian Branch of the Australian Nurses Federation, explained that nurses took advantage of the offer because they could get the buyout and then leave the public sector to work in private-sector hospitals.

Although the nurses' union, which is strong in public-sector acute care hospitals, was able to block use of unlicensed personnel as RN replacements, nurses were replaced by patient-care assistants with minimal training throughout the private eldercare sector, which is funded by the federal government not the respective state governments. These cuts to the nursing workforce, when combined with the fact that nurses caring for the elderly in the private eldercare sector in Victoria may receive up to 20 percent less pay than nurses in the acute sector, created a major shortage of RNs in care for the elderly in Victoria.

On top of direct cuts in the nursing workforce were cuts in public health expenditure, including for nurses. By 1994, through implementation of a funding formula called "case-mix," the public hospital system also lost $190 million in funding. As in the United States, the system began to use rigid diagnosis-related categories. Rather than receiving funding based on the resources they actually used, they received funding on the basis of the proportion of particular types of patients, and thus DRGs, they treated.

A Weighted Inlier Equivalent Separation (WIES) is used to calculate the proportion of funding a hospital receives. A patient's WIES value is determined by the time they stay in hospital compared to other patients with similar conditions. It also takes into account the relative cost of treating that illness compared with other illnesses (in other words, a cost relativity). The formula has been criticized for being inflexible and for failing to take into account complications, atypical patient experience, and the unforeseen—or the fact that some DRGs receive lower funding even though patients need higher levels of care. For example, new mothers and older, frail patients were given less funding because they failed to neatly fit into clearly defined DRGs. Implementation of this model had several direct consequences for the delivery of health care. Because funding was cut across the board, hospitals simply got less money. To manage with less funding, hospitals had to devise their own accounting and reallocation models in order to manage the reduced budgets.

Phase Two: Squeezing Nurses Away from the Bedside

With smaller budgets and fewer nurses, care management regimes were redesigned to meet changing patient needs. Norrish and Rundall have documented how this trend played out in the United States and other countries and convincingly argue that nursing work was left profoundly altered by these processes.[12] The experience of nurses in Victoria confirms these observations.

Nationally, the number of acute hospital beds decreased from 5.2 beds per thousand people in 1987–88 to 4 beds per thousand people in 1998–99. This had cascading impacts for the rest of the services delivered in a public-hospital environment. Nurses in other wards were expected to deliver care to patients whose acuity constantly increased. Ironically, even though these patients are "sicker," the public-management model dictates that hospital stays decrease. Nationally, the average length of stay in the hospital decreased significantly in the five years preceding the peak of the labor crisis in Victoria.

In government documents submitted to an official public inquiry, in 1993–94 the average length of patient stay was 4.6 days. In 1998–99, this declined to 3.7 days.[13] At the beginning of 1999, a state government commission released an audit of the public hospital system to evaluate the impact of the funding model that had governed operations since 1992. The commission's agenda was to commercialize and to advocate the corporatization of the public hospital system.[14] The auditor's report nonetheless found that most of the public-hospital networks operating in Victoria were operating at a significant loss (in the order of millions), with about two-thirds being bankrupt.[15] The report seemed to implicitly question the wisdom of the new managerialist approach, since the system was so starved of funds that some hospitals could not even pay their permanent staff.

The Legacies of New Funding and Management Models: Agency Nursing, Quality of Health Service, and Fragmentation of Care

The end results of these changes were profound dysfunctions in both the nursing labor market and the provision of health services. A good example of the former was the deepening reliance on agency nurses as a source of labor. An example of the latter was the degrading of the infection-control system and the fragmentation and erosion of quality nursing care.

Agency Nurse Problems

The Kennett government implemented a radical program of decentralized management, in which individual business units became responsible for the management of employment arrangements. Middle managers became directly responsible for recruitment, rostering, and human resource management. Unfortunately, managers were no longer supported—either financially or clinically—by a large and well-resourced centralized human resources division. To keep shifts staffed, hospital managers increasingly turned to quicker and more expedient means to maintain labor supply—this meant using agency nurses. The government was supportive of this strategy because it believed this would limit public-sector employment and thus expenditure. In fact, reliance on agency nurses further undermined both financial and workforce stability. Belinda Morieson argues that the use of agency nurses created a vicious spiral in Victoria's hospitals. "Agencies were paying their nurses three times the amount of money permanent staff were getting," Morieson explained. "So more and more nurses left permanent work in the hospital and went and worked agency." The government paid for these agency nurses who ended up costing a great deal of extra money.

If they stayed on the job, nurses at the unit level were increasingly demoralized by the fact that so many of their daily encounters were with former colleagues who had gone to work in an agency. Jenny Withers*, who has been a registered nurse in a range of public hospital wards over the past twenty years, recalls the 1990s:

> We were heading towards a totally casual staffing profile where I worked. We had a bidding war. Across the sector it felt like millions and millions of dollars

were being devoted to agency nurses. There were three of us RNs who started at about the same time, who were at about the same stage of our careers. The other two on either side of me left, and I stayed like the piggy in the middle. I don't blame them for going. They said they just couldn't take the pressure, but they returned the next month as agency, being paid double the amount (and in some cases triple). Do you have any idea how heartbreaking, how utterly disheartening it is for those of us that stayed behind? I felt like they were just laughing in my face. Leaving to do agency, though, allowed them to have more control over when and how they worked. It just seemed so unfair.

Nurses giving care on the units weren't the only ones who were becoming increasingly alarmed at the use of agency nurses. Directors and managers were as well, as Marie Wilson, chief nursing officer at Western Health, recounted:

We had a migration of our workforce into agency. So, a permanent, full-time nurse saw that on the same shift that she was working, she could get triple her own rate by working agency in the organization. Our staff reduced their hours from full-time to, say, two days a week, knowing that they could well pick up their normal roster of work as agency staff. They'd still stay permanent, but if they worked five days a week, normally, they would go back to two days a week. They would then pick the other three up on their own ward in their own environment on an agency.

No policies or procedures prevented that. I was just so angry at the fact that I couldn't control my own workforce within my own environment, and that the amount of money being paid to agencies per month at Western Health was $950,000—a month. Our own staff within the health service at nurse unit manager level and at the associate nurse unit manager level were very demoralized. Staff were having to work with a significantly casualized workforce, and that meant issues of clinical risk, constant orientation of staff, and a lack of continuity of care.

Degraded Infection Control and Undermining Standards of Care

By the mid-1990s, the public health system in Victoria had been running on depleted resources and low staffing levels for three years. This produced two clearly observable results—problems with quality of service, notably degraded infection control, and fragmentation of nursing care. Nurses are guided by two core principles—preserving patient safety and caring for the "whole patient," not just treating the disease, and the erosion of quality in these areas was symptomatic of what many considered to be a total crisis in nursing care.

In 1997, the public broadcasting network, ABC television, ran a national exposé on the state of health-care delivery in Victoria.[16] The story included interviews with a wide range of doctors and nurses whistleblowing on the public health risk created by declining standards of care and cleanliness in hospitals. The health-care professionals interviewed complained of infestations of vermin and insects as well as the fact that staff could no longer follow, much less improve, existing infection-control procedures. Those interviewed attributed the problem to budget cuts and inadequate nurse-to-patient ratios. In desperation, many staff attempted to buffer these challenges by monitoring and completing infection-control procedures and by filling out supporting documentation on their own time.

Although all staff—doctors, nurses, contract cleaning staff, and attendants— share responsibility for infection control in hospitals, it is generally agreed that nurses face unique pressures in this area. Nurses face higher risks of personal exposure because of the high degree of patient contact. In the only comparative study of its kind, U.S. research has documented that nurses, more than any others in the health-care field, have the greatest risk of acquiring infectious diseases in the workplace. They are in direct contact with infected blood and body fluids, and they are at risk from needlestick injuries and when a patient sneezes or coughs and sprays their mouths or eyes. As one study identified, working conditions and infection rates often have an inverse relationship. Put simply, infection rates for patients and staff rise when the working conditions of staff (particularly nurses) decline.[17]

Nurses also face risks in transmission, because of the hands-on nature of many nursing tasks that involve touching wounds and surgical sites. In recent years this has become a particularly important issue for hospitals with the documented rise of multiple antibiotic-resistant organisms. Indeed, Linda Aiken, one of the most prominent nursing workforce researchers in the world, now argues that hospitals in industrialized countries are as dangerous as they were when Florence Nightingale began her crusade to reform the modern hospital in the nineteenth century. Aiken attributes many of these dangers directly to inadequate nursing resources.[18]

Infection control has been described as one of the silent aspects of nurse and hospital procedural work that is often squeezed by other more pressing duties and responsibilities. To be comprehensively effective, thorough infection-control protocols often contain a precise sequence of repetitive, time-consuming, and highly specific steps. Short staffing can mean that staff are quickly shifted from one task to another, or they may have to withdraw from one task to cope with an emergency. This is particularly the case when nurses are running between seven, eight, or ten patients.

Nurses are also the first line of defense in containing infection risks. In spite of this critical fact, in 1999 a special task force on infection rates and control surveillance in major metropolitan hospitals throughout Victoria found that a pressured work environment had produced several alarming practices.[19] Among coronary-bypass patients, for example, postsurgery infection rates were found to vary greatly depending on the conditions prevailing at the workplace. Over 80 percent of the hospitals in Victoria did not have an adequate number of infection-control nurses on staff. As one spokesperson for the project noted, this level did not conform to even the most lenient and outdated recommendations for effective infection control. A 1985 standard, formulated in the United States, recommended a ratio of one infection-control practitioner to every 250 beds. In those Victoria hospitals with the highest infection rates, the rate recorded was almost double the rates of infection reported in comparable U.S hospitals over the same period. Many of these Victoria hospitals were found to have poorly developed duty statements and staffing procedures for recruiting, both internally and externally, infection-control nurses and managing infection-control protocols appropriately.

As one of the largest hospitals in the state, Alfred Hospital in Melbourne, took a leading role in both identifying and monitoring the status of infection risks in Australian hospitals. Work by professor Denis Spelman, conducted in the infectious diseases unit, highlighted the link between hospital workplace practices and hospital-acquired organism risk in order to identify and improve current and future responses to infection control. The study outlined the sources of transmission of hospital-acquired organisms. The report found that microbial flora of colonized or infected patients were passed in most cases by direct contact with the hands of staff or contact with medical devices.[20] Inadequate disinfection of hospital equipment and direct staff contact with hospital devices or patients can result in the transmission of highly dangerous organisms.[21] These infections included the highly resistant strain *Staphylococcus aureus* or enterococci that resulted when staff inspected a wound or touched a site with contaminated fingertips or hands.

Endoscopy represented another area where less-than-vigilant infection control had adverse consequences. The device used to visually examine the esophagus, stomach, duodenum and jejunum, or the colon, may be hospital owned, but it is increasingly used on loan from a medical supplier because of the expense associated with its purchase. Patients undergoing endoscopy are at risk of infection because a single piece of equipment is reprocessed after each procedure, to be used on any number of patients in a day. To prevent infection, strict infection control and cleaning regimes must be used. Strict observance of these processing procedures is extremely important to ensure the equipment is decontaminated. The procedures, knowledge, and skills involved in infection control mean that training is essential. If a patient should contract an infection, staff must be able to identify all possible trails of transmission. Nurses must, therefore, keep highly detailed notes on the individual endoscope, the procedures undertaken and by whom, the patients treated, and the disinfection steps used. To cut costs, hospitals may reduce the training provided, or they may simply not provide dedicated personnel who can scrutinize infection-control procedures as a major part of their duty statement.[22]

In other cases, staff either did not adhere to disinfection protocols or were unable to revise these protocols quickly enough to respond to additional and heightened infection risks. When nurses are required to do their activities more quickly, or when they are responding to an emergency, they simply do not have time to take the precautions necessary to prevent the spread of infection. Telling people to work smarter, not harder, as managers did during this period, is clearly not an adequate enough infection-prevention protocol.

Patients were not only suffering because of hospital-acquired infections. Anne-Marie Scully, a Victoria nurse who worked for the Department of Health and Human Services as well as the Victoria Branch of the Australian Nurses Federation, researched fifty-five deaths that triggered coroners' inquiries in Victoria between 1990 and 2000. Seventeen were from medication errors. Of these, two occurred because patients didn't get their antibiotics, and the others resulted from faulty administration of drugs that require cautious administration. Other deaths resulted from lack of communication between doctors and nurses or between nurses and patients, and three deaths were the result of poor use of restraints that had been placed on patients. Scully found that these deaths were produced by a complex constellation of factors that included inadequate nurse staffing. "Management and organizations failed to provide appropriate numbers of nurses to deliver safe nursing care," she said. "They failed to provide enough experienced staff. Nurses who had no experience on a unit were nonetheless placed on that unit even though they didn't have the competence or confidence to do the necessary work. What is more, they weren't given policies or procedures that would guide them in the area in which they were working."

Nurses, she said, didn't have enough information and education to do their job, particularly when it concerned new medical equipment, medications, or treatments. In one case, physical restraints were placed on a patient, but neither nurses nor doctors were taught the basics of their safe use and the patient died. The manufacturer of the restraints had provided the facility with a video on how to manipulate the restraints safely, but no one ever bothered to show nurses and doctors the video. The manufacturer also warned that patients had to be constantly watched when restrained, but again nurses weren't told about this warning. Even if they had been, Scully added, they wouldn't have had the time to comply with the instruction.[23]

Fragmentation of Care and Erosion
of Professional Integrity

When nurses are unable to take basic precautions to prevent infections and patients become sicker as a result, nurses begin to question their very raison d'être. Victoria nurses described a qualitative and intrinsic change in their practice that was gradually stripping away the sense of professional discipline and integrity that had once previously defined their role. In qualitative interviews nurses vividly described what it felt like when the care they gave was compromised.

The issue of overwork also altered the qualitative nature of the care that nurses could provide. Nurses said they no longer had time to talk with patients and listen to their concerns, to answer their questions, or to educate them about their illness, their medications, or how to cope with infirmity and disability. For many nurses the loss of the "human face of nursing" or what some have called "the emotional competencies" of nursing work became the defining professional issue. Employers, nurses said, considered this work to be discretionary, and it therefore could be eliminated, while nurses consider these tasks to be central and defining to their identity as professionals.

Nurses thus began to feel that their work had become as routinized as someone working on an assembly line. Barbara Reid°, a registered nurse in a large metropolitan hospital, explained that while patient hygiene regimes were maintained and medication administered, nurses had little time to personally invest with the patient. As she put it, "You might have eight patients; I wouldn't know their names, but I would know an antibiotic was due at 11 a.m."

For Paula Hilton°, a nurse unit manager, being able to hear patients' concerns, answer questions, and provide education allows for a more comprehensive and proactive analysis of the patient's situation. This can mean that long-term problems are averted and return hospital visits avoided because the nurse can help design an appropriate postdischarge plan. This increases the chances for and speed of recovery. For Kelli Fisher°, a registered nurse, a pressured work environment also means that nurses cannot provide needed emotional support and care to either the patient or family:

> If you have too many patients, you just can't do the job properly. . . . What happened to us in Victoria in that period, well, it cut us, it broke us down. Nurses treat and deal with people at a time in their life when they are most vulnerable. If you have any professional pride at all you have to be able to invest time to give that support, that cup of tea, provide kind words to a family that may be grieving, crying, dealing with a loss or a crisis. To lose that ability is to lose sight of who we are as professionals.

The Nexus of Poor Staffing Ratios, Low Staff Morale, and Workplace Stress

By the late 1990s Victoria nurses had tried for over seven years to preserve patient care and protect individual patients from the consequences of inadequate staffing by working unpaid overtime, working through rest and meal breaks, and foregoing equipment and professional training in order to "stay on the ward." These strategies had, in fact, worked to provide a buffer zone between patients and the system the Kennett government had created. Nonetheless, many nurses simply could not cope with their lost faith in the system's ability to preserve a safe working environment for either patients or nurses. This set the stage as the Victorian Branch of the ANF membership and leadership prepared for the 1999–2000 round of enterprise bargaining negotiations. Both the membership and leadership were in no mood for haggling over wages. A far more comprehensive agenda for bargaining was expected and in preparation.

7

Winning Ratios in Victoria

By August 2002 nurse-staffing arrangements in public hospitals in Victoria had been transformed. Gone were the days when managers could make arbitrary—often purely budget based—decisions on staffing levels. Nurse unit managers could no longer simply tell a nurse who protested about workloads to "cope." Governments and hospital executives had handled their prerogative over nurse-staffing levels so badly that an Australian Industrial Relations Commission (AIRC) ruling inscribed mandatory staffing requirements in Victoria into Australian labor law.

This now meant that in a general surgical ward in a large teaching hospital, there had to be a minimum of one nurse for four patients on morning and afternoon shifts and one for eight patients on night shifts. The new staffing arrangements differ significantly from prior staffing arrangements. For example, in 1999–2000 during the preratios era, on a morning or afternoon shift in a general surgical ward in a level 1 hospital (better known as a large teaching hospital) the prevailing ratio typically fell within the range of one nurse for every four to six, or often more, patients. On night duty in 1999–2000, a ratio of one nurse for every twelve patients was not uncommon. At smaller hospitals obligatory staff levels were typically one nurse to six patients during the day, and one nurse to ten patients during the night. With the new ratios the Victoria government, as the funding body affected, was required to recruit over seventeen hundred extra nurses to ensure that these staffing requirements were met. While this still did not match the estimated two thousand nursing positions abolished by the previous Kennett-led government, it would make a huge difference to nursing staff on the ground. Where extra staff could not be found, vacant hospital beds were not to be filled.

A striking feature of the ratios was their level of comprehensive detail. Managers were not given general guidelines to follow on staffing levels. Rather, quite precise stipulations along similar lines were made for over a dozen different practice areas including accident and emergency departments, neonatal intensive care units, high-dependency units, and operating theaters. Where relevant, the ratios sometimes varied by shift and class of hospital.

How was such a dramatic change achieved? How did the idea for the ratios emerge, and why were ratios successfully won and implemented during this particular round of enterprise bargaining?

ANF Victoria: Key Advocate of the Ratio Principle

To understand the ratio model in Victoria, it is important to appreciate the role and history of its key, and on occasions only, advocate—the Victorian ANF. The evolution of the ratio principle in Victoria is deeply embedded in the changing culture of this union.

Historically, nursing has developed a separate and unique culture that, while essential to successful clinical treatment, was not recognized as such or even defined as a distinct profession. Indeed, as many sociologists and historians have documented, from the late nineteenth century and up to the mid-twentieth century the field was not even recognized as a skilled sector of work. Doctors were perceived as clinical practitioners, and nurses were generically defined as caregivers who had little knowledge and functioned as physician handmaidens. In this era (and even up to the 1970s) nurses were generally required to live in dormitories (nursing quarters) attached to their hospital employer, and they were often expected to work very long hours for very little pay. Both the culture of nursing and the operating environment of hospitals in the 1950s and up to the 1960s were more rigid both socially and culturally than most modern hospitals. Madsen describes it as "a distinct culture that was a compilation of work, moral and traditional elements,"[1] and Bloomfield explains it as a vocational training ensuring "installation of morals and manners."[2]

It could be argued that nursing was not just a vocation, it was a lifestyle.[3] This cultural tradition shaped the working environment, and a senior nurse or "matron" closely managed and allocated the workload within a health-care unit. The strict code of conduct also meant that nurses conformed to stringent demarcations governing both duties and behavior. This highly stratified structure is often described as the "Nightingale" method or model. It influenced the way nurses were trained, how their duties were circumscribed, and how the nursing hierarchy was structured within hospitals throughout much of the Western world until as late as the 1960s[4] (and in Australia until the 1980s) when nursing education was formally transferred to the university sector.[5]

The Victorian Branch of the ANF, which was founded more than one hundred years ago with the formation of the Victorian Trained Nurses' Association (VTNA) in 1901, initially rallied around the issue of protecting vulnerable workers. In the early days the movement focused on improving pay and basic working conditions.

As the Victorian ANF and other Australian nursing unions evolved in the 1940s and 1950s, their demands primarily concerned "bread and butter" issues. Improving the very low wages of nurses was, for example, a key focal point of union campaigning. The second wave of cultural change within the Victorian ANF might be described as the professionalization of the union. Influenced by the second-wave feminist movement, throughout the 1970s and 1980s the union invested its efforts in gaining equal pay for equal work and in elevating the status of nursing as a profession. Linked to this strategy, the movement lobbied for greater access to more formal training and education. These efforts were successful in 1984 when the federal government approved the transfer of nurse education out of hospitals and into the tertiary-education sector.

The 1980s also became a significant period in nursing because of changes in the mode of care delivery at major hospitals. Accounts of the social history of nurses in the mid- to late 1980s not only point to dramatic changes in nursing practice and delivery but foreshadow elements of the staffing crises that nurses would face a decade later. In the 1980s, Victoria hospitals (like public hospitals in other states) began to deliver patient care in highly specialized units, and these required more staff, particularly nurses.

Technological advances also began to have a significant effect on the practice of nursing. Feminist researchers Chinn and Wheeler, as well as Sandelowski, noted that nurses assumed a broader range of more complex activities. As doctors concentrated on the expanding and ever more prestigious task of diagnosing, researching, and treating diseases, more complex equipment and constant patient monitoring became central to medical practice. Doctors delegated to nurses the task of manipulating this equipment in a process of intense patient monitoring.[6] For nurses this represented a double-edged sword. Nurses gained greater recognition as a professional group of clinical practitioners in their own right. But the expansion of their work also created work intensification and added to nurses' workload. The effects of this would be felt all too clearly a decade or so later.

The emergence of the union in its modern form (ANF Victoria) occurred in the 1980s, during this period of work intensification and workload expansion. The union removed its no-strike rule, and in 1985 nurses took industrial action for the first time in their history. This was a precursor to the historic strike in 1986 that lasted fifty days. In this action the ANF defined itself not only as a union that represented the professional interests of nurses but also as an industrial union. The strike action was a definitive and comprehensive campaign that dealt with working conditions, labor shortages, slow wage growth, and career and professional development. Later in the 1990s, following the Kennett government's election, the Victorian ANF developed its tactical reputation for strong and effective campaigning, which rallied equally strong public support for nurses. Nurses were able to utilize this public support to win more favorable collective agreements. In particular, the union became known for its skillful execution of the bed-closure tactic.

Rather than engaging in full-blown industrywide strikes and walk-offs the union instead used an isolated strike tactic, which was crucial in the 2000 ANF campaign for ratios.[7] These bed closures occur in solitary areas or services while wider health-care services are maintained. Alternatively, reduced or skeleton staff schedules are used so that emergency patients can still be treated, but beds are closed to less urgent or elective surgery cases. Industrial action was also typically deployed around certain job tasks. For example, tasks involving direct patient care remained largely unaffected, but nurses cut back on administrative, paperwork, and processing tasks. Hannah Sellers, an organizer during the 1980s and ANF assistant secretary during the 1990s, describes these forms of action: "It's an easier way of taking industrial action than it is to strike. You still achieve an outcome—it certainly brings the message home to the management. But it doesn't put nurses or the community through the terrible emotional trauma of having to take the ultimate [strike] action."[8]

Even though the ANF represented nurses at all public-sector hospitals in Victoria, nurses were not obliged to be union members, pay union dues, or participate in union activities, including mass meetings or strikes. The fact that large numbers of nurses participated in the union's first strike and later bed closures thus suggested a high level of commitment to professional and workplace concerns. Although the union had always been structured to allow any member to put forward motions and then participate in debating these motions, it was not until the 1980s that members began to exercise greater influence over everything from negotiating proposals to campaign strategy. For example, in the 1986 strike, nurses at one hospital organized themselves to resign en masse because they felt patient safety had been so compromised by the poor working conditions that they could not, in good conscience, continue to practice.[9] Although the leadership of the union did not support the strategy it stood behind the members when a majority of them voted to resign. One delegate described the union culture in the following way: "Irene [Bolger, ANF Victoria leader at the time] is our employee. We tell her what to do."[10]

During this period, more rank-and-file union members also began to attend mass meetings. Some traveled great distances to participate in statewide meetings in which broader professional concerns were discussed. It was not unusual for five to six thousand members to attend such gatherings. Some of these were stop-work meetings where thousands of nurses voted to walk off the job. This level of commitment to union activity, even activity that could have significant financial consequences for nurses themselves, remains high to this day and was instrumental in nurses' ability to mobilize a successful campaign for staffing ratios.

Throughout the 1990s, the Victorian ANF continued to maintain a high profile and stable growth in union membership. This ran counter to the trend in many other Australian unions, which experienced significant membership decline in this period. By early 2000, the Victorian ANF represented approximately 60 percent of the public sector or thirty-two thousand government-employed nurses. It is against this backdrop that negotiations with the state government, as sole funder of nurses across the state, for an enterprise agreement claim began in early 2000.

The Early Genesis of the Ratio Model in Victoria

In July 2000, for the first time, the ANF Victoria's formal demands of the Victorian Department of Human Services (VDHS) included nurse-to-patient ratios in the formal log of bargaining claims. This was an extraordinary step, given that no clause pertaining to ratios existed elsewhere in any Australian nursing award (sectorwide employment agreement).

Although the 2000 enterprise bargaining agreement was the first time that nurse-to-patient ratios had been formally included in negotiations, the notion of a ratio as a workload tool actually has a long history in the nursing labor movement.

Since the turn of the last century nurses in Australia have debated whether and how a nurse-to-patient ratio could contribute to both patient safety and nurse competence. For much of the twentieth century, nursing resolved this issue by allowing managers at local hospitals to use their professional judgment in allocating staff. Managers evaluated the complex issue of how individual workers, with variable skill and experience levels, coped with variable patient workload as well as the inevitable unforeseen aspects of patient care. Although there were isolated occasions in which ratios played some role in nursing practice, historically the hospital matron (a formidable figure in the hospital system) was given the power to oversee the workload allocation process.

This situation changed again in the early 1940s and through the 1950s when a government authority known as the State Wages Board in Victoria prescribed a workload ratio for nurses in the public sector. The wages board system operated in Victoria until the early 1990s, after which the Employment Relations Act of 1992 replaced them with a judicial institution—the Employee Relations Commission (ERC).[11] The boards were originally established to protect the most vulnerable workers in the community. Each trade or craft had a separate board that set wage and employment levels and defined detailed conditions including everything from clothing allowances to board and lodging to transport claims.[12] The boards were typically composed of an independent arbiter (chair) and employee- and employer-elected representatives (two each in most cases).

Nurses were considered to be among the class of workers that included hotel workers, cleaners, and unskilled factory workers who required board protection.[13] The Hospital Nurses' Board (the State Wages Board for nursing workers) had authority under the State Factories and Shops Act to determine basic rates of pay and entitlements for the two broad categories of "certificated" and "trainee" nurses in public hospitals. However, these early industrial (and legally binding) board determinations did more than set pay. The documents they produced provided hospitals with a detailed account of the wages, conditions, night duty and other allowances (e.g. uniform and accommodation), and leave entitlements that applied to nurses in public and private hospitals, community hospitals, and convalescent homes.

In the 1940s, the board also made determinations regarding a "reasonable" workload for nurses by setting a nurse-to-patient ratio. At this time, the ratio of a day-shift nurse was one nurse to ten patients. A night-shift nurse was required to work to a ratio of fifteen patients.[14] When we consider that nurses in the 1990s in some settings were taking care of a similar number of patients with more complex health problems and while manipulating more complex technology, the extent of work intensification in the sector becomes even more stark.

Although it may appear that these 1940s ratios represented a significant precedent, their effect appears to have been minimal. Many historians doubt that wage board determinations had any real clout. The process of board decision making was far from transparent. Board meetings were closed to both the media and the public, and the board was not required to provide a reason or supporting rationale for its determinations. As Gahan notes, although the decisions of these boards were technically binding, individual employers had multiple options to appeal decisions they considered unrealistic or unfair. Appeals to the state government minister for labor allowed board determinations to be rescinded, and abolitions of board determinations were common.[15] So, while a ratio may have existed as an abstract or ideal industry standard, individual employers could opt out of this process if they submitted documentation for an exemption.

Ratios again resurfaced during the 1986 strike when the Victoria nursing union challenged the idea that ratios were a local workplace issue by including a reference to the viability of ratios in its bargaining claims. The pivotal issues during this lengthy dispute were related to wage raises. The union claimed that the Victoria government had reneged on previous commitments to make pay raises retroactive and to change the career structure for nurses and make it more secure. The union's ability to reduce nurses' workload and further explore nurse-to-patient ratios as a workable model was severely compromised when the Labor Party state government, led by Premier John Cain Jr., decided to recruit nurses from England and Ireland—at an estimated cost of $6 million—to meet the staff shortages.[16]

Prior agreements (awards) covering public-sector nurses in Victoria have also included isolated references to the staffing arrangements that should apply in particular settings. The Nurses (Victorian Health Services) Award 1992 included a "proportion on duty" clause that dealt directly with the minimum proportion of nurses assigned to a maximum number of patients, in other words, a nurse-to-patient ratio.[17] In 1996, however, the Federal Workplace Relations and Other Legislation Amendment Act was approved and it directed that all federal awards be "simplified." In real terms this meant that the scope of issues and matters that awards could cover were severely restricted. A full bench of the Commission in August 1999 found all clauses pertaining to staffing (i.e., nurse-to-patient) ratios to be "nonallowable matters" under section 89A of the act.[18] Ratios were thus removed. As a result, no other nursing award in Australia has established nurse-to-patient ratios within its terms and conditions to this day. When the ratio campaign strategy of the Victorian ANF in 2000 is viewed in this hostile industrial context, it makes the victory all the more remarkable.

Formation of the 2000 Ratio Claim

Belinda Morieson, secretary of the Victorian ANF in 2000, is often publicly credited with the idea of introducing a ratio claim to the bargaining negotiations. Morieson was clearly influenced by debates within the nursing union movement at the time as well as the struggle for ratios in California. Indeed, there is strong evidence that the notion of a mandated ratio as the workload management tool preferred by working nurses emerged from the union membership itself. In a historic set of mass meetings that occurred before the 2000 campaign (and which informed the 2000 agreement list of claims), a motion to include ward-appropriate nurse-to-patient ratios was presented on the floor of the meeting. A majority vote directed ANF Victorian Branch officials to include as a centerpiece of bargaining a claim for nurse-to-patient ratios in the total list of 105 claims that covered issues such as wages, training, extended leave for long periods of service, shift length, ongoing professional development, and a wide range of entitlements designed to improve day-to-day working conditions in wards.

As the union prepared to present its case to management, the rank-and-file members voted to give direction on workload management solutions. The union provided the administrative support to collect and collate data on workable ratios from nurses across the sector. At local union meetings, delegates collected data from members identifying optimal and workable ratios in their practice environment. This information was fed back to the union head office so the state branch leadership already had at its fingertips the statistical evidence needed to mount a well-prepared case for ratios during the negotiations. Union staff also collected data about ratios.

As Morieson explained, twenty staffers in the Melbourne headquarters conducted a telephone survey of about two hundred charge nurses and nurse unit managers:

> These nurses were all asked the same question: "If you have a twenty-bed ward, and you're in charge and you don't have any patients that you yourself are caring for, how many additional nurses do you need?" We told them that the number should include a range of nursing staff because we knew it would be too complicated to create a ratio that was filled with X number of nurses with two years' experience, and X number of nurses with ten years' experience, and X number of nurses with five years' experience. It would be impossible for managers to roster [schedule] like that.
>
> We also said, "We're not saying that every nurse will have four patients, what we're saying is, there will be some flexibility." Finally, we told them, "Look, it's us you're talking to so please don't give us an ambit claim [Australian for an exaggerated demand]." We didn't want them to do the rostering equivalent of wanting a ten dollar raise but asking for a twenty dollar raise. We told them to ask for the number that they needed and assume that would be what they would get. The union surveyors spent a fair amount of time talking informally with each manager because they wanted to be sure the managers understood the issues. The surveyors asked the question about morning, evening, and night-duty shifts. And the answers were all pretty much the same.

Morieson and union members pitched the idea of ratios as a worker-retention issue that also had positive financial ramifications. Morieson believed firmly that people had to understand and support the ratio proposal. "It had to be transparent," Morieson argued, "so that people could understand it and it could not be manipulated either by the nurses or the management."

This idea resonated with nurses, the public, and ultimately with the Australian Industrial Relations Commission when it was called in to arbitrate the dispute. The ANF clearly explained the cost to the system of hiring agency nurses. Its work intensification campaign defined the greatest threat to professional renewal as the fragmentation of the labor force through expanding agency employment, rather than from professional encroachment. The ANF recognized that the use of agency work was actually driving committed permanent nursing staff to leave the health sector completely, and in the long term, this would undermine the professional integrity of nursing and the supply of nurses overall. The ANF therefore campaigned for a cap on the use of agency employment across the sector.

The union convincingly depicted the restriction and regulation of the growth in agency contract firms (the intermediaries between the funder and employee) and casual employment as a major way to enhance the long-term health of the profession. In some cases, as noted in the previous chapter, agency staff received more than three times the wages of permanent staff and, beyond putting in an individual shift, they personally invested little in the workplace. As one permanent RN in a Melbourne inner-city hospital who had remained with the system throughout the 1990s described it, "This was utterly disheartening for those of us that chose to stay."

Risky Business

The ANF Victoria strategy to deal with the issue of work intensification was unique in both historical and sectoral terms. Since the 1980s, Australian unions have been under great pressure to justify wage and condition claims on the basis of economic efficiency.[19] Indeed, the need to justify wage growth on the basis of productivity improvements—with a "quality" or "optimal" wage outcome often defined as the most cost-effective one—has shaped the form and strategy associated with collective agreements in both the private and public sector for almost twenty years.[20] As Buchanan and Considine note, employer groups as well as employee representatives promoted the imperative of economic efficiency and actively mobilized this discourse to leverage better wage outcomes.[21]

In the context of Australian industrial relations, the ANF rejected twenty years of pressure to highlight the "price competitiveness" of their agreements in three key ways. First, the union did not steer the debate toward "health service efficiency" but toward issues of sustainability and professional renewal. More dominant unions and pace-setting blue-collar unions, such as those in the metals sector, continued to rally around industry competitiveness. The ANF garnered support from both its members and the public by focusing on the notion of sustainable efficiency. Under the campaign slogan "Nursing the System Back to Health" all its literature and other campaign material emphasized the importance of a health system with sufficient labor and skills to maintain high standards of patient care. This allowed the ANF to tap into nurses' professional allegiance as a driving force for the campaign. "Defining objectives in terms of sustainability helps redefine the terms of debate and mobilisation," Buchanan and Briggs note. "The nurses were neither for nor against competition. Rather they saw it as a constraint that had to be recognised and responded to. The health system was losing in the competition for quality health professionals."[22]

Second, the ANF structured its campaign around preserving the integrity and renewing the professional aspirations of the nursing profession. That professional groups seek to defend their skill base in the face of management control is not new. Other Australian research explains that the corporate culture of health-care systems has forced a range of medical professions to respond defensively to encroachment on professional territory.[23] Historically, for example, there have been disputes over professional territory between doctors and nurses or more recently between patient-care assistants and nurses.

In the context of this campaign, working conditions and issues of professional preservation took priority over wage claims. For the union, this was a risky strategy. Nursing, like teaching, has developed a reputation as a white-collar professional ghetto for women, in which the high level of skill and competence required is both underpaid and undervalued relative to some male-dominated occupations (e.g., building trades). Australian nursing union strategy throughout the 1970s and 1980s was heavily influenced by principles of gender equity and the "equal pay for work of equal value" movement. Wage improvements in nursing were long given a high priority because of the need to address these basic gender inequities and thus attract future generations of workers to nursing. Strong wage growth, it was argued, acknowledged the inherent challenges—shift work that keeps nurses from having a normal social life, high levels of stress and burnout, to name just few—of a nursing career.

The ANF (Victoria) claim of 2000 was not only distinctive because of its focus on creating a sustainable public hospital system and promoting professional renewal by winding back and reducing the degree of managerial prerogative in that system. Compared with nursing unions in other Australian states it broke new ground in proposing a highly prescriptive approach to the setting of staffing levels. During this period, nurses Australia-wide were increasingly concerned about the issue of work intensification. However, each state union branch pursued slightly different strategies to alleviate the problem. In Queensland, the introduction of case-mix (DRGs) and changes to funding incentive measures, which were tied to narrowly defined performance outcomes, had also escalated work intensification in public hospitals.[24] For this reason, in their bargaining with the state government in 2000 the Queensland union rallied around the role of performance management and its impact on working life. The union sought significant and unconditional

wage improvements by seeking to break the hold of benchmarks and performance targets over wage growth in the sector. The union also pursued improvements in job security for the public-sector nursing workforce. Dealing
with the issue of workload management through promotion of the "best practice" principle, the union argued that this would have a greater influence on
public-sector employer behavior because employers would seek to emulate
"employers of choice."

In New South Wales (NSW), the nurses' union also ran a strong campaign
that focused on the heavy workloads and the need to improve pay. The union
initiated work bans and strikes with the use of skeleton staff to protect patient
care across the state. Local workload-management teams took responsibility
for monitoring and making recommendations on staffing levels and workload
concerns. This strategy emphasized that local teams would be best able to understand and identify the ratios required in specific health settings.

In other state-based campaigns, for example the one in South Australia,
nursing unions addressed the issue of work intensification through implementation of computerized workload programs. These programs would give nurses
the ability to manage and monitor workload on a day-to-day basis and to gather
more detailed data so that hot-spot workload issues might be identified early
on. Willis conducted an evaluation of the enterprise agreement negotiated in
South Australia.[25] In this case, the union successfully negotiated to get the
State Department of Human Services to use a computerized nursing-workload
product (Excelcare) and commit to operate shifts using its staffing profile.

Because nurses had been working with the system for some years, the situation in South Australia was different from that in many other states. Union
strategy could be uniquely informed by the years of experience piloting and
working with the system. Willis argues that South Australian nurses did not
struggle for the implementation of Excelcare because they believed in its su-
periority and accuracy. Rather, the union contended that with the inclusion of
appropriate clauses in the agreement, the Excelcare system provided the best
opportunity to ensure senior management compliance with a consistent
staffing practice based on objective workload formulas.

While modest wage improvements formed part of the 2000 claim in Victoria, the ANF (Victorian Branch) made workload and redressing nurse "overwork" its top priority. The means the union proposal for achieving this was
distinctively clear and unambiguous.

The Claim and the Process

From the outset of negotiations in March until just prior to the final Commission decision in August 2000, both the Department of Human Services

(the state government employer) and the Victorian Hospitals Industrial Association (VHIA, the hospital employer representative) opposed the ratio claim. The nurses, however, would not budge. Rather than shut down the system, nurses used ongoing and persistent industrial action and work bans to continually remind the public (and employers) of the importance of the staffing and workload issue. As Morieson recalled, "First we closed one in six beds, and we sat at the negotiating table. We didn't get anywhere, so we closed one in five beds. This was all done over a period of months with statewide stop-work meetings. We then closed one in four beds."

At Bendigo Hospital in regional Victoria, the state had invested significant funds in expanding the number of accident and emergency cubicles but gave no commitment to provide any additional staff to service these cubicles. Nursing staff continued to provide the same level of service for the existing patient load but refused to open the new beds until adequate staffing could be provided. Nurses employed in all hospitals closed one in every five beds. This decision had important sector-wide effects, as bed closures meant elective surgeries had to be cancelled.

Asking for improvements in wages and benefits has often been difficult for nurses. Whenever they raise such issues, they risk compromising the trust of a public that considers nurses to be altruistic and self-denying. These concerns multiply when nurses use trade union strategies—bed closures, work bans, strikes—to press their issues. They are often accused of patient abandonment, which is both a legal and moral category to which they are both personally sensitive and for which they can be held professionally liable.

The prolonged nature of the dispute and the ANF's reluctance to acquiesce on the ratio issue led to the dispute being taken to the Australian Industrial Relations Commission for resolution and private arbitration. The AIRC is a national tribunal that has the authority to make rulings with legal authority on issues pertaining to working conditions. The most common issues that the AIRC adjudicates are claims by employees of unfair dismissal, resolution of disputes that have reached a point of impasse, and in some cases the setting and determination of pay and conditions of employment.[26] The final decision of the AIRC was made under what is known as "private arbitration." Under provision s111AA of the Workplace Relations Act of 1996, parties in a position of negotiating stalemate agree to participate in an arbitration process and to fully abide by the decision handed down. In such private arbitrations, a commissioner meets with the parties and comes to a binding decision that cannot, unlike in other private meetings, be appealed to the full bench of the Industrial Relations Commission. The use of this private arbitration process to resolve the union–state government stalemate came about, to a large extent, because of an unexpected change of government. When the campaign commenced, the union was opposed by the conservative Liberal-National coalition state government led by Jeff Kennett. Halfway through the campaign for nurse-to-patient ratios, this government unexpectedly lost power. The new Labor government, led by Steve Bracks, had been elected on a program of social renewal directed at rebuilding services cut as a result of the aggressive neoliberal policies pursued by the Kennett government. In a public radio speech, Premier Bracks said that his government would abide by private arbitration at the Industrial Relations Commission. Once this decision was announced, the new premier would have lost face if he had backed away from this very public commitment.

The case the Victorian ANF put to the Australian Industrial Relations Commission relied on quantitative evidence in the form of independent sectorwide workload evaluations, which were commissioned by the union. The case also presented detailed qualitative accounts from nurses who, under oath, gave hundreds of key witness statements that provided raw accounts of what the day-to-day life of a Victoria hospital ward had become for both patient and worker. This was a particularly effective strategy because it allowed the message of overwork to be repeatedly reinforced, but it also ensured that patient safety remained center stage in the discussions surrounding workloads.

In all of these statements, the issue of poor workload management was a common thread that connected the key problems of staff shortages, workplace stress, and poor patient care—all of which affected hospitals in metropolitan, regional, and remote settings alike. Nurses from the accident and emergency units at Royal Melbourne described their heartbreak on seeing rushed and inadequate patient assessments and elderly patients wetting the bed because they could not be taken to the toilet. Nurses from a regional acute hospital in Geelong argued that the most basic tasks—assisting patients to bed, hygiene, and nutrition—went unattended because of staff shortages. One nurse argued that the culture in hospitals marginalized and harassed nurses who chose to speak out against the poor working conditions. Another nurse testified about a patient who had been fed while sitting on a commode so nurses could save time and complete the round of duties expected within a shift. In wound-care units, nurses spoke about the effect of inadequate staffing for bedsore care and outlined the serious infections that resulted when nurses didn't have time to turn, properly bathe, or take patients to the toilet. The testimony of neonatal intensive care unit nurses was particularly persuasive. On these high-risk units, where nurses care for ventilator-dependent babies, nurses generally care for only one baby. But nurses testified that they had, on occasions, been forced to abandon this standard and care for more than one dangerously ill infant.

Nurses' testimony was so dramatic and compelling that even employers began to acknowledge the need to address the issue of workload and its influence on nurse professionalism and patient safety. In statements of evidence given to a public inquiry, a senior official of the VDHS characterized the union campaign: "It was not primarily about incomes that the ANF came to us; it was about nurse patient ratios. It was work related. That is a consequence of the shortage of nurses. We have had nurses working harder and seeing more patients, and eventually it blows. They said 'no more.' "[27]

The union convincingly asserted that a systemwide problem of work intensification called for a systemwide solution. Systemic pressures that create work intensification, the ANF contended, cannot be solved using a workplace-by-workplace approach. Although this realization is not a new one to the union movement, the ANF Victoria was in the fortuitous position of being strategically well placed to pursue a sectorwide campaign that clearly highlighted both the system issues and a proposed solution. Hospital administrators recognized that a workplace-based recruitment strategy, no matter how well designed, cannot combat widespread nurse disaffection with the sector. The union convincingly argued that it had a long-term plan that would provide sectorwide sustainability, skill growth, and staff retention. As Jill Iliffe, the national secretary of ANF, described the campaign at the time, "We do not have a shortage of nurses. We have a shortage of nurses who are willing to work in a system where staffing levels have been reduced to the point where patient care and professional integrity is compromised."[28]

Finally, the union made a financial argument to support their case, by showing that ratios could have a positive impact on the overuse of temporary agency staff. In her discussions with the Commission, Morieson linked the issue of ratios to the cost of using agency staff: "I told the Commission and we told the public, 'Look, we're two thousand nurses down; nurses are leaving in droves. If you don't resolve the workload issue you will have nothing but agency nurses in this state, and they're costing you three times as much. You put in ratios and it will cost you less and you'll get a more stable workforce.' "

The union also described why the increasing use of agency staff exacerbated the long-term problem of recruiting and retaining nurses. They debunked the idea that computerized and automated workload analysis systems posed a viable solution to the labor crisis, because these systems leave management structures and power unchallenged. The union contended that management was a key factor in exacerbating the labor shortage and sought sanctions relating to how, where, and why agency staff should be used to fill staffing vacancies.

The Management Case

Even after six months of intense negotiation, and ultimately stalemate with the union, the employers continued to reject any argument in support of a ratios model. The employers contended that ratios were an inappropriate solution to the labor shortage of the 1990s, for a number of reasons.

Ratios Limit the Ability of Workers to Remain Flexible

Both the government of Victoria (Department of Human Services) and the hospital administrators asserted that ratios were unworkable because they needed to maintain maximum flexibility. Employers insisted that ratios raised flexibility concerns and would offer an artificial protection from the labor crisis. In his statement to the Commission, Dr. Michael Walsh, chief executive officer of Alfred Hospital, said, "We must endeavour to equip those partici pating in or entering into the workforce to expect change and to respond positively to it. Artificial protection against the impacts of change appears futile and doomed to failure."[29] This flexibility would be compromised if the system attempted to offer any of the key health professions, nurses included, any certainty in the workload they could reasonably expect when they arrived to work a shift.

As a key witness for the VHIA during the Commission proceedings, Dr. Walsh spoke about the "tremendous amount of volatility in terms of what is actually happening at the clinical bedside . . . which involves not only nurses but all professions." However, during cross-examination, the ANF team exposed a number of flaws in the employer case about flexibility. In particular, the ANF zeroed in on what it considered to be management's myopic focus on flexibility at any cost—a stance that implied that employers had no obligation to measure workload. At one point during the cross-examination of key witnesses, Dr. Walsh conceded that "it is a source of some concern that in the year 2000 we still have not come to grips with a proper measurement of workload at the patient level so that we can't bring those sorts of facts to the debate."[30] When Walsh essentially acknowledged that hospitals had changed the work environment without seriously considering the impact of these changes on their largest workforce, it was a pivotal moment in the presentation of evidence.

Hospitals Don't Care for Patients, They Treat Them

In presenting their case, employers justified their position by pointing out that the hospital was no longer the primary locus of patient care. Because home and community-based care now played a much greater role in the provision of patient care, to constrain a hospital system with ratios would reduce the system's ability to respond to the needs of patients. Similarly, employers argued that health-care work had been broken down into a set of specialized services that form part of a total care episode. If hospital admission had, at one time, been defined by a "bundling" of diagnosis, treatment, and recuperation, the modern hospital had disassembled these components.

Diagnosis now typically occurs before admission (for example, by ambulance officers). Recuperation increasingly occurs at home or in post–acute care institutions. Treatment had become the key role of acute institutions—and this was overwhelmingly delivered in a "same day service" (for example, dialysis, chemotherapy, and endoscopy examinations).

What employers failed to acknowledge or address was the fallout of this fragmentation on nurses or patients. The ANF acknowledged that shorter hospital stays were indeed a growing trend, one that created significant work intensification for nurses. It pointed out that the paperwork, admission, and discharge procedures combined with the volume of patients expected to be processed had not reduced but had, in fact, increased nurses' workloads.[31]

Ratios Don't Take Patient Acuity and Complexities of Care into Account

Employers further asserted that care had changed and is always changing and that a ratio would effectively lock them into a workload model that would inevitably become irrelevant. A ratio, they stated, does not take into account differences in patient acuity or specific patient considerations. During the Commission proceedings, employer representatives repudiated a " 'one size fits all' approach that appears to us to characterise the ANF approach. Hospitals are extraordinarily diverse and complex and that is clearly reflected in the diversity of working arrangements and they shouldn't be repudiated in favour of a 'one size fits all' model."[32] Demand is not constant across beds, shifts, or facilities, nor can a ratio take nursing expertise or differences in skill mix into account. In concluding statements, employers warned that ratios would result in dire consequences—increases in patient waiting lists for elective surgery, increases in episodes of ambulance bypass, and prolonged emergency waiting times.[33]

During the presentation of evidence and ensuing negotiations, the union focused on the weaknesses in an employer case that rested on an absolute resistance to even consider the concept of a minimum ratio as a viable workload management model. In discussions with Commissioner Wayne Blair, Morieson presented independent research reports providing quantitative workload studies, in addition to qualitative evidence in the form of hundreds of detailed key witness statements by nurses themselves, that documented just how much workload had increased for nurses.[34] The employer response to this was simply to argue that they did not measure workload so they had no supporting evidence.

In its final judgment the Commission stated:

> Therefore the Commission cannot ignore the issue of a nurse patient ratio mix. It is obvious to the Commission that whatever measures (if any) that have been put in place by the hospital networks to address the recruitment and retention issues, have failed. During the s.111AA process and the conciliation conferences, there was ample opportunity for the hospital networks to provide alternatives to the nurse patient ratio mix proposed by the ANF and this did not eventuate.

This stands in contrast to the ANF case, which included sectorwide documentation and feedback from nurses justifying why ratios could work and how they would help to alleviate some of the workload excesses crippling the system.

When Commissioner Blair asked the employers to offer suggestions to deal with the health labor crisis, they proposed no alternative model for a comprehensive systemwide solution for workload management. Instead, they offered a list of disparate and disjointed measures: a review of staffing levels; a grievance procedure and protocols for nurses to complain if they felt a workload problem had emerged; an inventory of priority equipment for immediate purchase (cordless phones, wheelchairs, electric beds); and the employment of more nonnursing staff (ward clerks) and patient-care assistants to help ease the workload of nurses.[35] Although clearly not the intention, this approach appeared to sideline the workload issue entirely and dismiss the compelling accounts nurses presented to the Commission. When the chief executive officer of the VHIA, Dr. Alex Djoneff, examined the hospital association's own key witness, Susan Williams, chief nursing officer at Royal Melbourne, this disregard for the significance of the workload issue became clear.

Dr. Djoneff asked Williams if and why there was no "simple solution to the workload issue," and what alternatives she proposed:

> I think that there's no quick fix. . . . There are things we can do in the immediate term that would have an immediate impact on nurses at the coal face and I think in the immediate term we need to purchase equipment to make life easier. We need to get beds, we need to get wheelchairs . . . commode chairs, blood pressure machines, more IT and training in IT. The other things that the nurses have said that they want is they want simple things. They want nurses—additional nurses to escort patients to radiology.[36]

When the ANF lead negotiator, Bob Burrows, cross-examined another VHIA witness, Dr. Walsh, he pointed out that the administrator had, in a previous response, conceded that the system did not adequately measure nurses' workloads.

"I think it's more correct to say that there are many measurements," Walsh replied. "A number of measurements are used in different organisations, none of them are used at a policy level to start to inform, for example, . . . the case mix funding price."

"I thought your words were, and I haven't obviously got the transcript, but it's not a proper measurement of workload levels," Burrows said. "In other words, not an accepted one?"

"There are multiple measures but none of them have . . . been given a State-wide application," Walsh acknowledged.[37]

The ANF Victoria cross-examination also raised suspicion that hospital management would have allowed the issue of workload measurement "ambiguity" to continue because its targets of higher patient throughput and worker productivity had essentially been met.

In the last week of August 2000, the final week of evidence, the ANF continued to drive home the point that a viable systemwide workload tool was the only technique that would bring systemwide relief. In her statement, the assistant state secretary of the ANF, Hannah Sellers, identified senior managers' complicity in the workload and staffing crisis. Managers, Sellers explained, were either complicit because they were so constrained by financial accounting disciplines or so resistant to change:

> In the absence of any other manner of measuring workload, and whilst it [nurse-to-patient ratios] may not be the absolute ideal, it is in fact necessary as a minimum to ensure that nursing workloads can be managed. I am not aware of any hospital, or indeed any management who has taken pro-active measures to ensure that the workload is managed appropriately to ensure that patients are cared for in a safe manner, and to ensure that the nurses' workload is able to be conducted professionally and safely. . . . I am not aware of any hospital that has taken a series, or implemented a range of strategies in the last few years to accommodate the concerns of nurses. There is absolutely no doubt that nursing management, if not general management, are aware of the stresses that nurses have been working under for some considerable period of time.[38]

In closing arguments, the ANF presented a picture of employers who were absolutely resistant to remedying the problem of workload management. In summing up, Bob Burrows concluded: "In our view, the employers have not provided any alternative, workable solution to the problems that are commonly admitted and the problems have existed for at least seven or eight years. The VHIA describe our solution as simplistic. We think it is better described just as a simple solution. It is a transparent and obvious solution to the nurses who are actually facing the problem."[39]

The failure to acknowledge the voice and authority of nurses as experts in health care also weakened the employer case.[40] For example, when Ella Lowe, executive director of Nursing Peninsula Health and a witness for the employers, was giving evidence, Commissioner Blair interjected with the following comments:

> COMMISSIONER: I take the point that you have made about being able to—
> the benefit of being able to—step back and look at the way in which things are
> carried out—workloads. . . . To see whether or not there are better methods,
> who does the challenging?
>
> MS. LOWE: Nurses generally. Nurses are very good at sitting round a table
> and saying "This is the problem. What sort of solutions can we pool together
> that will make this work better?"
>
> COMMISSIONER: But that implies that there is a receptive person to listen to
> those views constructively?
>
> MS. LOWE: Yes.
>
> COMMISSIONER: And what has been presented to the Commission so far, as
> part of the evidence, is that that's not necessarily the case, that there are peo-
> ple within the structure who frown upon nurses challenging or having some
> view that may be different to that—to the person they are challenging.[41]

The commissioner seemed to view the ratios as more than a workload management tool. He believed the public health system needed to ensure nurses had the ability to exercise some judgment over staffing decisions and give feedback on the impact for patients. This, in the opinion of Commissioner Blair, needed to include a systemwide ability for nurses to be heard by all levels of management—the nursing fraternity (directors and assistant directors of nursing) and hospital administrators (senior management). Indeed, on August 31, 2000, the Industrial Relations Commission ruled that nurse-to-patient ratios represent the most effective response to both the workload and staffing crises facing the Victoria health sector. "He gave us the most outstanding deal," Belinda Morieson concluded. "We got back so much we'd lost. We got additional nurse educators, we got additional senior nurse clinician additions, we got qualification allowance if you went back to university and got additional qualifications. We got additional night duty allowance. We got study leave paid, and seminar leave. It was extraordinary." On September 1, nurses in the ANF held a mass meeting to consider the AIRC's decision and, with a standing ovation, overwhelmingly endorsed it.

The Commission stipulated that the government should maintain discretion over the introduction of ratios. It strongly recommended, however, that implementing mandatory nurse-to-patient ratios was an urgent matter and that the first wave of ratios be introduced in December of that year. "There is a crisis in nurse recruitment and retention and workload to the extent that if it is not addressed now, with measures to deal with the short term issues as well as providing some measures to deal with the long term issues, then the nursing crisis will get worse," Commissioner Blair stated bluntly in his decision.

"Those who choose to say that there is not a nursing crisis, in the Commission's view, are in a state of denial."[42]

In establishing the ratio principle the Commission said that hospitals must ensure "the number of nurses available is commensurate with the number of patients requiring care."[43] Put more simply, minimum mandated nurse-to-patient ratios are calculated on *actual* numbers of patients in a particular care or unit setting. The ANF also decided to quickly survey the state's hospitals to establish the level of vacancies that were reported before the ratios took effect and discovered that there were thirteen hundred unfunded positions vacant.

In determining the appropriate ratios that should apply, the Commission relied on data presented by the ANF on patient presentation patterns collected over a twelve-month period and disaggregated by unit. The Commission chose this method because the ANF had argued that *average* occupancy alone could not shed light on the important variations in patient numbers and would therefore not ensure that suitable levels of staff would be available to meet peak periods of demand.

This premise is critical to the implementation of ratios. It means that a hospital ward must enforce a staffing policy that is responsive to both "occupied bed" levels and "capacity bed" levels. For example, if a ward has thirty beds and twenty-six of these beds are usually occupied, then the four vacant beds cannot be opened unless additional staff are engaged in line with the ratio requirement that applies. This approach has a profound impact on containing workloads for nurses, because management cannot keep beds open (that is, continue to admit patients) with an assurance that nurse-staffing levels will be increased at some undefined point in the future.

To determine the appropriate nurse-to-patient ratio that should apply, the Commission considered the intersection of three main factors in shaping nurse workload: the work context or practice setting in which care is delivered; the composition of skill and experience level within the nursing team; and the characteristics of the patient, including aggregate patient numbers, patient acuity, and the profile of the patient. (A summary of what the ratios are, by type of hospital and areas of practice, is included in the appendix.)

Key Elements of the Decision

The Commission stepped beyond the issue of immediate staffing problems and gave direction on the way in which ratios could be staffed in a sustainable way. On the issue of the use of agency staff, the Commission gave strong support for the union's plan for sector renewal and included a cap on the use of agency staff, with only "bank staff" (casuals engaged directly by the hospital, without use of an intermediary) to be used. In addition, these staff could only be used to cover unforeseen absences (such as sick leave).

Double handover or staff "overlap" (a two-hour handover with a long shift regime) was also an important supporting condition to ensure that ratios could be met throughout the course of a shift. In practical terms this means that during the day there is a two-hour overlap between when one shift nurse finishes and the next shift nurse begins.[44] The preservation of this handover system would improve the operating systems in the hospital by ensuring that routine maintenance and infection-control procedures were preserved and promote ongoing training and professional development for nursing staff.

As the AIRC defined them, ratios specify the minimum nurse-staffing levels required to operate across a range of different health-care settings and for different shift rotations. Because these ratios are based on an award, made under the AIRC power of private arbitration, these ratios have the force of law in Victoria.[45] If hospitals don't have enough nurses to staff beds, those hospitals risk being forced to close beds.

The Commission's ratio decision is constructed around a hospital classification system that is recognized and applied by the Victorian Department of Human Services. The categories are used to provide a framework through which the demands on nursing staff can be better explained and understood. The four categories relate to the numbers of beds the hospital maintains; total patient capacity; and the range and scope of services provided by the particular facility. In other words, ratios depend on understanding whether a hospital has, for example, an oncology ward, provides specialist services for transplant patients, or is a leading teaching hospital. Each category reflects several complex factors that influence how care is provided and the service expectations associated with the hospital because of its geographical location. The determination of ratios depends on factors including whether the facility is large or small; whether it is centrally located or in a remote area; whether its facilities and patients are geographically dispersed across a wide area; and the number of specialized and generic care services provided by the facility overall.

The Commission's Division of Victoria's Hospitals

Level 1 Hospitals

Level 1 hospitals are large and highly consolidated facilities that represent the main teaching and research hospitals and are the major referral points for care across the state. The descriptor "large" is appropriate because these hospitals, as single employers, employ substantial numbers of medical personnel (nurses, doctors, surgeons, anesthetists, physiotherapists). These level 1 hospitals are also physically and geographically large. They have extensive facilities and grounds and access to large-scale diagnostic and treatment equipment. As major referral centers, level 1 hospitals also serve a vast number of patients. Specialized care in the fields of trauma, transplant, oncology, neuroscience, cardiac, obstetrics, pediatrics, and acute surgical and medical services are all provided within level 1 facilities. The Royal Melbourne, Monash, and Alfred hospitals are included in this category.

Level 2 Hospitals

Level 2 hospitals include large metropolitan and country base hospitals. These hospitals are also impressive in size with a large staff, and they are expected to serve a significant number of patients and thus are under pressure to rapidly admit and discharge patients. However, level 2 facilities do not typically provide the breadth of specialized services level 1 hospitals provide. The teaching and referral responsibilities associated with these hospitals are also less extensive. Large country base hospitals do act as referral points for the smaller and more remote country base hospitals. Goulburn Valley and Wangaratta hospitals fall into this category.

Level 3 Hospitals

Level 3 hospitals include small to medium metropolitan and country base hospitals. These hospitals typically process fewer aggregate patients annually but often serve a population that is more geographically dispersed.

The level 3A category includes medium-sized country hospitals. These facilities are located outside the metropolitan and urban area and typically have a patient capacity of two hundred beds or fewer. Frontline medical care is provided, including some maternity care, but other, more specialized forms of care are referred to larger and more extensively resourced hospitals. The line between a 3 and 3A category hospital is blurred, with often very little distinction between the two categories. Wodonga hospital in the north of the state is a fairly typical level 3 hospital.

Small Country Hospitals

Facilities within the "small country hospital" category are among the smallest hospitals in the state, with thirty beds or fewer and limited operating theater sessions. These bases are typically established to provide some form of frontline emergency and medical care to the most rural and remote regions of the state. Myrtleford Hospital, with a capacity of about thirteen acute beds, a dialysis unit, midwifery, and an attached senior-care facility, is fairly typical of this category.

Understanding Nurse Classifications

As we explained earlier, in Victoria nurses are divided into two broad classifications—division 1 and division 2, or div 1 and div 2 in common parlance. Both are regulated by the Nurses' Board of Victoria. Division 1 registered nurses (commonly known as RNs) have completed a three-year bachelor's degree in nursing at the university level through the higher education system. The division 1 nurse in Australia is similar to the RN in the United States except that they are all university trained. Division 2 registered nurses have been trained through the vocational training stream (TAFE or technical colleges) in twelve-month programs. They are similar to the licensed practical or vocational nurse in the United States. Historically in Victoria, division 2s were known as enrolled nurses or ENs. This term is still commonly used in some Australian states.

The broad scope of duties undertaken by division 1 and 2 nurses is very similar. The main distinction between these two classifications is the degree of responsibility associated with each position. Enrolled nurses assist patients (dress, shower, walk, lift, or move patients to increase comfort levels), monitor (take temperature, pulse, blood pressure readings), change dressings, and care for and emotionally support patients. Although registered nurses also undertake these responsibilities, they can do so without supervision. Enrolled nurses can contribute to patient notes and administer a very limited range of medications, but they are required to work under the close direction of a registered nurse.

To minimize workload problems for the nurses on a particular shift, the Commission's ratio decision acknowledges the need for an appropriate level of experience and skill among the nursing staff. The Commission prescribed the level of division nurses that should be assigned, taking into account the hospital classification and the care setting. In the major acute hospitals no more than one division 2 nurse, per ward per shift, can be scheduled to meet the ratios. This is because their limited scope of education and more restricted scope of practice would make it inappropriate for them to take on more advanced patient-care responsibilities. In eldercare and smaller rural hospitals more division 2 nurses may be scheduled in to meet the ratios, but this must be determined by local agreement with the nursing staff in individual wards.

The ratios that were ultimately determined gave the ANF most, but not all, of what it had lobbied for. During the process, debates continued to rage about ratios in small country hospitals and on labor and delivery units. Lisa Fitzpatrick, the secretary of the Victorian ANF, explained that the ANF's midwife members originally wanted one midwife to each labor-and-delivery suite. Instead, a compromise position was three midwives to two birthing suites. The union also wanted a better skill mix in the ratios. The ANF wanted the ratios filled with one-third division 1 nurses with more on-the-job experience; one-third less-experienced division 2 nurses; and one-third with a mix of new graduates and division 2 nurses. The precise mix of skill and experience for each shift remained at workplace discretion; however, the skill mix principle provided a guideline against which staffing decisions could be made. The skill mix was put in writing in the agreement as a goal but not as an enforceable entitlement.

The issue of staffing in small country hospitals was also controversial. Managers in smaller hospitals insisted that their patients weren't as sick and thus didn't require as much nursing care as those in larger metropolitan hospitals, thus fewer nurses were needed. The union countered that small country hospitals lack the infrastructure and ancillary support that can support the nurse as he or she undertakes daily activities, as Fitzpatrick explained:

> You've got nurses who will be a nurse in the ward but also the stomal-therapist nurse or infection-control nurse. There won't be a pharmacist out of hours. Plus, nurses don't have the luxury of being able to specialize in one field, but have to be able to smoothly and efficiently move from patients who have very different problems. You don't have fifty orthopedic patients in a ward every day. You're caring for adult patients, pediatric patients, cardiology and psych patients. If the nurse is fulfilling multiple roles, the work may feel even more intense. Plus, the idea that if you have diabetes in the country it won't be as serious as diabetes in the city, and that you won't need diabetes education, nutrition counseling, and other services, is ludicrous.

Consider, for example, how Greg Hopkins*, a registered nurse working in a small regional hospital, described the workload. The hospital has a small acute ward, some day and overnight surgery each week, an accident and emergency department, and a midwifery unit. Even though the hospital is much smaller than a hospital in Melbourne, he can be run ragged. He said, "You might be delivering a baby in the morning, then help out with dialysis in the afternoon, then deal with a road accident that night. In the case of emergencies, yes, we do often have to refer on to a bigger hospital, but that still means the patient has to be stabilized before referral. The crisis is still yours to deal with at the time it occurs."

A Matter of Law and a Funded Mandate

Once the AIRC ruled in favor of ratios, they operated as part of Australia's system of labor law. Although this system has been changed dramatically in recent years, decisions of the AIRC tribunal result in the formulation of "awards" (see appendix).[46] These can be legally enforced, initially by unions. Indeed, one of the main reasons for union (and employer association) recognition in Australia is that they are agencies with delegated authority to enforce award standards. If unions do not achieve compliance they can refer the matter to a specialized enforcement agency of the government, the Office of Workplace Services.[47] Should negotiations with this group fail, prosecutions can then be launched in the Federal Magistrates Court to ensure compliance with award provisions, enforced as delegated pieces of legislation—much like regulations of the Tax Office are enforced in local courts when these is low-level noncompliance. Use of this machinery is rare. The threat of its use provides the sanctions necessary to achieve effective compliance with award standards.

Unlike the California law, ratios in the state of Victoria allow managers a certain amount of flexibility in their shift-by-shift implementation. The rule is that medical/surgical units must have five nurses to twenty patients, not four patients to each nurse. As Lisa Fitzpatrick explained it, "In essence the ratio is not a hard and fast 1:4 nurse-to-patient ratio. One nurse might be looking after five patients, and I am looking after three. That's because my three might be very sick and her five are less sick—say three of them might be just about to go home." Nor has there been a battle, as there was in California, about applying ratios strictly at all times—during breaks and mealtimes.

One reason ratios have not been as contentious in Victoria is that, once stipulated, they became a funded mandate. In the Victoria public health–care system the newly elected Labor government agreed to fund the nursing positions required to comply with the outcome of the arbitration proceedings that it proposed. Once wages and benefits were settled the government had to then set aside money to pay for enough staff to fill ratios. Although there may not be funds set aside to hire staff above the ratios, there is money to fund the ratios. This money is earmarked for nursing and nursing alone and cannot be raided by other hospital departments or other clinical disciplines. Thus physicians cannot argue that they need another piece of high-tech equipment and go to the nursing budget to finance it. Nor can administrators poach from the nursing budget to fund an administrative scheme.

In 2000, therefore, the government allocated $198 million to fund the ratio positions.[48] In 2001, it became apparent that the government had not set aside sufficient funds to fill the ratios, and the union and government entered another set of negotiations known as the 2001 compromise. During these negotiations, the government set aside another $300 million to better fund the ratios.

It was at this time that the union and government negotiated another compromise known as the 50 percent rule, which we will explore in more depth in the next chapter. In brief, the 50 percent rule is intended to deal with units that are not neatly divisible by four. If a unit has twenty-two beds, rather than twenty, and the ratio is five to twenty, which works out to one to four, then what happens? Do managers add another nurse and "round up," or do the five nurses deal with the twenty-two patients? According to the 50 percent rule, the union members and managers bargain about whether another nurse is added. The 50 percent rule usually results in a "rounding down" in the number of nurses. Only rarely are staffing levels set in excess of those specified in the ratios.

The Role of the Commission

The arbiter of the ratio debate, the Australian Industrial Relations Commission, did not simply help determine what the ratios would be. It also took an active and instrumental role in ensuring that the ratios plan would be viable and committed to an ongoing monitoring role. The adjudicating commissioner, Wayne Blair, required both the VHIA and the VDHS to comply not just with a stand-alone decision but also with an ongoing process that would change the way in which workforce issues would be managed across the sector. This monitoring exercise solidified and legitimized a place for the union in these negotiations through a heads-of-agreement monitoring committee. This committee comprised the key players from each of the negotiating teams, hospital management (executives of the Victorian Hospitals Industrial Association), and the ANF Victoria leadership.

This committee was charged with the responsibility of ongoing discussion and negotiation to oversee and iron out disputes that might arise during ratio implementation, which took between six months to a year. This forum of negotiation proved to be pivotal to the successful implementation of ratios because it affirmed not only the rights but also the responsibilities of all parties. The union could raise issues of noncompliance. At the same time, employers could exert leverage over the process through requests that work bans be lifted while they negotiated with unions over these issues. All the while, this process was scrutinized by the Commission to ensure that all parties continued to behave in good faith and to remain truly invested in the process of ratio implementation.

This process of ongoing monitoring gave the ratios model the best chance of success because it acknowledged the inherent difficulties associated with developing and orchestrating a systemwide workload model. The commissioner instructed the heads-of-agreement committee to keep him informed of progress through status reports. Instructions were also given on the use of "local implementation committees," which were made up of nurses elected or nominated from local work units, employer representatives, and union representatives (job reps and delegates). In practical terms, this heads-of-agreement process offered an effective way to anticipate, manage, and resolve both local and systemwide obstacles to effective ratio implementation. The local implementation committees allowed nurses on the ground to shape the way in which ratios were implemented across the system.

Across the public hospital system, the heads-of-agreement committee process allowed employers to negotiate with the state government to ensure sufficient funding would be available to meet the ratios—in other words, it bought them time. The process also allowed the unions to have a say over the aggregate number of positions required to fill the ratios, while giving hospital managers time without threat of industrial action from the nursing union to phase in the ratios. Meetings of the heads-of-agreement monitoring committee covered all aspects of the ratio, including revision of the efficacy of supporting recruitment strategies; management of attrition; establishment of relevant staffing profiles for divisions and shifts; and development of an overarching timetable for implementing of ratios.

Statements the Commission made in December stipulated that ratios should be phased in. If ratios were to work over the long term, all wards and units would need time to both introduce and adapt to this new staffing arrangement. Management was given the opportunity to table evidence with the Commission about the specific units or wards in which ratios could not be met before December 1, 2000. In effect, management had to outline to the commissioner how the ratios had been met and, if they had not been met, to present a robust case explaining how these ratios would be met within an extended time frame.

It is worth underscoring the importance of this process. The Commission did not establish a system that would invite ceaseless conflicts over ratio methodology or procedure—thus designing a system destined to fail or to be awash in endless conflict. Instead, it created a contingency plan that the parties involved could use to manage the disputes that would inevitably arise during implementation of such a complex and politically sensitive system. Nurses widely recognize the role Commissioner Wayne Blair played as a "patron" or agent of change for the ratio model. Indeed, they often informally refer to the ratio decision and its components as "Wayne's World." This might suggest that nurses felt the Commission was squarely in their corner. However, the commissioner's response to the problems encountered during the implementation process show that Blair was determined to assert the Commission's judicial independence and leadership on the issue.

The Commission's role as a nonpartisan agent that did not favor or prejudge either of the presenting parties (employer or union) was asserted again in March 2001. The ANF Victoria had challenged the state health department's claim that the number of nurses it had committed to fill the ratios was adequate. The VDHS put in a request for a cap of thirteen hundred new positions, while the ANF argued that this cap would be inadequate to meet the existing shortage plus growth. Commissioner Blair directed the state to fill funded vacancies that existed before August 31, 2000, recruit an additional thirteen hundred equivalent full-time nurses, and recruit an additional four hundred equivalent full-time nurses for growth including new services. He also, however, threatened to withdraw the entire decision (ratios as well as all other negotiated entitlements) if the Victorian ANF did not abide by the original decision. In a ruling on March 27, 2001, Commissioner Blair stated, "If the Commission is of the view that the ANF have abandoned their commitment then there is a strong possibility that the recommendations in their entirety may be withdrawn by this Commission."[49]

In June 2001, the ANF again challenged the thirteen hundred cap for new nursing positions. The union insisted that the department of health was misusing money allocated to fill the ratios and diverting it to fund other expenses. In addition, the ANF pressed for an additional claim—that additional ratios should apply beyond those contained in the original Commission decision (in particular the extension of ratios to specialist areas). To push its claim, the union held statewide stop-work meetings and voted to initiate work bans. Blair met the ANF challenge with a similar firm response.

"In terms of the ANF resolutions . . . the ANF should understand very clearly that the Commission does not welcome these resolutions," the Commission stated. "If at any point in time the Commission felt, as indicated earlier, that there was an abandonment of these commitments, not only by the ANF but by any of the parties, then it would seriously have to withdraw as indicated all those recommendations, not only the nurse/patient ratio issue."[50]

The Commission continued to insist that the parties remain committed to the process of negotiation. In July 2001 Commissioner Blair took the controversial step of "ordering" nurses back to work, vehemently stating that the ANF could not implement resolutions to close beds, even though these had been voted for at a mass meeting in the same month. The union objected strongly to the severity of the commissioner's sanction. The severity of the Commission's reprimand was unequivocal. The Commission threatened to withdraw all rulings, not just the nurse-to-patient ratio issue and refer the matter to a full bench of the Commission for resolution. In July the Commission did not hold back and communicated its "extreme" and "total disappointment" with the ANF because it appeared to be willing to jeopardize the contents of the decision. "I find it extremely difficult to come to grips with and extremely disappointing given the amount of time that the Commission, as currently constituted, has spent with the parties," Blair wrote.[51]

The Commission's "order" that nurses return to work was one of the most controversial elements of the decision process. The union argued that the Commission bowed to pressure from the state, which alleged that the failure to keep beds open might cause a public health calamity and that committing additional money for more positions beyond the thirteen hundred would cause a financial crisis. The Commission argued that ANF Victoria, through the conference process with the employers, had been offered every opportunity to nominate the number of staff required to meet ratios and had agreed that the allocation of thirteen hundred equivalent full-time staff (with an additional four hundred for growth) would be sufficient to meet these ratios. This agreement could not, in the view of the Commission, be altered in retrospect: "The parties accept that any additional ratios must fall within the 1300 EFT cap and that no other ratios will be sought."[52] The commissioner strongly implied to the ANF Victoria that disputing the allocation of thirteen hundred nurses could not be used as a way to lever an extension of the ratios beyond what had been agreed.

The severity of the Commission's statements surrounding the ratio-related bed closures must be considered in the context of the significant (and highly sensitive) legal processes being undertaken. Commissioner Blair determined that the ANF action to close beds would jeopardize the entire consent basis of the s111AA private arbitration process. In this process, the State of Victoria used Commonwealth of Australia provisions under the Workplace Relations Act of 1996. These private arbitration processes rarely occur, as indicated by the commissioner: "When the Commission undertook the process of s111AA in this particular matter it was not an insignificant matter that it was undertaking."[53] If either party, employer or union, appeared to be dismissing the significance of these arbitration processes, the Commission had to be swift to reprimand, otherwise the future enforceability of these processes would be undermined.

A Unique Convergence

When researchers and other observers analyze the ANF's successful ratio campaign, they often point to the creativity of union leaders and union members' commitment to alleviate their workload pressures. Other commentators might highlight the role of Commissioner Blair in ensuring conciliatory working relationships between the parties during the formulation of the ratios. Alternatively, the success of the ANF might simply be explained by a weak employer case. These factors alone cannot explain why nurses in Victoria won ratios when they did.[54] Several unique factors converged that created a favorable environment for a systemwide and state-sanctioned model to emerge. In an environment dominated by new managerialism and cost control, the union succeeded in breaking the trajectory of the chronic nurse shortage only with the backing of other stakeholders. The government was necessary to fund the staffing of ratios, the media also played a key role, as did the general public.

One critical fact that influenced the ratio outcome was the degree of public despair over the failing health system. By the late 1990s this despair had reached a peak. The media had run a highly successful campaign exposing the declining standards in patient care, the pressures on an overworked nursing labor force, and long hospital waiting lists.[55] Several public inquiries at the federal and state levels helped illuminate the depth and breadth of the challenges hospitals faced in recruiting and retaining nurses. Public inquiries in Victoria, New South Wales, and Queensland all separately found that, in each state, the public sector faced severe difficulties in recruiting and retaining nurses.[56]

Ironically, the fact that the public and nurses themselves were faced with a relentless barrage of bad news produced a heightened sense of despondency over the scale of the crisis. As the Queensland Nursing Council described it, "The nursing profession . . . is heartily sick of the number of inquiries which are held, but from which governments rarely implement any innovative recommendations and strategies."[57] In the most comprehensive Australia-wide nursing inquiry to date, the inquiry conductors themselves acknowledged the failure of coordinated policy reform by stating in the final report that "structural changes and reforms to overcome the major issues were slow in occurring."[58]

Another critical factor that influenced the outcome was the union's ability to draw on long-held public respect for and trust in the nursing profession. Throughout the late 1990s, the media ran an aggressive campaign against the government. Story after story exposed the extent and results of cuts to funding for the public sector. Although this reinforced public cynicism about the ability of the public health system to cope, it did not undermine support for and trust in nurses to deliver a high standard of care. In Australia-wide public opinion polls conducted around the time of the ratio campaign (1999 and 2000), nurses were ranked highest for ethics and honesty, above more than twenty-eight other professions.[59] Nurses were ranked higher than doctors (ranked third) and members of parliament (ranked twenty-first).

This high level of public trust in nurses and nursing allowed the ANF to show leadership, which promoted its remedy to the labor crisis in a convincing and nonpartisan way. In her public statements Belinda Morieson consistently highlighted the connection between staffing ratios and patient care: *"The minimum mandated numbers as ordered by the Commission is the only way the Victorian public can be confident that nurses will be able to provide their legal duty of care to patients."*[60] When the public was faced with a choice between nurses and Members of Parliament, they placed their trust in nurses to propose a strategy that would protect the interests of patients.

Another key factor that improved the nurses' bargaining position was the local labor market conditions within Victoria. This created a highly favorable environment for a systemwide response to the labor shortage. Both an ANF survey of directors of nursing across the health sector (conducted in 1996) and a national skills shortage census prepared by the federal Department of Education[61] found critical shortages in accident and emergency, critical and intensive care, operating room, midwifery, renal dialysis, geriatric nursing, and psychiatric care. Indeed, the nursing labor shortage permeated every pocket of the public health sector. This gave the union significant leverage in their negotiations because union members could be mobilized for work bans and industrial action in every conceivable health-care setting.

Finally, the union engaged in a struggle with a state government eager for resolution of the public health crisis and willing to accede to state-based independent adjudication. As we mentioned before, the Labor government under Bracks was elected on a program of social renewal. In particular, Bracks promised to rebuild the health system and address the nurse shortage. The government had already identified or framed itself as directly answerable should the shortage persist. During the course of the dispute Premier Bracks stated that he hoped the AIRC would quickly resolve the union claims. Before the arbitration even began, the government agreed to fund the final outcome. In August 2000, ANF members agreed in good faith to this process, and work bans were lifted. While the government was not actively supportive of the ratio principle, it was at least neutral and submitted to the arbitration process and outcome.[62] When Premier Bracks suggested that the matter be referred for private arbitration and agreed to abide by and fund the final outcome of the Commission decision, it was a definitive turning point in the ratios decision. Although the premier may not have anticipated that a minimum mandated-ratios model would emerge, once committed the government was locked into the process and would have publicly lost face had it reneged on its commitment.

The government of Victoria also recognized that the deregulated and privatized model for workforce management (strongly advocated by the federal government) would have been utterly ineffectual at the local level. At the federal level, under the leadership of the Liberal John Howard, government legislative change in industrial relations over the last decade has focused on encouraging workplace-level bargaining. Howard's workplace reform agenda focuses on encouraging individual enterprises to be responsible for formulating their own local solutions to recruitment and retention, working arrangements, and workload management. Liberals insist that, in a tight labor market, employers will "race to the top" by offering continual improvements to working arrangements in order to retain staff. For this reason "employer of choice" models and "family-friendly" schemes have played center stage in this approach. Using this logic, it is assumed that benevolent employers who offer employees the best deal will be most successful in retaining staff.

However, this free market model, which encourages employers to compete for the existing pool of workers, was unable to respond to the scale of the crisis faced by the Victorian government. When working conditions have deteriorated to this extent, positive behavior by a single employer will not be sufficient to convince nurses en masse to return to the system. To respond effectively, the government needed to increase the aggregate pool of labor by recruiting more people into nursing and enticing inactive nurses to return to work. If the government instead pursued an approach that encouraged individual private and public hospitals to compete against each other, both within their respective sectors and between sectors, then all it would have achieved was a shuffling of nurses between and among public and private hospital employers. This would not systematically encourage a mass return of nurses to the system.

The simplicity of the ratio principle also provided the government with an expedient marketing strategy that could be used to reassure the public that the nursing crisis was "in hand." To do this, in 2001 the Victorian government ran an extensive recruitment campaign built entirely on the ratios as the lure for burned-out nurses. The VDHS committed $1 million to advertising ratios on television and radio and $6 million to the provision of free refresher and reentry courses. The advertisements featured photographs of hospital wards or surgical environments with a group of nurses working closely together (affirming that the ratios would bring a sense of teamwork back to nursing). At the same time, the deputy premier wrote to each of the seventy-one thousand nurses registered in the state of Victoria to reassure current workers that the ratios would stabilize the system and encourage the nonpracticing nurse that a different and better working environment would await them.[63]

The ratios achieved in Victoria's public hospitals took years to devise. They were only implemented after an intense industrial dispute that had widespread public support, and they were only finally adopted after a newly elected Labor government agreed to abide by the decision of an independent industrial arbitration tribunal. A key feature of the arbitrator's decision was his attention to detail. The ratios he supported were not a crude one-size-fits-all number assumed to be relevant for all practice settings. The ratios vary by type of hospital, domain of nursing, and time of day. Unlike in California, the ratio goes up on medical/surgical in the third, p.m. shift (see appendix). Equally important, the arbitrated decision provided carefully formulated ideas for how the system would be implemented in practice. Central to the success in devising them were Australia's systems of funding public hospitals and a long tradition of active state involvement in managing relations at work. These settings ensured that, once adopted, the implementation of the ratios could occur in an environment in which there was an established infrastructure of funding and enforcement that maximized their chances of operating successfully. The next question therefore becomes: Just how *have* they operated in practice?

8

Evaluating the Impact of Ratios:
An Imperfect Experiment

Rachael Duncan, the neurological nurse we met in the introduction to this section, has described what it was like to work without ratios. Her story illuminates the way that many nurses have responded to working with ratios. Exhausted and stressed out by work overload, Duncan took a maternity leave, then returned to work in spring 2003. Of course she had heard about ratios and their impact, but she had never experienced working under a full supplement of ratio-scheduled RNs. The difference was remarkable. Her experience is not an isolated one. Countless nurses in Victoria public hospitals have similar stories to tell.

In seeking to understand the operation and impact of the ratios, researchers face several challenges. To start with, there is a dearth of data. Add to this the fact that the system continues to face recruitment and retention problems as well as ever-increasing challenges in the volume and complexity of patient demand. This means that the ratio experiment in Victoria could not be conducted under what scientists might describe as controlled conditions. Nonetheless, by 2006 two evaluations of the ratios had been conducted, both of which were commissioned and driven largely by the ANF Victoria. In the latter part of 2003 the ANF Victoria commissioned us (and colleagues from the University of Sydney) to study the working conditions of its members in the Victoria public health system. This was the ANF Victoria Work/Time/Life survey.[1] In 2006 the Workplace Research Centre also conducted a study on the impact of ratios for nursing work, using both survey and qualitative methods. These studies document that ratios have helped to foster a renaissance in the profession.

How Nurses View the Ratios

In 2003 and 2006 we surveyed nurses employed in the public-sector health system in Victoria. The sample was drawn from the ANF Victoria membership, which represents the majority (roughly 60%) of Victoria's public-sector nurses.[2] The selected sample reflected the profile and composition of the membership of the ANF (and therefore the public-sector nursing workforce) at the time. Approximately four thousand copies of the questionnaire were printed and distributed to public-sector members. In both 2003 and 2006 we received a response rate of just under 50 percent. In both survey rounds we sought to discover whether and how ratios had transformed the way hospitals staff their units. For consistency and to ensure we could compare the data, the surveys for 2003 and 2006 explored the same issues. We asked very concrete questions about whether managers assigned more nurses to more wards to cover nearly every shift. The nurses we queried were those who had worked with the ratios since their introduction. Using this technique ensured that nurses gave an account based on their *actual* experience with ratios not perceptions of ratios that may have been generated by impressions or propaganda surrounding the ratio debate. This is important because the use of rigor in the survey and sampling design means that the perceptions of nurses we describe does indeed provide an accurate account of what the majority of the nursing public-sector workforce felt about ratios and their impact at the time.[3]

In broad terms, the introduction of ratios did lead to an increase in staffing levels. To capture this, we specifically asked nurses who had worked in the same ward for three years or more, and could therefore directly compare the pre- and post-ratio environments, to comment on any change in staffing levels. These nurses (whose ward placement and substantive position had remained constant over this three-year period) represented just over 40 percent of all nurses surveyed. Over half of these nurses (51%) reported that ratios had led to an increase in staffing levels. Thirty percent said the number of nurses working in the ward had remained the same, and less than 10 percent thought that ratios had contributed to staffing cuts.

When reflecting on the experiences of the ratios it is important to remember that some nurses—even in public hospitals—are not covered by them. This includes areas where workloads are harder to measure such as community nursing, dialysis, and medical imaging, as well as those involving a high degree of supervisory or clerical work. Thus, one way of assessing the impact of the ratios is to compare the perceptions of how workloads are increasing for nurses covered by the ratios with those who are not covered.

Overall, 58 percent of nurses who worked without ratios said their workload kept increasing "year after year." Nurses with ratios still saw workload as a problem, but fewer indicated an "escalation" in workload in the previous year (47%).[4] When we asked nurses whether ratios were essential for ensuring manageable workloads, the overwhelming majority of respondents (96%) said that mandated ratios were essential to effective workload management.[5]

Although nurses still cope with many other problems, they nonetheless express strong support for the ongoing use of mandated ratios. Looking more closely at the effect of ratios on workload management practices at the unit level gives some insight why this is so. More than half of all nurses working with the ratios reported they were now able to take entitled rest breaks, and almost half reported less stress and fatigue in the postratio environment. Over 37 percent said they had more time for team building, 35 percent said there was a better skill mix where they worked, and more than 25 percent reported that fewer nurses were out on sick leave. Although this is a significant improvement, it is also a clear indication that staff shortages are still influencing the volume of work that staff members are expected to undertake during their shifts.

Nurses also gave ratios high marks because they thought that their implementation had improved quality of care. More than 47 percent said patients receive their medications on time more often than they did when nurses were racing between too many patients. Over 67 percent said they had more time for the personal care of patients, and more than 51 percent said they now had time to talk with relatives of the patients. More than 59 percent said they had more time to complete the cascading amounts of paperwork that have become such a ubiquitous feature of nurses' work.[6]

Given the sheer volume of work, and the ongoing staff shortages, ratios alone were not enough to improve patient care to the degree the nurses believed was necessary. The most important benefits have clearly been more time for the personal care of patients, greater ease and personal discretion in prioritizing and managing workloads, and more time to complete necessary documentation.

A distinctive feature of the ratios has been the sensitivity nurses have shown in their application. Although the ratios have changed underlying staffing levels they have not been implemented in a dogmatic, one-size-fits-all way. This is evident in the variety of personnel involved in enforcing them at the workplace level. In many places implementation has become part of the daily practice, with nurse unit managers (44.8%) or nurses themselves (32.6%) being responsible for their enforcement.

Ratios, Certainty, and the Limits of Rival Workload Management Systems

In principle, mandated ratios should create a stable and predictable staffing base. The ratios have indeed provided nurses with a sense of certainty in their day-to-day work. Their workload may still be taxing, but when they come to work they will not have to cope with the uncertainty of never knowing how many patients they will have to care for. They can rest assured that there will be at least some minimum staff threshold of nurses on the unit. In our qualitative interviews to assess the impact of the ratios, these outcomes are among the most important noted. As an acute care nurse in a large metropolitan hospital described it: "It has taken the anxiety out of it. I now anticipate a shift really differently to what I used to. At least I know what I have to deal with to some extent, whereas before I really could not tell if I would face a situation that was completely out of control." Another nurse in a metropolitan hospital in the inner city commented that "at least a ratio gives you an assurance you will have a minimum number of staff for the entire shift, it gives you some certainty. . . . It's basic, but it's there."

The nurses also valued this newfound certainty because they feared that management would try to introduce an alternative system—some sort of computerized patient acuity system—that would create wide variation in the number of staff from shift to shift. Their fears were well-founded. In 2003, the Labor government announced that, in the next enterprise bargaining agreement, which would take place in 2004, it would seek to replace ratios with a nurse staff allocating system—a patient dependency system. Advocates of these systems contend that they can more accurately distribute nursing hours according to patient acuity level. The government chose a system called TrendCare.

TrendCare Systems, an Australian company, produces what it calls "Advanced Nursing Management Systems that are used in Australia, New Zealand and some hospitals in Southeast Asia." The company's patient acuity/patient-nurse dependency system promises to "measure patient acuity related to clinical hours required for care, predict labour hours required, distribute equitable workloads" and identify acuity and efficiency trends, among other things.[7] Advocates of TrendCare and other patient-acuity measurement systems such as those used in California, claim that they provide a much more accurate picture of workflow and provide predictable data on which to base projections of staffing needs. Those who recommend the use of TrendCare and other acuity systems believe that a flexible workforce is the most efficient workforce and that top-level or unit-based management can—from above—determine how to allocate either total hospital or unit hospital resources in a way that saves money and enhances quality.

Critics of such systems, as we've seen in California, believe that these systems do not accurately assess the immediate needs of patients and that the ideal of a flexible workforce turns the nurse into a servant of computer-generated algorithms and not actual patient need. Because acuity systems depend on nurses to input their activities, many nurses feel that inputting data represents yet another onerous burden. Moreover, nurses are concerned that the main purpose of such systems is to cut costs, not improve patient care.

During the course of our qualitative interviews, nurses expressed all these concerns and more. As one nurse explained, "TrendCare has a retrospective element. It can tell you how many staff members you should have had on last shift. It also doesn't give you an assurance you can have those staff." The computer might identify a need for extra staff, but nurses had no lever to pull to produce an extra nurse. Nurse unit managers said they would have to go through the cumbersome process of entering the data required by staffing profiles, yet work intensification on the unit would be unaffected. Nurses thought that computerized systems could not provide them the sense of professional security, the safety net of staff that could help them deal with the predictably unpredictable, which is a hallmark of nursing work.

For example, a patient who has just been monitored may appear fine. In the following half an hour, a phlebotomist may enter the room and note that the patient appears confused. Or a patient receiving an infusion of platelets after a bone marrow transplant may appear stable when an oncology nurse checks his status. Yet ten minutes later an enrolled nurse may discover that he's complaining of feeling cold—the first sign of an adverse platelet reaction that can, if not reversed, be fatal. These are everyday occurrences for nurses. No nurse can predict when one of these—or thousands of other variants on the theme—will happen. What she or he can predict is that some time, perhaps multiple times, on his or her shift an urgent or emergent situation will occur that cannot have been foreseen.

Nurses need to know that when these predictably unpredictable events do occur there will at least be a stable threshold of staff to help the unit and the individual nurse deal with the ensuing stress, without creating chaos. If modern nursing has made hospitals safe by creating order out of chaos, nurses fear that understaffing and the technologies that often seem to accompany the phenomenon will create chaos out of order.

Many nurses insist that computerized systems radically underestimate how many staff will be needed because they fail to consider the breadth and complexity of nurses' actual work. Lisa Fitzpatrick, Victorian Branch secretary of the ANF, explained why so many nurses believe patient dependency systems give an inaccurate account of a typical nursing shift:

> These systems are built on a very narrow view of the nurses' work. Like management in general, they only assess what a nurse does when a patient is *in* a hospital bed. They forget about the additional things nurses do in order to perform their work every day. Nurses have to check, stock, and restock equipment. We have to educate the patient. We have to talk to the relatives and find out about the patient and family's life at home. Do they need a district [home

health] nurse when they get home? Do they need bath rails? Do they have a shower, or only a bath at home? Do they have enough to eat, someone who can help them get to the bathroom? All of this is what a nurse does when he or she talks to and cares for the patient. It takes time. And you can't just hitch a number to each nursing activity—like half an hour to do a wound dressing or fifteen minutes to take vital signs. That's why so many nurses are so opposed to patient dependency systems.

Or consider this example of a nurse, Joan Shirley*, taking care of an elderly female patient in a public-hospital ward:

We had an old lady who only came in to have an abscess drained, a straightforward procedure, but she was required to fast. She also had only a very mild dementia but [with] the fasting she got hungry and started wandering round the ward for something to eat. She made her way to the canteen. We had three staff looking for her, and she was only missing for fifteen minutes, but it sent the whole routine out of whack. Now if we had relied on patient-acuity alone, that lady should have required minimal care, and we would not have had the staff we needed to deal with the crisis.

Concerns about TrendCare, variants of which are used in other states and in some private hospitals in Victoria, were so widespread that nurses vowed to take "industrial action" during the 2004 bargaining to oppose their introduction if they were to replace ratios. Unlike the government, nurses wanted not only to keep the ratios but to improve them. "We wanted to introduce nurse-patient ratios to areas such as dialysis, day-surgery units, and medical-imaging areas; and we wanted to improve them in regional and country hospitals," said Fitzpatrick.

To express their commitment to ratios, nurses devoted $500,000 to advertising and media activities to maintain public support for the ratios in 2004. The theme of the campaign was "5-4-20" (i.e., five nurses for every twenty patients). They plastered the state and especially the state's public hospitals with the campaign symbol—a pyramid made of small circles with five red circles going up the left side supporting the other twenty blue circles that made up the rest of the triangle. Fitzpatrick articulated the public message: "Victoria is the only state in Australia that does not have a severe nurse shortage, because the state government was the only one able to advertise nurse-patient ratios. We are taking this action to ensure patients have a mandated minimum number of nurses on each shift to provide a safe proper level of care."

Nurses were so committed to the ratios that within forty-eight hours they closed thirteen hundred hospital beds across the state. The government quickly capitulated, but it did not agree to improve ratios, as the union had petitioned. The nurses won only the maintenance of the status quo.

Challenges to Ratio Effectiveness

It is inarguable that most nurses support the staffing ratios. Nonetheless, they are also concerned about some of the problems that have occurred during their implementation. Lisa Fitzpatrick believes that government and employers would like to moderate the impact of ratios by having nurses work what are known as short shifts. When the Kennett government began to slash nursing budgets, hospitals introduced the six-hour or short shift. Unlike hospitals in the United States, hospitals in Victoria cannot by law (under the terms of the enterprise agreements) send nurses home to take vacation or personal days or sick days if the unit is not busy or the census is down. In Victoria, to cut costs, hospitals used nurses two fewer hours a day, which allowed hospitals to pay nurses less. Nurses were not universally pleased with this development. As Fitzpatrick explained, "Many times there wasn't time for proper handover and in-service education to take place, no time for people to take meal breaks. When some nurses finished afternoon shift at 1 or 1:30, afternoon nurses or remaining morning shift nurses had additional patients to look after, which escalated workloads."

In the 2000 negotiations the union set a limit on short shifts, as Fitzpatrick explained:

> You could only have one short shift in the morning and one in the afternoon, not three in the morning and three in the afternoon. Higher level hospital management would now like to temper the financial impact of the ratios by having no limits on how many nurses work short shifts and by winning the freedom to assign nurses to not just six-hour but four-hour shifts.
>
> Managers will try to bring someone in to the hospital, say from 1 p.m. to 5 p.m., for example, just after an orthopedic theater list is finished, and things get really busy. Then they tell the nurse that they don't really need her on a Friday afternoon because the unit isn't very busy or the patients [are] not that acute.

Although some nurses value short shifts if, for instance, they have childcare responsibilities or want to work a shorter schedule, many others feel this introduces unpredictability into their job. Fitzpatrick also argues that telling nurses they are needed only when patient loads are heavy or the unit is very busy fails to include activities such as education in the workplace, learning new policies and procedures, or keeping up with the latest nursing and medical research.

Jenny Withers° works full time at a large medical center in suburban Melbourne and has twenty years' experience in nursing. In addition to the ratios, Withers argues that long shifts (the double handover principle) and limits on the use of agency staff have all been important to supporting and giving strength to the benefits of ratios. In her work area, Withers explained, short shifts have been phased out. Now, nurses are scheduled for a longer shift that includes a two-hour handover:

> I cannot overestimate how important the link between ratios and longer shifts is. . . . We use that time for those really important tasks that we often don't have time to devote a shift to—because we need to spend time with patients. I can attend a seminar that updates my equipment training, or I can organize the med supplies. Can you imagine someone going into cardiac arrest and no one has restacked the cardio trolleys? If we didn't appropriately staff shifts [through the ratios] we wouldn't have the time during handover to do these kinds of critical, but basically hidden, tasks.

Management Discretion in Implementing the Ratios: The "50 Percent Rule"

While nurse unit managers are most often responsible for the enforcement of ratios, staff nurses are also active agents in the workload management process. Although opponents of ratios argue that ratios somehow represent a legislated ceiling of staffing, under the terms of the enterprise agreement, management can increase the level of staffing at any point. This was, in part, the rationale for the 50 percent rule, which the ANF and hospital management negotiated in 2001 to resolve the problems created by wards with bed numbers not divisible by the ratio.

For example, a 1:4 ratio in a thirty-bed ward would require seven nurses, plus half a nurse. The 50 percent rule deems that management has the discretion to respond to this anomaly by either rounding down (scheduling only seven nurses on a shift) or rounding up (scheduling eight nurses one a shift). Or if a twenty-bed unit had only seventeen patients, managers could round down, or if patient acuity was high enough they could also maintain the 5:20 ratio. To exercise its managerial discretion, management was under no legal obligation or pressure to round down rather than up in these cases. Nurses would argue that managers and administrators truly committed to the flexibility needed to provide high-quality patient care would round up—or view ratios as a minimum and ratios-plus as best practice.

This is not, many nurses argue, how it has worked out in reality. The 50 percent rule remains one of the most controversial issues associated with the mandated-ratio model in its current form. When asked in 2003 whether their managers usually dealt with the 50 percent rule by rounding up or down, two in three respondents (65%) in work areas with ratios reported that "my ward never rounds numbers up." Only 10 percent of nurses reported they worked in wards that "always round up." Nurses' general views about this rule were captured well by a respondent who reported: "We have a 50 percent rule, so on day shift we have four patients each but can have up to six patients to one nurse. On evening shift we have five patients to one nurse but can have up to seven patients to one nurse. Get rid of the 50 percent rule, please!"[8]

Respondents were also asked whether their work area closed beds if the ratios could not be staffed. Less than half, 48 percent, reported that this occurred.[9] Clearly, arbitrary enforcement is not the norm in many workplaces with ratios. Many nurses accommodated some deviations from the ratios. This flexibility, however, was not open-ended. Deviations from this norm do not, generally speaking, persist for long because nurses still seem to maintain clear standards about staffing levels. Even though, as we shall see, nurse unit managers and directors of nursing are generally very supportive of ratios, they are under constant pressure to provide more care to sicker patients who are, in escalating numbers, cycling through the system. This outcome appears to have arisen from the context within which the ratios have operated: one of continuing change and increasing workloads. Thus, in 2006, one nurse who works in an acute ward of a regional hospital described the way in which rounding down had been used as an ongoing strategy of ratio resistance by management and had allowed the perpetuation of workload problems: "Management refers to this fifth staff member as an 'extra.' Well, it's not an extra, it's an entitlement. This can mean at our hospital, say, on every shift, someone is picking up five, not four, patients."[10]

Is the Staffing Floor a De Facto Ceiling?

In some areas, particularly eldercare, the adequacy of ratios has always been—and continues to be—contested. Moreover, because eldercare in Australia, as in many other industrialized countries, remains poorly funded, management has used the ratios as a very clear ceiling. Nurses in public eldercare facilities discuss quite frankly how senior management can use the ratio to cap, rather than expand, permanent staffing levels. In the eldercare sector, workload problems continue to confront nurses, because it is generally agreed that the ratio of 1:7 is inadequate. The ANF had asked for ratios of "one to four—across the board" but did not get them. As one eldercare RN described it, "Our facility houses about fifty-four people. Just our usual morning routine the other week—that includes bathing, meds, dressing, etc.—we did not finish this until 1:30 in the afternoon. That is entirely due to the 1:7 rule. It is just not enough staff."

In 2006, the ANF reports that no eldercare facility in the public sector has staffing arrangements that are below the mandated ratio, despite the overwhelming evidence of persisting workload problems in the sector. As one eldercare RN in a metropolitan senior-care facility noted in 2006, before the introduction of the 2000 ratio many facilities operated on a principle of 1:5. The postratio environment has created an opportunity for management to justify staff cuts. "We always had 1:5, and I have worked here for fifteen years. As soon as the 1:7 came in, management got rid of the staff. Nothing else changed—it is not like we had less residents. Doesn't matter how hard we have fought this, we will never get them back." It is important to understand that the ratio decision did not dictate or require that eldercare facilities lay off staff. The government chose not to fund ratios at the previous level, and this created a way for employers to reduce costs by cutting staff, rather than seeking other ways to maintain funding and revenue levels.

In hospitals, the use of ratios as a de facto staff ceiling is also evident in the onerous requirements often placed on nurse unit managers should they wish to lobby for extra positions beyond the ratio limit. In another 2006 interview, a nurse unit manager argued that staff beyond the recommended ratio level are needed and described the situation confronting her: "We will need about twenty properly prepared incident reports before senior management will even listen. In order to justify a claim for overtime a few years ago, we had to properly prepare, file, and lodge six hundred incident reports before senior managers would address the problem. They did in the end, but it took that amount. The same trick is being used with the ratio issue." For a nurse unit manager who is already responsible for supervision and management of staff, accounting, administration, and education, preparing a stack of incident reports over and over again hardly alleviates a burdensome managerial workload.

Ruminating on Life without Ratios

The 2003 survey indicated that nurses overwhelmingly believed that working life would have been worse had ratios not been introduced. Eighty-one percent of nurses who had worked to ratios for three or more years said the quality of patient care would have declined without them. Eighty-four percent reported that nurses' working conditions would be worse.[11]

Nurses working in areas with ratios were asked what they would do if the ratios were abolished. The responses indicate that the shortage of nurse labor would increase profoundly. Fewer than one in six (14%) of the nurses reported they would not make any changes if the ratios were abolished. Over half (53%) said that if the ratios were altered they would reduce the amount of time they worked as nurses: 24 percent would consider leaving nursing altogether; 20 percent would consider cutting their hours; and 9 percent would consider retiring early.[12] The degree to which ratios continue to directly affect decisions on staff flight is illustrated by this 2006 comment from one nurse, who works at an outer suburban Melbourne hospital: "God help us if we hadn't had them. I would have long since gone. It is the only thing that has kept me nursing."

Ratios: Facilitating a Professional Renaissance?

Opponents of ratios argue that ratios deprofessionalize nursing, making the profession less appealing by reducing the level of judgment and discretion associated with professional practice. Contrary to these assertions, our research has revealed that ratios are contributing to the rebuilding of the profession. The aggregate number of nurses entering the public health system to practice has increased each year since the introduction of ratios. This growth has been attributed, in large part, to nurses returning to the system from which they had previously fled. The Department of Human Services in Victoria reports that within twelve months of the introduction of ratios, twenty-three hundred nurses returned to the public hospital system (a 10% increase overall). This growth is particularly significant when compared with the typical numbers of nurses who either come into the profession for the first time or reenter after an absence. Before ratios, four hundred or fewer nurses entered or returned to the profession each year.[13]

While senior hospital management and government officials voice an uneasy acceptance of ratios and continue to advocate computerized workload management models (TrendCare), they also acknowledge the role that ratios have played in encouraging the return of nurses. As the executive director of Metropolitan and Aged Care Services in VDHS, Shane Solomon, noted twelve months after the introduction of ratios, "We also introduced pre-determined nurse patient ratios, which was I think the single biggest step toward improving nurses lives' at the ward level."[14]

Because there has been a constant stream of nurses returning to the system each year since their introduction, the ratios continue to stabilize the health system in Victoria. In 2007, the Victorian government claimed that around seven thousand nurses have returned to the system overall since 2001.[15] State nursing unions also claim that the improved working conditions for nurses in Victoria have created an "interstate drainage" effect. Both the Tasmanian and Queensland branches of the ANF argue in their respective annual reports that the emergence of better working conditions in Victoria has contributed to the migration of members to Victoria in the postratio period. The state union branches claim they can document this migration because their affiliation with the ANF nationally allows the union to track membership transfer between the states.[16]

In extended interviews with nurses across a range of practice settings, nurses maintain that ratios have improved their status as professionals.

Ratios, they insist, have given them opportunities to exercise autonomy within a team-based work model; helped them have more time to engage in psychosocial or "emotional work" during which they can hear patients concerns, answer questions, and provide education; and enhanced their sense of certainty and stability in the patient-care environment. Nurses insist that this has reaffirmed the role of nurses as clinicians who have a unique professional contribution to make within the health system.

"Emotional" Work

It is well documented that providing psychosocial services and emotional support during their work in direct patient care—and the complexity of the skills required to do so—is the most immeasurable area of nursing care.[17] Nurses still insist that they struggle as professionals to gain recognition for these duties as credible components of their work. However, nurses argue that ratios have offered them a chance to create more time at work to perform these important roles than had previously been the case.

This type of work represents one of the most important elements of the discretionary tasks that define nurses as professionals. Nurses argue that before ratios, high patient load meant that perfunctory and routinized elements of care (maintaining patient hygiene, administering medication) would occur, but time pressure would simply not permit the personal element of work to occur.

Not surprising, nurses expressed concerns over computerized workload management models in the context of discussions over the psychosocial roles nurses perform. As one inner-city RN describes it, the time that might be needed to support and manage a patient's needs cannot always be factored in to workloads in a systematic way: "Some of technically the 'sickest' patients may need little in the way of this emotional support because they may be out of it, while others may need more support but be undergoing a relatively simple procedure." For this reason, this nurse vehemently contended that ratios represent the preferred workload management model. Ratios permit nurses to make decisions about where and how psychosocial work should be performed, and to retain responsibility for the decisions made.

Building and Maintaining the Professional Nursing Team

Five years after the introduction of ratios, nurses say that the ratios have permitted the team-based nature of nursing work to again play a role in patient care. As one nurse in an acute care team at a public hospital in Melbourne described it:

I had to go up to theater with a patient, and I was gone much longer than I expected. As I was heading back down to the ward, I braced myself . . . I thought here we go, I will have a huge catch-up. I expected everything else I had to do for my other patients would have fallen behind. But it hadn't. The other nurses had at least made sure that my patients had received their meds and had kept it ticking over [had continued to conduct observations and attend to other patients' needs]. . . . That was never possible before ratios. Ratios just mean we have less patients, so we can help each other out, and the nurses really can work as a team.

Enhancing the Clinician Role

Nurses' ability to exercise their professional judgment as clinical practitioners has also been improved under the ratio system. In interviews with nurses in 2006, interviewees argued that having fewer patients per nurse gives them greater scope to assess, plan, and manage a patient's recuperation and rehabilitation. Jenny Withers describes herself as a "nurse for life," but she was not sure how long that "life" would have lasted before ratios. "The ratios are the single most important thing to have happened in nursing since the beginning of my career at least. . . . They have changed how we work so much. I can honestly say that within six months of their implementation for those of us on acute care wards, work was totally transformed. It was that powerful, that quick," she said. Withers also argues that ratios bring a sense of pride back to nursing:

A lot of people talk about the magnet hospital or the magnet ward as being a strategy that is separate or distinct from the ratios. Like you can't have one without the other, or that somehow these approaches aren't compatible. I don't believe that. NUMs should all aim to make their ward a place where people want to work. Ratios actually let us do that better, because they give us a lever as managers to think about our skill mix and roster effectively with nurses who are committed and willing to invest in the system.

In this postratio environment nurses—at least those nurses in the public sector who have been able to work to reasonable ratios—say they experience a sense of professional reawakening. For nurses who had worked through the deepest periods of crisis in the 1990s (which included extended hours and high patient load), the opportunity to revisit and understand what it means to nurse "people" rather than "illness" is welcomed and valued. As Paula Hilton°, a nurse unit manager working in an outer suburban hospital argued, the nurse role had become so routinized that it was undermining the integrity and unique contribution of nurses: "We were heading down a path that I think would have changed nursing forever, because we were no longer able to do what had defined us as nurses." Again, nurses saw the introduction of computerized systems (specifically TrendCare) as a major threat to the exercise of this clinical role. "I believe these systems undervalue and underestimate what nurses can bring to a clinical environment," Hilton said. A more manageable workload, even in a system that is still facing a number of staffing challenges, allows nurses to explore and consider their clinical contribution in a more meaningful way. "I believe we can now practice what we teach," Hilton said. "We can truly practice what we have been trained for."

In a more formal sense, there is also evidence that the supporting arrangements for ratios (including the two-hour handover and long-shift arrangements) have, in many places, restored the access to in-service education programs. In the independent evaluation of ratios released in 2004, researchers found that access to professional development programs and in-service education, including updating training on equipment and procedures, had improved.[18]

Implications for Managers

In the United States, nurse managers at the middle and senior levels have been among the strongest critics of ratios. This has not been the case in Victoria. Many nurse unit managers and directors of nursing have appreciated the support the ratios give them in carrying out their managerial responsibilities. Although not all have embraced them, nurse unit managers as a group are the single largest group involved in enforcing them. Why and how this occurred was uncovered in semistructured interviews done with nurse unit managers and directors of nursing for the studies we have undertaken during the course of our research on this issue.

Nurse Unit Managers: Ratios, Patient Dependency Systems, and Discretion

For the nurse unit managers interviewed in late 2006, ratios had significant implications for their role as managers and in the elevation of this role in the public-hospital hierarchy. Since the 1990s, the shift toward decentralization has meant that nurse unit managers have been required to undertake a greater share of the administrative work, including managing supplies and equipment, education, assuming responsibility and accountability for the wages bill, and developing retention strategies and recruiting staff, all in addition to managing and supervising staff. As one nurse unit manager in a metropolitan hospital described it, the mandatory nature of the ratios means that there is certainty over at least one aspect of their responsibilities: "It deflects the angst between the senior manager and ward staff, with the NUM caught between. It is still a stressful job, but ratios take just that one important point of consternation away. That one issue of conflict is removed because the ratio is known and understood." As another nurse unit manager in a regional hospital argued, "The bean counters and the CEO have most of the say. This is one small way that nurses themselves get to at least be heard."

In the minds of nurse unit managers, working with ratios and the certainty of a staffing threshold allows them to distil, define, and practice what the role of nurse manager actually is. Kristy Spencer, a nurse unit manager in a large inner-city hospital, insisted that ratios allow managers not just to manage but to manage well:

> As a manager, I like the certainty of ratios. I actually think they help define what the role of a manager in nursing is all about—making decisions about your team, their experience, what they need to cope, and be supported, and to know how to roster effectively. A patient dependency system can't do that. The argy-bargy now is over the skill mix—and I think that is what defines the very job of the NUM—to manage people, and to look at what they need from shift to shift, and be responsive to that.

In interviews with a group of nurse unit managers in the summer of 2004, we found them very supportive of ratios and highly critical of patient dependency systems such as TrendCare. The following commentaries, provided by nurse unit managers—Clare McGinness, a NUM of a respiratory medical ward at Monash Medical Centre, Delia Comodo, a NUM of a Hematology Stem Cell unit at the Peter McCallum Cancer Centre, and Kate Ireland, NUM of a liver transplant and general surgery unit at Austin Health in Melbourne—give insights into the positive ways in which nurse unit managers have worked with ratios.

Delia Comodo described the stresses of working under the preratio system. She was what is known as an ANUM, associate nurse unit manager (or a charge nurse in the U.S. system), which meant that, unlike the nurse unit manager, who was often not on the floor, she was not only on the floor but also taking a load of patients as well as managing the other nurses and patients.[19] When she looks back on it, she says, she can not believe she managed the workload:

> You took a patient load as well as running a ward. I now wonder how I did it. When you're looking after four sick neutropenic patients and you had to actually physically look at all the other patients to see what the skill mix was, it was impossible. A lot of time I would get the sickest patients because I was the most senior person. We had four patients each, including a charge person taking four patients.

Now, Comodo says, the ratio is five to twenty, plus one who isn't taking patients:

> This makes a huge difference from the point of view of the NUMs and ANUMs, because it allows the ANUMs to actually go and see patients, to work out who's the sickest, who of your staff needs more support on a particular shift and who doesn't, who's going to struggle at night and is going to need a bit of a hand. If you've got an agency nurse who isn't familiar with the unit [you've got somebody] to oversee [them].

Kate Ireland does not believe that the ratios are inflexible and insists that they provide nurse managers with the foundation of security they need to use their judgment in assessing the skill mix necessary to deal with shifting patient acuity:

> With the ratios, what it comes down to—is using your judgment. You use your ratios with relation to patient acuity and how you're going to run the shift but also in relation to the skill mix you have. Some days, you look at your roster and it's diabolical, you have a junior grade, two years experience, and you. You're in an area like pain or liver transplant and you have people who are, on paper, less skilled but who are competent and safe and good team players. Well, you'd rather have them than somebody who's a senior nurse who knows it all but is not going to be a team player on a shift that might require that.

McGinness echoes these sentiments:

> The ratios are not set in concrete. As a NUM you have the flexibility to play with it. Today on my ward I have one nurse with two patients. All the other nurses have picked up the other patients to accommodate that. Why does she have two patients? Because they are the two sickest with the highest acuity. I haven't changed anything with the ratios. I haven't got extra staff, I've just manipulated it so that the work flow is better and the actual patient care is directed in the way it should be. The more acute patients requiring the more intense patient care got one nurse between them. You can play with it. It's up to the judgment of the NUM.

Clare McGinness also says that the legal obligation of fulfilling the ratios and not overloading nurses allows her not only to "play with the work flow within the ratios" but also to just say no when she feels the unit cannot handle another patient:

> We regularly do that. We did that last week. We don't have an emergency department. A patient presented at 4:30 in the afternoon needing a bed. There were no beds in the hospital, which meant this person might have had to go to another casualty hospital. They asked us to take the other patient. I said, "I'm sorry, normally I'm happy to take more patients but not with the skill mix and the patient acuity I have on today."

I had two patients post-ICU. I said, "This is crazy, it's dangerous, I can't take another patient." It turned out this patient had a pneumothorax as well. I said, "I can't take another that's quite unwell. We have two patients back from ICU, a patient who's having blood products who's in DIC"—disseminated in intravascular coagulation. I had a grad, a couple of agency nurses on. When someone is requiring that level of care and the skill mix doesn't allow you to care for them, that one extra patient would tip that whole balance over.

All three nurses were angry because of what they described as a government line against ratios. "The thing that irks me," said Kate Ireland, "is that the government and some nurse executives push this line that ratios are inflexible, and that's what the public is led to believe. But the clinical nurse manager determines what is done with the nurses that are provided to the shift according to the ratios."

Ireland believes that some nurses, like government bureaucrats, fail to grasp the flexibility of the five to twenty scheme. "Sometimes bedside nurses think inflexibly that one to four means you're actually only looking after four patients, so when a NUM assigns a nurse six patients because they are not so acute they may believe it's unfair. But that's where we, as NUMS, use the flexibility within the ratios to manage the differences in acuity of patients on the ward," she said.

All three nurse unit managers insisted that ratios gave them more control over their units and enhanced unit morale. According to Clare McGinness, it would be difficult to create an appropriate schedule of—and for—nurses without ratios:

As a manager, without having a ratio to work with, you don't know how many staff you're going to need. How do you roster? How do you put people on annual leave? How do you plan in advance? We have to have rosters done six weeks in advance. With the ratios we have what we need night, afternoon, and morning. You can't put people off on annual leave with a day's notice, that's just crazy."

Delia Comodo argued that ratios were the logical extension of good nursing management and the nursing philosophy of providing care under difficult and often unpredictable circumstances:

Even before the ratios NUMs took into consideration skill mix, acuity—this is just a way of putting it in writing that allows us on a daily basis to work out what we should always have. NUMs have always done that. This is just formalizing it. We've always had nurses who would have a harder patient and other nurses would pick up lighter patients. That's the nature of nursing. It's the fact that nursing changes minute to minute.

Like many of their colleagues, several of these managers were adamantly opposed to the introduction of patient acuity systems such as TrendCare.

They insisted that the data inputted into patient dependency systems could be manipulated and did not reflect actual practice on their units. "A lot of nurses," said McGinness, "couldn't see the value of it because they felt it didn't reflect what was going on in the unit and you had to sit and enter data into the system all the time when it didn't always really equate to what was happening."

These systems, McGinness insists, did not capture what, say, a cancer nurse did and the acuity of patients with whom she or he was working. TrendCare would assign the number of nurses based on, for example, the fact that some patients were determined to be "ambulatory." But what does ambulatory really mean, she asked. "Yes, a patient may be ambulatory and on self-care but may be having a very complex regime of chemotherapy which may take some time to give. These systems don't factor the education that was required if this was the first time the patient has had the chemotherapy. If they're a newly diagnosed patient . . . it doesn't capture any emotional or psychosocial work you do."

Although many advocates of computerized patient acuity systems contrast them to the specter of impersonal, bottom-line government bureaucrats dictating nursing care, these nurse unit managers believe that TrendCare and other patient acuity systems represent an equally impersonal and bureaucratic-corporate, computer-based control over their professional judgment and staff nurses' professional practice.

Clare McGinness explained that her unit at Monash Medical Centre was a pilot unit for TrendCare following the enterprise bargaining agreement of 2000:

> I went to a lot of the training sessions, and it was insulting. The person who ran the training session said they believed all the psychosocial time was factored in. All the timings were done so well that they accounted for everything. I didn't believe it and one of my night staff actually told me it wasn't reflecting the care-giving at night. It was quite insulting and humiliating. It was time consuming for us as well. Everyone had to have a computer password, be trained up—it was time consuming even setting it up.

The system, McGinness said, would tell her how much time she, as a nurse unit manager, had to spend on her particular duties. It would also tell her what her ward's workload looked like, say, in the afternoon, and how much time she should spend dealing with staff or other duties:

> The system would say, "This is what your workload is this afternoon," which was actually taking away my own clinical judgment. It would tell me who the busy patients were, so it was actually saying, "Well, you don't know what's going on on the ward. I'm here to tell you." If it says you need more or less staff, I'm not going to

tell one person to take the day off. I always felt that was the driving force to get us to tell someone, "Well, I'm going to give you annual leave this afternoon."

Nurses also complained about how much time it took them in the morning to enter data about what they planned to do that afternoon and then to "actualize" the system by entering what they actually did that afternoon. "When nurses have to come in to work and enter data into the computer about what they plan to do during the day and then, later on, 'actualize'—entering more data about what care they actually delivered, this time feeding data to the technology—it takes away from time caring for real patients," McGinnes added. "But that, promoters of TrendCare say, is how nursing should be actualized."

Directors of Nursing: Ratios and the Management Function

Unlike directors of nursing in the United States, who tend to fiercely oppose any government regulation and the introduction of ratios, some—although certainly not all—directors of nursing in Victoria embrace ratios.

Danny Rathgeber, then director of nursing of the Royal Melbourne Hospital, was one the chief nurse executives who were very supportive of ratios. In 2004, when the ANF was lobbying to maintain and extend the ratios and was fending off the government's attempt to remove them, Rathgeber went on record opposing the patient dependency system the government wanted to introduce. "We think what works in this organization is ratios plus," Rathgeber explained. "We think ratios work once a year at the financial time to set the minimal level budget. And then when you truly understand your workforce, you truly know what that means—you've analyzed every department and you know that the ratios are reasonable ratios and aren't the issue. It takes ratios plus to maintain safe nursing care."

"We haven't been in a dispute with the ANF at all," Rathgeber elaborated. "We're working with them. We think they've done us justice in not always going back to zero in a debate over the baseline of the budget and not discussing ratios, but starting discussing what we also need."

From the point of view of the director of nursing, Rathgeber explained what it was like to function in the preratio environment:

> Before, in management, you always went back to zero in your budget discussions. So you had a thirty-bed ward and you're talking to the finance people and you'd be back to zero—that's your starting point trying to get staff. If you've got ratios then you actually start at that level of five to twenty, as long as you accept that tool. That's where I see a huge advantage with ratios. Where I see a disadvantage with ratios is that we will [need to] be flexible, because, as I said, the

average is one to three, not one to four, but there are times when I would say
maintaining safe standards you can go one to five, easy.

Rathgeber said he does not believe nurses should be turned off and on like
hot and cold running water and that they need stability to practice safely. That
is why he is not a fan of patient acuity systems:

> It amazed me when I was in New York and went around to some of the hospi-
> tals, the lack of systems and processes that were there because I don't believe
> that you can measure a nurse's workload. You might be able to measure it for
> that point in time while you're there, but five seconds later it could be totally
> different—and why is it the shift before measures the workload for the shift
> that's coming on? It's not real time and even if it's real time it's not accurate
> anyway—[it tells you nothing about] what's going to happen in the next eight
> hours of the shift. That's what you need to measure, what you need to know to
> measure what staffing level you need. We don't get engineers involved who
> understand flow and physics to measure workload. My view is all we do is cre-
> ate project people who collect all this data. It's so big and so awkward that all
> we do is give all these consultants who come in more opportunity to discredit
> the data. It's not practical enough and so it becomes a target. [The] ratios [sys-
> tem] has helped us but it hasn't been the real reason we've succeeded. The
> fact is the real reason is we understand every ward, every department right
> down to what the workload is and what the staff supply needs to be to work
> with that.

Rathgeber explained that "we build up from that. Ratios plus means understanding your workforce in a complex environment and saying what is safe.
We bring it back to standard of nursing care. Instead of allowing the clinicians
to use it, we've adopted the approach that management should use it, and it's
a win–win."

Marie Wilson is the director of nursing at Western Health. Wilson's comment about ratios also illuminated how managers and nurse executives can
use them to build trust and to tackle issues they were unable to consider
under alternative systems.

Wilson said that one of the major things ratios and the Nurses 2000 EBA
agreement did was help her to address the radical overuse of agency nurses.
Before ratios, there was no incentive for those loyal to the health service to remain in permanent employment. Part of the rationale for the ratios articulated in the Blair decision was the cost of agency nurses. In implementing
ratios, hospitals would cap their use of agency nurses. Wilson was an early advocate of implementing this cap in her hospital. She did this by developing a
policy she called management of nursing vacancies. Under this policy no
nurse who was employed within Western Health was allowed to work for an
agency at the same time:

Our specialist nurses, who received the highest rate of pay, balked at this. They threatened to leave, which made the divisional directors who managed the workforce very, very worried. They came to me en masse, as a posse, to say, "Don't go down that track, they're going to migrate out." They insisted that if we were the only ones in Victoria restricting agency nurses, we wouldn't be able to get needed staff.

Wilson thought:

We have to send our permanent employees a strong message that we support them. The nurses did not leave en masse. Once they recognized that nobody in our health service could work agency here anymore, they all came back on board, because the reality was they knew their shift routines; they knew their policies and procedures; they were comfortable in their working environments, and that was what I called them on. I didn't believe that they would want to work elsewhere where they'd have to be new employees and be orientated to a new environment. I knew that they wanted to be loyal to the health service underneath it all. And having done this in about October of 2001, we quickly saw our own nursing workforce start improving. People who had only worked part-time came to work full-time; people who were inactive returned to work.

Wilson quickly adopted a strict policy about filling vacancies. Staff were first offered overtime, and as a last resort agency nurses would be called. Only a few months later, Wilson said, "the Department of Human Services amended the Health Services Act to prevent nurses in any health service working agency in their health services. So, they mimicked our policy on a more global scale throughout Victoria."

Next, Wilson used the ratios to develop a stronger relationship with undergraduate nursing students who were potential recruits to the hospital. Western Health, she said, always had a graduate nursing program. This program is for nurses who have just graduated from nursing school after three years and who work one extra year on the wards in a special apprenticeship program. Western Health increased the number of graduates from twenty-five to seventy-six a year. These graduates work on wards and have four patients, but in addition they have a special clinical support staff assigned to them to help orient them to their new work. To make Western Health more attractive to undergraduates, Wilson assigned special preceptors and mentors and tried to align the clinical rotations to track the stage of theory they were studying in their undergraduate curriculum.

The most serious problem Wilson addressed was a shortage of specialty nurses—those educated in intensive care, accident, emergency, coronary care, and operating theaters:

We had a seventy EFT [effective full time] gap in our workforce in those areas. Here again, we said, OK, it's a feeder issue. Every recruitment strategy should have feeders into the system. People aren't going into critical care because of two reasons: One is that they can't afford the postgraduate fees, and the second one is that they're too scared to dip their toes into the area, because it's such an intimidating, frightening environment.

To entice nurses into specialty areas, Western Health created a six-month postgraduate discovery program that allowed staff to get experience in a specialty area by working as an extra nurse on what were called "education days" and "clinical competency days." An educator worked with them, and, if they liked the environment, they could enter a postgraduate course. The system quickly began to offer nurses scholarships for these courses. As long as a nurse committed to work at Western Health for a year after the course, the hospital paid 50 percent of their fee. Nurses who entered the program and didn't like the specialty area were guaranteed not to lose their job. Now, said Wilson, the postgraduate discovery program has become a significant feeder into the postgraduate diplomas in specialty nursing.

Wilson believes that ratios have led managers to be more creative and that they have certainly brought more nurses back into the system: "Ratios were giving nurses the opportunity to work in an environment where they had adequate numbers of nurses on the floor that allowed them to carry clinical components of their work that weren't adequately prescribed by a dependency system."

Wilson expressed only two concerns about the ratios. The first concerned finding nurses to fill them. She is dealing with this through initiatives of the kind noted above. The second, she says, regards some nurses who are rigid about ratio interpretation: "Belinda Morieson and then subsequently Lisa Fitzpatrick were big advocates of five nurses for twenty patients, but the nurse on the floor saw it as one per four patients." Rather than taking care of a patient with high acuity and letting other nurses take care of less acute patients, she says, nurses will ask for a "workload special," that is, an extra nurse.

To deal with what she described as a "hands-up" phenomenon—a nurse who raises his or her hand to say "I need a special"—Wilson requires any nurse unit manager requesting a workload special to get the approval of their divisional director, who is their senior manager. "This manager will then say, 'Why do you need this special? Have you considered a reallocation of workload within your five nurses for twenty patients, rather than automatically going to a special?' "

Wilson believes that ratios solve some, but not all, of the problems in nursing. Among other things, she believes nursing must accommodate the needs of people who want a social life and do not want to constantly work evenings, weekends, and holidays. She believes some nurses should be able to work shorter shifts of six hours to accommodate their child-care or other needs. She also believes nurse managers need to be more supportive and flexible. Wilson insisted that ratios have not only enhanced nurse morale but they have also increased trust between nurses at the bedside and those who manage their work. Although some hospital administrators were initially opposed to ratios, most now work constructively with them. She said the mandating of ratios has had the following effects:

> Our nurse unit managers sent a very strong message back to our teams that management cares about us; they're trying to rectify the situation of the gap that's caused by ratios. They're supportive of ratios, and they want to bridge that gap. We've told our nurse unit managers, graduate nurses, and experienced nurses: we're putting money into your postgraduate scholarships; we're putting money into your postgraduate discovery program; we are insuring that we are staffing to that ratio. Certainly, I think that in itself attracted people back in Western Health.
>
> Once it was signed off that ratios were going to be in situ, we as managers were able to say, OK, we've got ratios now, what are we going to do to address this gap and make your environments more attractive to have a permanent workforce in, rather than this casualized workforce? And once we had committed to doing that, and once we actually delivered on it, we gained a significant amount of credibility with our staff.

Quality of Working Life in the Postratio Workplace

From nurses' point of view, ratios in Victoria are *part* of the solution to a complex problem. They are not the entire solution, nor are they a panacea. On the issue of working conditions and work overload, the story is one of improvement, but not resolution.

When, in 2003, we took a snapshot of the postratio workplace in Victoria, we found distinct improvements to some areas of working life for nurses but not resolution of ongoing workload problems facing the health sector. The 2003 ANF Work/Time/Life survey data indicates that workload remains a significant and ongoing concern, even after the introduction of ratios. Overtime remains a common feature of the working experience of nurses in Victoria. The survey of nurses in Victoria that was concluded in 1999 found that 65 percent worked overtime on a regular (weekly) basis. In the postratio environment, the ANF Work/Time/Life survey found that 63 percent of nurses still worked overtime on a regular basis.[20] The state health system continues to rely on a high level of commitment from the nursing labor force in order to meet workload expectations in excess of current staffing levels.

Why So Much Overtime?

The 2003 survey asked nurses who worked overtime to identify the most important reason they worked longer hours. Only 5 percent of public-sector nurses surveyed reported that they worked additional hours on an entirely voluntary basis. This is noteworthy because the endemic level of overtime does not appear to be the result of a culture of workaholism. More than half of the entire workforce believes that overtime is necessary to deliver the most basic standards of care. More than 10 percent of managers said overtime is an expected part of their work, and 5.6 percent said they worked overtime voluntarily but that peers and managers expected them to do so.[21]

The 2003 survey collected data in the management of, and decision-making processes surrounding, overtime. The results show a fragmented approach to the absorption of overtime hours across the sector. Management clearly relies on these additional hours to maintain standards of care, yet it shows no systemwide nor consistent response in acknowledging these hours.

Nurses were asked to describe custom and practice surrounding reimbursement of overtime and the quantity or scale of overtime hours that the system is absorbing. Overtime is not handled or processed in a consistent manner across care environments, even though payment for overtime is a legal entitlement according to the sectorwide enterprise bargaining agreement. Almost 40 percent of nurses said their overtime was treated differently by the organization on each occasion. Less than 15 percent said that they always received payment for overtime. More than one in five reported that the overtime they worked was always left unpaid. These data form a cumulative picture of a system that relies heavily on the good will of nurses in order to maintain standards of care. Although managers are clearly attempting to acknowledge and compensate for these additional hours in some form, there still appear to be significant funding constraints on the ability of work units to financially reimburse for overtime worked.[22]

Superficially, it would appear that ratios have not solved two critical and detrimental impacts associated with excess workload—a high incidence of overtime and workplace practice that absorbs and conceals additional hours rather than recognizing and compensating workers for these additional hours. This raises the obvious question: Do nurses believe that ratios have had any impact on reducing workload and has this improved the quality of their working lives?

Ongoing Challenges to Renewal

Ratios, although broadly effective, also create new challenges for nursing staff. The greatest challenges appear to be associated with the formulation of what represents an appropriate staffing level and ratio compliance. In areas where ratios are generally considered inadequate, the situation for nurses can only be described as conflicted at best. Surprisingly, the findings of our most recent qualitative study suggest that outright avoidance or evasion of the ratios is not widespread. Instead, employer resistance to ratios appears to take the form of what might be described as "hypercompliance." This hypercompliance occurs through strict adherence to a 50 percent rule, using the ratios as a staffing ceiling rather than a staffing floor. Resistance also takes place when senior management insist that highly detailed and onerous documentation be prepared at the unit level to justify any lifting of the ratio.

In pockets of the public health sector, the ratios that currently apply appear to be inadequate. The ratios currently applying to postnatal (1:5 on an a.m. shift), maternity wards (ratio determined by size and location of facility), public eldercare facilities (1:7), and regional and remote areas (1:5 or 1:6 depending on hospital classifications) are the most controversial. In the most comprehensive postratio workload evaluation conducted, the greatest workload problems were still found in these areas.[23] In regional and remote areas, it is well understood that the challenges facing nursing staff are different than those in larger metropolitan facilities. In remote areas, nurses are typically expected to manage a wider range of high-dependency problems within one care setting, because a single facility is expected to take care of a whole range of medical emergencies.[24]

In addition to areas with particular problems there is the continually changing nature of nursing work. Although the ratios have stabilized a deteriorating situation, the underlying pressures that precipitated the call for ratios in the first place have continued. This was an issue noted in the qualitative interviews undertaken in the lead up to finalizing the 2003 survey instrument. Nurses in focus groups and one-on-one interviews that were conducted to refine the questionnaire noted that these continuing changes often overwhelmed or partly offset the positive impact of the ratios. Two nurses spoke for many when they observed that "Management sees more nurses as a means for more jobs to be allocated to them."

The major changes affecting nurses have been in their working environment (reported by 68% of relevant respondents), the intensity of their work (49%), and the nature of the nursing workforce (27%). We realize that these categories are not mutually exclusive. We devised them on the basis of what nurses reported.[25] The most widespread changes have been in the operating environment, with 43 percent reporting increasing workflows and work demands such as extra paper work or computer use (noted by 24%) and increased patient throughput (12%). Typical comments about changes in the operating environment were as follows:

- "An increase in high dependency residents has dramatically increased the workload as has a change to improve care plans . . . paperwork has gone mad."
- "Hospital has no HDU [High Dependency Unit] so ICU [Intensive Care Unit] discharges straight out to wards and HDU ratio not applied, only normal 1:4 or 1:8 ratio given. Very stressful."
- "[In the past patients sent to rehab were ready for it]. Patients coming to re-habilitation now are usually complex medical problems and not ready for rehab. Patients are often sent back to acute hospital day of admission or soon after."
- "Combined midwifery ward with Acute Surgical. Dreadful situation!!!! For all concerned!"
- "Patients are in for less time, but still require same amount of care."

Just under half (49%) of nurses reporting change noted issues associated with work intensification. Just over a quarter (26%) noted it had fallen, and one in five (20%) said that it had risen. Of the 4 percent who reported it was the same, the overwhelming majority reported that this did not represent sta-sis but rather that gains in terms of declining work intensification were offset by increased activities that increased workloads. Typical comments about work intensification included:

- "As acting-in-charge, I have no patient load, therefore more time to 'manage' WD for shift."
- "Allocated three cubicles now, not 4–5 cubicles in 2000. Easier to get breaks as staff available to cover. More job satisfaction as able to care for patients fully, not just the 'urgent must-do' tasks."
- "The most recent change has been the nurse-patient ratio, and it has improved nursing care and the morale in my area of nursing has in-creased. The hospital tries hard to maintain the ratios. I can keep up a little more with ongoing education, which improves nursing practice and quality patient care."
- "Not responsible for total patient care—assembly-line mentality introduced—faster patient turnover—more patients through unit daily—sick leave is not replaced."

Over one in four (27%) reported that there had been a change in the nurs-ing workforce. The single biggest change concerned negative changes in skill mix, that is, 12 percent reported that while the number of staff per patient may have been stable or risen, the depth of skill in any one ward at any partic-ular time was less. Typical comments about this issue included:

- "The employment of division 2s [enrolled nurses] in place of division 1s [registered nurses] has added to the workload."
- "Difficulty fulfilling ratios, therefore less experienced staff rostered. Stress increases when supervising these staff and also having to constantly worry where the staff for the next shift will be found."
- "Loss of senior experienced staff plus increase in junior, less-experienced staff equals an inadequate mix for the complexity and acuity of care required, and increases stress on all staff."
- "We have not been able to fill the extra positions with experienced staff."

The 2006 study confirmed that mandated ratios have worked to help stabilize the workload challenges nurses face but that the system still confronts a number of complex problems—patient demand, continuing technological change, nurse labor supply, appropriate skill mix, and financial cost cutting.[26] Of those who had been in the same job between 2003 and 2006 most reported that their workloads had increased. The three most commonly reported causes of workload increase were: increased administrative tasks (noted by 90% of respondents), patient turnover (noted by 76%), and rising levels of patient acuity (noted by 70%). If ratios are to remain relevant, they will need to be regularly adjusted in light of the changed circumstances in which they operate.

The Need to Regularly Recalibrate the Ratios

The ratios, emerging as they did from an enterprise agreement negotiation, have been altered from the form the union originally intended and for which it continually advocated, particularly in the 2004 enterprise bargaining round. Despite this difficult context and the compromises that were made in negotiations, the ratios have made a significant difference to many bedside nurses, managers, and even directors of nursing. At the time of this writing in early 2006, their implementation has been widespread and flexible. They do not operate as a universal straitjacket tying up the system. They are enforced by the people responsible for day-to-day patient care—nurse unit managers and nurses. The most tangible results have been more time for patient care, more effective management of stress, and better documentation for patients.

The union organized their 2004 bargaining claim around extension of the ratios. Management, in contrast, wished to abolish them and have a patient dependency system introduced. The outcome of these negotiations was that the ratios would be maintained as settled in 2001, but they would not be augmented in the light of changed workplace conditions. Preliminary results from a third evaluation of the impact of ratios conducted in 2006 indicate that while ratios are good, they are not good enough. The ratios require what might be best described as a recalibration.

In noting the need to regularly recalibrate the ratios our research also shows that this will probably require continued industrial action by nurses or intervention by third parties such as industrial tribunals. This is because of the practice of managers applying the ratios inflexibly. They do this not because they necessarily wish to be inflexible. Rather, their hands are tied. Tight budgetary controls often mean they have little discretion on the matter of staffing levels other than to cut them. This creates a major challenge for the maintenance of sustainable staff levels. The demands on nurses (and others involved in the health system) continue to rise because of the demands created by an aging population and the introduction of new medical technologies. Changes such as these mean that the acuity level of patients rises continually. The only way service levels can be maintained in this environment is if the ratios for particular types of work are regularly recalibrated in the light of changing circumstances. This was the key finding of the 2006 evaluation of the ratios in action. The future success of the ratios will turn on whether an effective mechanism for their regular recalibration is devised.

Until now in Victoria, contract negotiations between the nurses' union and the state government have provided a de facto recalibration mechanism. Although in 2004 that mechanism failed, it succeeded in fall 2007 when the union and government negotiated the latest Enterprise Bargaining Agreement. Nurses wanted to improve the ratios. The Victorian Labor government wanted to replace them and hold wages down. On October 25, 2007, a new four-year agreement was reached between the Victorian Branch of the ANF and the Victorian Hospitals Industrial Association. It provided for wage rises of between 3.6 and 6 percent per year and improvements in a range of employment conditions.[27] The most important was preserving, and in some case up-grading, the nurse-to-patient ratios. Under the agreements, five hundred new nurses will be added to the system. According to Lisa Fitzpatrick, the majority of these new nurses will go to effectively eliminating the 50 percent rule on the morning and afternoon shifts of the 184 units to which the rule has applied. This will improve care on units that abused the 50 percent rule, particularly in targeted areas such as geriatric care, palliative care, rehabilitation, and some medical and surgical units. Two hundred of the new positions will be allocated to increasing the number of nurses per patient in emergency departments and post- and antenatal areas. In emergency departments, nurses will be added to triage and resuscitation. In post- and antenatal areas the ratios will be improved to 1:4 on morning and afternoon shifts and 1:6 on night shifts. Two country hospitals will also have improved staffing.

This settlement was only achieved, however, after nine days of intense industrial action. This occurred after months of negotiations failed to result in any agreement. In the lead-up to the dispute, employers would offer only 3.25 percent per year for wage increase with anything extra requiring "productivity offsets." Employers also sought more "flexibility" in staffing arrangements. When the old agreement expired in late September 2007 nurses decided to hold unauthorized stop-work meetings where thousands of nurses met to endorse work bans, the temporary closure of 900 beds and the cancellation of 1,000 elective surgeries.[28] All action taken was illegal and exposed the union and its members to significant fines and legal sanctions. This was because in 2006 new labor laws—known as *Work Choices*—were passed by a Federal conservative government that had recently been reelected in the lower house and unexpectedly gained control of the upper house. These laws radically reduced unions' bargaining rights and the capacity of industrial tribunals to settle industrial disputes.[29] In essence *Work Choices* consolidated employer power by buttressing managerial prerogatives. This was achieved by a variety of means, the most important of which was requiring all agreements to be enterprise based, banning pattern bargaining and confining industrial tribunals arbitration power to very limited circumstances on a very narrow range of issues. *Work Choices* made industrywide agreements almost impossible and prevented industrial tribunals dealing with staffing matters. Innovations such as nurse-to-patient ratios that operate on a multiemployer basis and limit managerial discretion are essentially illegal and can prevail only if management agrees to their operation site by site. The only way the ratios could have been saved in this context was by illegal direct action.

The union's success can be attributed to three factors. First, members of the ANF were absolutely resolute in their support and extremely well organized. The venue hired to hold the mass stop-work meeting to endorse industrial action could not accommodate the more than 4,000 members who attended. The motion proposing action was endorsed unanimously. The bed closures and cancellations of elective surgery began the next day. This support reflected nurses' growing frustration with wages and workloads that had been documented in the latest study of the ratios in action.[30] The union had been informing members for months about the slow progress in negotiations. When the call for action came, the entire membership knew what was at stake.

The second factor underpinning the union's success was the widespread support enjoyed by those nurses both within the health system and the community at large. On the day the bans were announced the Australian Medical Association (the professional association representing doctors) publicly backed the nurses on both the wage and ratio issues. All segments of the media reported the dispute in a manner sympathetic to the nurses. Melbourne's most popular daily tabloid, Rupert Murdoch's *Herald Sun*, even wrote an editorial in support. While not supporting industrial action, it noted nurses were underpaid and overworked and called for rapid settlement of their reasonable claims.

The third, and probably most decisive, factor behind the nurses' victory was the political context of the dispute. The mass meeting endorsing industrial action occurred two days after the 2007 federal election date was announced. Arguably the key issue of this election was the conservative federal government's highly controversial *Work Choices* industrial laws. These laws had generated significant concern in the community. The federal government and state opposition opportunistically exploited the dispute. They called on the state labor government to give the nurses what they claimed and urged hospital employers to turn a blind eye to the *Work Choices* antiunion, antiindustrial labor law regime.[31] At the same time, federal government agencies reportedly behind the scenes sent inspectors out to ensure the law was being followed.[32] As the dispute reached its ninth day, pressure grew on the state labor government to settle. A prolonged dispute in the middle of an election campaign was not good for labor federally. The dispute was finally ended with direct intervention by the premier, John Brumby.

The legacy of the dispute was the creation of a new generation of nurses committed to the ratios, a strengthening of the union, and the unsettling of workplace industrial relations. Over 1,900 new members joined the Victorian Branch of the ANF in September and October 2007. Over members 2,000 lodged complaints with the union about management intimidation and harassment that occurred during the dispute. The docking of pay, active threats to impose fines for industrial action, and threats to dismiss nurses who spoke to the press poisoned relations at several hospitals.[33] These actions ensured this was a dispute with a lasting impact. Throughout it all, nurses had continued to provide core services to the public. Management tactics were all legal. Relations at work, however, require more than adherence to the strict letter of law. Ironically, the nurses won a major victory by actively breaking central elements of federal labor law. Management found itself isolated, both within the health system and the broader community, by playing within the rules. In this way the dispute highlighted fundamental problems within the *Work Choices* federal labor law regime as well as fundamental problems concerning wages and work overload in the public health system.

Ratios: The only answer?

When reaching conclusions about the operation and impact of the ratios it is worth reflecting on a quasi-natural test concerning their impact on recruitment and retention levels. The two largest populated states in Australia are Victoria and New South Wales. They share a border along the Murray River. According to ANF organizers and workplace representatives hospitals on the Victoria side of river have less difficulty finding staff than those in NSW. This conclusion needs, however, to be augmented by two additional pieces of information. First, most hospitals are on the Victoria side of the border. Second, the best place to make a direct comparison is the largest human settlement on the river—the twin cities of Albury and Wodonga (located side by side). Locals argue that the hospital in Wodonga (located on the Victorian side of the border and hence covered by ratios) has less difficulties overall, in recruiting and holding staff, when compared with the Albury hospital. According to union sources ratios have contributed to this outcome—but they are not the sole cause. Differences between the management approaches taken by local hospitals also contribute to this outcome. The example of this quasi-natural experiment captures nicely our key findings about the operation and impact of the ratios to date.

Like the comparison between Albury and Wodonga, any assessment of the impact of ratios must take account of the context in which they have been implemented. The introduction of the ratios has not been the only change in the Victoria public health system in recent times. Nurses must contend with more paperwork, rising levels of patient acuity, and new computer technology. Most important, the national nurse shortage also continues to profoundly influence the public health system in Victoria. Insufficient staffing levels across the system continue to be the system's greatest challenge. Ratios close off the easy management "solution" of work intensification from shift to shift. On their own, however, they cannot neutralize the negative consequences of many other changes affecting nurses, nor can they end the nursing shortage. Nonetheless, they have been a crucial advance. Even the Victoria government that still opposes them recently acknowledged in a press release that since the Labor government took office in 1999, over seventy-six hundred nurses have come back into the workforce.[34] What is very clear from both the quantitative and qualitative work on ratios is that the Victoria public-hospital system would have been far worse without them. As such, the evidence points to the following simple proposition: Although ratios are not the sole answer to work intensification (and its negative implications for recruitment and retention), there can be no solution to the current nursing crisis without them.

PART III

Arguments and Alternatives

9

What We Know about Nurse Staffing

When Governor Gray Davis received a barrage of letters urging him to veto AB 394, almost all the hospital administrators who wrote him argued that no scientific research had systematically evaluated the appropriate ratio of nurses that should be utilized on hospital wards. In Australia, the Victorian Branch of the Australian Nursing Federation believes the appropriate ratio of nurses to patients on medical/surgical units is 1:4. The California Nurses Association argued that a more appropriate ratio would be 1:3 registered nurses to patients. The California Hospital Association insisted that patients would be perfectly safe with staffing at 1:10 and that either RNs or LVNs could fill the ratios. The state of California ultimately settled on a phased-in 1:5 ratio, and Victoria implemented 5:20 ratios on its medical/surgical floors in 2001. But how do we know whether the minimum number of nurses that guarantees safety on medical/surgical floors is 1:3, 1:4, 1:5, 1:10, or for that matter 1:100?

The fact is, we don't. No studies have established the correct "therapeutic dose" of nursing care that should be administered on particular units. Industrialized countries have the most assiduously researched system of care known to humankind, yet the dose of human labor that patients need to survive high-tech medical treatments in hospitals and other health facilities remains a matter of intense debate in some fields and of little or no debate in others. Do we, for example, know how many patients an internist can safely see in one day? Do we know how many operations—on eyes, knees, hearts, or hands—a surgeon can safely perform? We know it's best to go to a surgeon who has performed a particular operation numerous times. We don't know how many times that surgeon should safely perform that operation in one day or one week.

Nursing is thus at the forefront of a discussion that should probably be held in many fields in health care. What research underpins the idea that nurse staffing affects patient care and that there is a quantitative relationship between nurse staffing and quality patient care?

As of this writing, we have analyzed over sixty articles and studies that consider the relationship of nurse staffing to patient care. By the time this book appears in print, more studies will have appeared, and many more will follow. Many of these studies were prompted by the comments in the 1996 Institute of Medicine report that found a "serious paucity of recent research on the definitive aspects of structural measures, such as specific staffing ratios, on the quality of patient care in terms of patient outcomes when controlling for all other likely explanatory or confounding variables."[1]

It has not been easy for researchers to rectify this problem. Isolating the contribution of nursing care to patient outcomes and quality of care is complicated by the fact that, as Sean Clarke has elegantly elaborated, so many complex phenomena influence patient care.[2] Research must overcome structural differences among hospitals (hospital teaching status, technology, unit layout, and size). Researchers lack standard tools to assess patient acuity and have limited access to unit-level outcome data. Unit-level data allows researchers to adjust for severity of disease if, for example, the patient is in the ICU versus an acute medical/surgical unit. Without controlling for confounding patient and hospital characteristics, the effect of nurse-staffing levels may be over- or underestimated. Researchers designing studies must also take into consideration factors such as the proportion of RNs among licensed nursing staff, support-staff levels, experience, nurse specialization, and education.

In addition to patient outcomes, studies also need to focus on the impact of workload on nurses' health. Indeed, some studies have found an association between high nurse-to-patient ratios and burnout, stress, absenteeism, musculoskeletal injuries, and poor job satisfaction among nurses. Nonetheless, for a variety of complex reasons that will be elaborated below, over ten years later research has still not been able to identify the ideal ratio of patients for every nurse necessary to provide optimal care. Research has, however, shown a clear link between nursing care and patient outcomes and health care costs. Research also connects staffing to nurses' health.

The following review of the literature discusses the effects that have been found between nurse-staffing levels and patient outcomes, including mortality, failure to rescue, morbidity, and other complications. In most studies, mortality is typically measured by whether or not the patient died while in the hospital whereas some studies use a measure of thirty-day mortality, following the patient for thirty days after hospital admission. Failure to rescue is defined as death following an adverse occurrence or, as Jeffrey Silber and his collaborators elaborate, a hospital's inability to prevent death following an adverse occurrence.[3] An adverse occurrence is a complication that occurs after a patient is admitted to the hospital.[4] Silber goes on to explain that "because only adverse occurrences can become failures, and because the quality of care may affect the number of adverse occurrences, one cannot fully understand a hospital's failure rate without also examining its adverse occurrence rate and its death rate."[5] Researchers have found links between the following outcomes and nurse staffing: mortality,[6] failure to rescue,[7] pneumonia,[8] pulmonary compromise,[9] pressure ulcers (bedsores), urinary tract infections,[10] falls,[11] medication errors,[12] patient complaints,[13] thrombosis,[14] sepsis, shock or cardiac arrest,[15] and upper gastrointestinal bleeding.[16] Nurse staffing is also correlated with patient length of hospital stay. Studies have shown that many dimensions of nurse staffing have an impact on quality of care, as well as the cost of patient care.

Role of Nurse Staffing on Patient Mortality, Failure to Rescue, and Adverse Outcomes

Before the IOM report in 1995, Jeffrey H. Silber and his research team at the University of Pennsylvania School of Medicine sought to determine whether certain patient outcomes could be predicted by differences in hospital characteristics.[17] They studied three patient outcomes (death, adverse occurrences, and failure to rescue) in a sample of 73,174 patient admissions in 1990 and 1991 at 137 hospitals. After adjusting for patient acuity, the authors found that hospitals with a high ratio of registered nurses per bed had lower death and failure-to-rescue rates. Silber notes that a limitation of the mortality measure employed is that deaths of patients who died soon after leaving the hospital were not counted.

In a follow-up study in 2000, Silber and his associates examined outcomes for general surgery and orthopedic procedures in elderly patients between 1991 and 1994 in 245 Pennsylvania hospitals.[18] They reviewed Medicare claims data for 217,440 procedures and again found that a higher RN-to-bed ratio was associated with reduced death and failure to rescue rates within thirty days of hospital admission.

In a widely publicized 2002 study, Linda Aiken and her colleagues, including Jeffrey Silber, analyzed data from surveys of 10,814 staff registered nurses and the outcomes for 232,342 general, orthopedic, and vascular surgery patients from 168 hospitals in Pennsylvania.[19] The researchers found that "each additional patient per nurse was associated with a 7% increase in the likelihood of dying within 30 days of admission and a 7% increase in the odds of failure-to-rescue."[20] The study considered patient and hospital characteristics, including size, teaching status, and level of technology. The results imply that if a nurse goes from having four patients to six patients, the odds of dying are increased by 14 percent. Their findings suggest that 2.3 more people would die per 1,000 patients and 8.7 more deaths would occur per 1,000 patients with complications if a nurse had to care for six patients instead of four. If the nurse's caseload is increased from four to eight patients, the study found that the increased chance of mortality is 31 percent (1.07 to the fourth power). While the findings are staggering, the authors did not directly recommend an ideal minimum ratio.

The study of the impact of nurse staffing on quality of care, and specifically adverse outcomes, is not new. Motivated by the ongoing restructuring of health care as well as the ongoing shortage of RNs, Christine Kovner and Peter Gergen used data from 1993 to conduct research on the impact of nurse staffing on adverse events among postsurgical patients in 506 acute care hospitals in the United States.[21] Controlling for hospital characteristics, they found a large inverse relationship between full-time equivalent RNs per adjusted patient day and urinary tract infections and pneumonia for patients who had undergone major surgery. They also found a significant but weaker association between RNs per adjusted patient day and the development of thrombosis and pulmonary compromise.

In a follow-up study, Kovner, Gergen, and other researchers again looked at quality indicators developed by the Healthcare Cost and Utilization Project (HCUP) that are sensitive to nursing care.[22] They studied outcome data from 1990 to 1996 and sought to improve on the adjustment for severity of illness among postsurgical patients in 530–570 hospitals in the United States. Again, analysis showed an inverse relationship between RN hours per adjusted patient day and pneumonia for routine as well as emergency patient admissions. A similar, though not statistically significant, relationship was found for other postoperative adverse events. Like other studies, this study confirms a relationship between nurse-staffing levels and adverse events. However, it does not address questions about the optimal level of nurse staffing for high-quality, cost-effective patient care.

In 2002, Jack Needleman, Peter Buerhaus, and their colleagues reported that they found no association between mortality and increased RN-staffing levels, but they did find associations among RN staffing and several other important patient outcomes.[23] Notably, the study did find a similar inverse relationship related to staffing by licensed practical nurses, which the authors found consistent with recent research. The study assessed quality of care in hospitals by examining administrative discharge data from 799 hospitals in eleven states of almost 6.2 million medical and surgical patients.[24] They found that for medical patients, a higher rate of hours of care provided by RNs and a greater number of hours provided by RNs each day were associated with a shorter length of stay and lower rates of urinary tract infections and upper gastrointestinal bleeding. When RNs provided a higher proportion of care patients had lower rates of pneumonia, shock, or cardiac arrest, and failure to rescue. Among surgical patients, more RN care was associated with lower rates of urinary tract infections, and a greater number of hours of care by RNs each day was associated with lower rates of failure to rescue.

In 2003, Sung-Hyun Cho et al. studied the impact of nurse-staffing levels on adverse events, morbidity, mortality, and medical costs among surgical patients who were in medical/surgical units (acute and intensive care) and coronary care units.[25] The study included 232 acute-care California hospitals and 124,204 patients. The effect of nurse staffing was analyzed three ways: total hours provided by licensed nursing personnel per patient day, total hours provided by registered nurses per patient day, and the proportion (or skill mix of) care provided by RNs (RN hours divided by hours worked by all licensed nursing personnel). The researchers examined patient falls/injuries, pressure ulcers (bedsores), adverse drug events, pneumonia, urinary tract infections, wound infections, and sepsis to determine whether nurse staffing had an effect on these adverse occurrences. They found that "an increase of 1 RN hour (hour worked by registered nurses per patient day) was associated with a decrease of 8.9% in the odds of pneumonia." The study also found that a 10 percent increase in the proportion of RNs providing nursing care was associated with a 9.5 percent decrease in the odds of pneumonia. Patients in the study who developed pneumonia, wound infection, or sepsis had a greater chance of dying during their hospital stay.

When considering pneumonia, the authors suggest that adequate RN-staffing levels would allow registered nurses to provide attentive lung care and adhere to standards of care that would in turn help prevent pneumonia. They advise that RN staffing would have more of an impact on the prevention of pneumonia than overall nursing care, because of the expertise required. This study only included adverse events that were not present when the surgical patient entered the hospital. Although the study had low rates of adverse events as a result, it enabled researchers to control for factors that were not attributable to nurse staffing.

Cho and her colleagues reported one surprising, although not unique, finding: as the overall number of hours of nursing care increased, the number of bedsores reported also increased. This challenges the claim that appropriate levels of nurse staffing contribute to the reduction and prevention of pressure ulcers. In 1998, Blegen, Goode, and Reed's study also found the same increase in pressure ulcers with higher nurse staffing.[26] Cho and colleagues noted that adverse events were associated with longer hospital stays and increased costs of medical care. For example, they found that developing pneumonia was "associated with an increase of 5.1–5.4 days" in the hospital, 4.67–5.55% in the probability of death, and $22,390–$28,505 in costs."

Cho suggests that the data may not allow them to adequately control for acuity at the unit and patient levels. The authors recommend further research that considers possible explanatory factors such as "immobility, malnutrition, operating time, and conditions on the operating table to isolate the effects of nurse staffing on pressure ulcers from those of patient risk factors." The authors do not disregard the finding and hypothesize that perhaps adequate nurse staffing may simply "enable nurses to assess the skin for bedsores more regularly and therefore detect them more often."[27]

This finding may also have to do with the fact that, as Joanne Spetz explained earlier, RNs may not be the most important personnel to influence bedsore prevention. If increases in RN staffing mean decreases in nursing assistants and basic physical care, then patients may, in fact, suffer more bedsores, not fewer.

In 1998, Blegen, Goode, and Reed studied the relationship between nurse staffing and adverse outcomes in forty-two inpatient care units.[28] They found that a higher proportion of RNs among the nursing skill mix was related to lower rates of medication errors, pressure ulcers, and patient complaints. The study also found that the total hours of nursing care from all nursing personnel were associated directly with pressure ulcers, patient complaints, and mortality. As mentioned above, they found an unanticipated increase in the number of bedsores reported as the number of nursing hours increased. Additionally, they found that the relationship between nurse staffing and adverse outcomes was not entirely linear. When the ratio of RNs in the skill mix of nursing personnel hit 87.5 percent, the rates of complications did not continue to decrease.

Blegen and Vaughn were concerned about the impact of replacing nursing staff with unlicensed assistive personnel as a result of hospital restructuring during the 1990s.[29] As the proportion of RNs on a hospital unit increased from 50 percent to 85 percent, medication errors decreased. Above 85 percent, the errors did not continue to decrease, suggesting a nonlinear relationship between nurse staffing and patient outcomes as seen previously. There also were fewer patient falls with an increased proportion of RNs. In a study published in 2004, Thomas A. Lange and four researchers reviewed several studies to see if peer-reviewed research supported "specific, minimum nurse-patient ratios for acute care hospitals and whether nurse staffing is associated with patient, nurse employee, or hospital outcomes." They found that "richer nurse staffing is associated with lower failure-to-rescue rates, lower inpatient mortality rates, and shorter hospital stays." They did not, however, find any support in the literature for a specific minimum nurse-to-patient ratio. This finding is hardly a surprise, since no random controlled studies have, to our knowledge, ever assessed different ratios of nurses to patients on similar units.[30]

In 2006, a multivariate study by Bruce E. Landon and his colleagues that was reported in the *Archives of Internal Medicine* addresses why, in spite of the fact that quality of care in hospitals is of essence when dealing with acute medical conditions such as acute myocardial infarctions, congestive heart failure, and pneumonia, data measuring the quality of care have been limited.[31] In January 2004, the Joint Commission on Accreditation of Healthcare Organizations (JCAHO) required hospitals it accredited to begin reporting monthly on various performance measures covering a handful of disease conditions. At the same time, the Medicare Modernization Act of 2003 began requiring hospitals to report ten performance measures relating to congestive heart failure, acute myocardial infarctions, and pneumonia to the Centers for Medicare and Medicaid Services (CMS). The CMS chose performance measures that would overlap with the ones reported to JCAHO and to indicate whether or not hospitals are carrying out recommended standards of care for each disease condition. Hospitals reported on process measures that ranged from diagnosis and treatment to prevention and counseling activities.

By linking newly collected information from the JCAHO and CMS for 3,627 hospitals, Landon and colleagues were able to measure and predict the quality of care. They were also able to control for hospital characteristics collected by the American Hospital Association in its National Hospital Panel Survey.

The analysis distinguishes among individual measures of quality indicators for each of the conditions. For example, the eight measures for acute myocardial infarctions included giving the patient aspirin within twenty-four hours after arrival at the hospital and prescribing aspirin at discharge. The four measures for congestive heart failure included providing the patient with detailed instructions regarding activity level, diet, medications, follow-up appointments, weight monitoring, and actions when the condition worsened. The five measures for pneumonia covered areas such as blood oxygenation assessment within twenty-four hours after arrival at the hospital and providing an initial dose of antibiotics within four hours of arrival.

In addition to these indicators of care by condition, two other aspects of quality were explored. These were treatment and diagnosis and counseling and prevention. For the purposes of this book, we focus on findings related to care provided by registered nurses versus licensed practical nurses. A higher proportion of nursing care provided by RNs is related to higher quality care for all three conditions. The study also found that hospitals with a higher level of LPN hours per patient day were associated with lower performance scores. These findings were true for the treatment and diagnosis as well as counseling and prevention. Overall, the findings show that good quality of care is more likely to occur in hospitals that invest in technology, that are nonprofit, and where the nursing staff has a high proportion of registered nurses. Although not noted by the authors, the need for highly trained nurses is likely to increase as more advanced technology is being used.

The majority of nurse-staffing research has focused on patient outcomes or adverse events. In the Landon study the researchers focused on the processes that are critical to delivering quality care. By showing that higher RN staffing levels are associated with better performance, the study is able to suggest "processes" through which high-quality care is delivered. The authors emphasize the role of nurses as an intermediary between the physicians and the patients. Citing their own findings and those of others, they point out the need for a sufficient size of highly trained nursing staff. Unfortunately, the study design does not allow the researchers to identify cause and effect. At the same time, it is one of the few studies among a large national sample of hospitals that explores the impact of the level of training of nursing staff as a predictor of the quality of care.

Nurse-staffing studies are, of course, a moving target, with more published each year. As of this writing, another Canadian study established yet another statistical documentation of the connection between nurse staffing and patient outcomes. In this case, researchers who analyzed nurse staffing in Ontario hospitals found that "a 10% increase in the proportion of Registered Nurses was associated with six fewer deaths for every 1000 discharged patients. . . . A 10% increase of baccalaureate-prepared nurses was associated with nine fewer deaths for every 1000 discharged patients."[32]

Just as we were completing this manuscript, a meta-analysis by the U.S. government Agency for Healthcare Research and Quality once again articulated the connection between nurse staffing and quality patient care, concluding that "increased nurse staffing in hospitals was associated with lower hospital-related mortality, failure to rescue, and other patient outcomes."[33] Similarly, a 2007 study of hospital nurse staffing in England published in the *International Journal of Nursing Studies* found that "patients and nurses in the quartile of hospitals with the most favorable staffing levels (the lowest patient-to-nurse ratios) had consistently better outcomes than those in hospitals with less favorable staffing. Patients in the hospitals with the highest patient to nurse ratios had 26% higher mortality."[34]

Finally, at a conference on nursing leadership in Boston in June 2007, Linda Aiken spoke about preliminary results of the study we mentioned in chapter 4 that Aiken, Sean Clarke, and other researchers recently conducted. The study—an extension of the ongoing international research program that looks at the consequences of hospital nurses' working conditions—surveyed 35 percent of nurses in California and Pennsylvania and 50 percent of nurses in New Jersey. The study included California, in part, because its staffing legislation has made it the site of one of the biggest natural experiments in nurse staffing that has ever occurred. The study tried to understand the causal link between nursing staffing and patient outcomes, to test the interaction between nursing staffing and the nursing work environment on patient outcomes and to examine the impact of better staffing on nurse satisfaction and burn-out and recruitment and retention.

Aiken explained that early results from the California mandated ratios showed that staffing ratios appear to be systematically lower in California than in the other states. For example, in the emergency department, nurses reported that ratios averaged 6.6 on all shifts, while in New Jersey they were 8.5 and in Pennsylvania 8.6. On medical/surgical units, in California they were 4.9, while in New Jersey 6.8 and in Pennsylvania 6.6. Because they had already been in place, ICU ratios were better in California. The researchers also wanted to know if acuity was different in the different states, and they found that there was a negligible difference in acuity in all three. This finding is important because one fewer patient per nurse may not represent a lower workload if the California patients were sicker over all. But they were not.

Thirty-seven percent of the nurses surveyed in California reported that after the implementation of ratios, they had fewer patients on their assignments, 71 percent said quality of care had improved, 65 percent said their workload was reduced, 64 percent said retention had improved, and 60 percent believed that nurses outside California were more likely to come to their state.

When the researchers compared the three states, they found that more nurses in California said they could take at least 30 minute breaks, had a reasonable workload most days, and did not believe that workload pressures would lead them to take a new job. By and large nurses said their hospitals did not use vocational nurses to fill the ratios, but instead hired relief nurses for breaks, increased floating, use of supplemental staff.

At this conference, Aiken was careful to insist that she did not advocate ratios. She also pointed out that it was too early to assess patient outcomes. Nonetheless, the research findings were clear. Comparisons with other states show that patient loads were reduced in California and nurses there were more satisfied with their job conditions than nurses in either Pennsylvania or New Jersey-two states without any systematic regulation of hospital nurse staffing.

Although none of these studies points to a certain number of nurses—specifically registered nurses—needed on particular units, they all document that there is a clear relationship between nurse staffing and a variety of important patient-care outcomes such as failure to rescue and mortality.

Nurses' Health

Most of the discussion about staffing ratios concerns the connection between sufficient numbers of nurses and patient outcomes. But what about the impact of staffing on nurses' own health? For centuries, the religious framing of nursing created the expectation that nurses should—and would—sacrifice their own health and welfare for that of their patients. This assumption of relentless self-sacrifice grew out of the fact that in the West, nursing, as an organized institutional intervention, developed as an integral part of Christian penitential practice. Nurses were first religious men and women who received their reward for their good deeds and self-sacrifice in the next life. When nursing became secularized in the nineteenth century, this expectation of self-sacrifice persisted. Although few contemporary men and women wish to sacrifice their own health on the job, documented studies of adverse health consequences linked to working conditions in the hospital suggest that the early Christian definition of the nurse is applicable, particularly when the issue is work overload.

Studies have documented that nurses suffer more depression and more stress-related illnesses than many other workers. Researchers Joel Hillhouse and Christine Adler found that "nurses experience higher rates of mortality, suicide, stress-related disease, psychiatric admissions, and general physical illness than does the general population."[35] Work overload heads the list of factors that influence nurses' job stress. This job stress often comes with a Siamese twin, burnout, which can be understood as "a psychological process in which chronic job stressors are translated into outward affective and physical symptomatology."[36] Burnout has also been described as "a prolonged response to chronic emotional and interpersonal stressors on the job, and is defined by the three dimensions of exhaustion, cynicism, and inefficiency."[37] RNs may perform poorly on the job, report to work late or not at all, and even abuse drugs or alcohol. Their resulting cynicism and exhaustion may make nurses appear to be discourteous or even callous toward their patients.

A report by Linda Aiken and her colleagues in her by-now-famous study published in the *Journal of the American Medical Association* found that patient loads correlated with burnout and job dissatisfaction. Of the 10,184 staff nurses surveyed and who reported that they felt burned out and complained of job dissatisfaction, 43 percent said they would leave their current job (though not leave nursing altogether) within twelve months. Aiken and her colleagues compared this with nurses who say they are satisfied with their job and found that of the latter group only 11 percent said they planned to leave their position within twelve months.[38]

A study done in the United Kingdom established a connection between workload and emotional exhaustion and job satisfaction. The authors initiated the study because of "concern about the impact of restructuring of nurse staffing and the reports of nurse shortages and work overload on nurse and patient outcomes."[39] The authors found that increased workload led to serious problems for nurses in England and Scotland. These problems occurred not only when nurses had too many patients but when they were burdened with clerical and administrative activities that had also increased. "This analysis," the authors wrote, "showed a highly statistically significant relationship between staffing and emotional exhaustion. . . . In the UK analysis, the odds ratios for burnout increased from 0.57 to 0.67 to 0.80 to 1.00 as the number of patients a nurse was responsible for increased from 0–4 to 5–8 to 9–12 to 13 or greater."[40] A 2007 study by Anne Marie Rafferty also found a connection between staffing and job satisfaction and burnout. The study found that nurses in hospitals with the highest patient-to-nurse ratios were approximately twice as likely to be dissatisfied with their jobs than nurses surveyed in hospitals with better patient-to-nurse ratios. These nurses also had high burnout levels.[41]

Studies have linked workload not only to burnout but also to problems that have a direct impact on both nurses' health and patient safety. This is because, as researchers have documented, working both longer and harder means that many nurses report getting less sleep than they need, being extremely tired at work, and even falling asleep on the job. This lack of sleep can create more errors and also have an impact on nurses' mood on the job.[42] Nurses also have a high risk for substance abuse, greater use of pain medication, and absenteeism.[43]

Nurses who carry too heavy a workload are also at greater risk for the kind of needlestick injuries that can have catastrophic—indeed lethal—consequences if they contract blood-borne illnesses such as hepatitis B and C and HIV/AIDS. Even if a nurse does not get a blood-borne illness she or he may be at risk from the side effects of prophylactic treatment. Whenever health-care professionals get a needlestick injury, they are prescribed a course of preventive medication that is as toxic as it is expensive. Either way, the nurse becomes a patient, which, in turn, may lead to absenteeism due to illness, worker's compensation and disability costs, and huge costs as the nurse deals with her own chronic, life-threatening illness.

Studies have clearly established that hospital staffing and organizational climate correlate with needlestick injuries. A 2002 study analyzed retrospective data from 732 nurses and prospective data (describing incidents as they happened) from 960 nurses on needlestick injuries and near misses on forty units in twenty hospitals. When a nurse worked on a unit with poor staffing ratios and a poor organizational climate, he or she was twice as likely to get a needlestick injury than a nurse who was well supported on a well-staffed unit. Since the article revealed that only one in four needlestick injuries is actually reported to hospital officials, the results of this study are sobering indeed.[44] This study took place before hospitals introduced protective equipment—safety-engineered needles, in the jargon—that makes it harder to get injured. Using 1998 data in another article, the investigators found that nurses were still getting stuck and that staffing and work climate made a difference. "Poor organizational climate and high workloads were associated with 50% to twofold increases in the likelihood of needlestick injuries and near misses to hospital nurses." Although safe-needle technology reduced the risk, the authors concluded that "nurse staffing and organizational climate are key determinants of needlestick risk and must be considered with the adoption of safety equipment to effectively reduce sharps [sharp-object] injuries."[45]

Finally, nurse staffing also exacerbates the epidemic of musculoskeletal injuries (MSDs) from which nurses have too long suffered. Nursing is hard physical labor, labor that produces more MSDs than those produced by construction work and even baggage handling, to cite only two examples. Alison Trinkoff, Jane Lipscomb, Jeanne Geiger-Brown, and Barbara Brady have spent years studying nurses' occupational health problems. They report that "for work-related musculoskeletal disorders in private industry, registered nurses ranked sixth overall with 12,400 reported injuries requiring a median of 5 days lost from work. Among all non-fatal occupational injuries, nursing and personal care facilities ranked second and hospitals ranked sixth." These nurses were also more likely to see a physician or other health care provider and to take medications to alleviate their pain and other symptoms: "In 1999, the rate of injuries in nursing and personal care facilities ranked second (incidence rate 13.8/100 workers), and the rate in hospitals was sixth among all industries (8.4/100 workers). Low back pain/injury is the most frequent MSD." This particular study reports that nurses also suffer from neck and shoulder injuries and that these "may contribute to nurse turnover. In a survey of over 43,000 nurses in five countries, 17 percent to 39 percent reported that they planned to leave their job in the next year due to the physical and psychological demands of the profession."[46]

It is ironic that health-care systems obsessed with cutting costs by cutting nursing care actually produce more people in need of medical attention. One of the University of Maryland studies documents that

> half of all MSD cases saw a provider for their problem. These nurses were often absent from work—which means they used sick leave or personal days that were, hopefully, paid for by their employer, thus wasting resources that could have been used to care for the sick or develop nurses themselves. They took a number of medications like non-steroidal anti-inflammatories, narcotic analgesics and muscle relaxants. Six percent of nurses with neck injuries, eight percent of those with shoulder injuries, and 11 percent with back injuries changed their jobs.[47]

When these researchers looked at the relationship between MSDs and workload, they found a distinct correlation. The harder nurses had to work, the more injuries they got. "As perceived level of demands increase, so did the odds of reported MSD. The associations were stronger among staff nurses, perhaps reflecting the high proportion of direct patient-care activities in staff nursing jobs."

In other words, if nurses have to work with eight rather than four patients, they will have to turn and lift twice as many patients, putting themselves at greater risk for back, neck, and shoulder injuries. Studies have similarly documented that nurses are at greater risk for substance abuse and stress-related illnesses because of the demands of their work. In a study published in 2006 in the *American Journal of Industrial Medicine*, the same University of Maryland researchers found a relationship between long hours and back, neck, and shoulder injuries. The demands of increased cost efficiencies, the researchers report, have resulted in reduced staffing and longer hours. "As a result, job demands and unhealthy scheduling practices such as overtime have been increasing." So have extended work schedules, like the twelve-hour day. Hospitals in the United States prefer to pay nurses overtime rather than pay the extra salary and benefits for hiring more staff. Sometimes nurses are forced to work what is known as mandatory overtime—an extra shift on top of the eight- or twelve-hour one they just finished. Or they may work voluntary overtime—a phenomenon that is not quite as voluntary as it looks when one considers that nurses' wages stagnated during the restructuring of the 1990s. When you combine the fact that most nurses in the United States are not only working harder—that is, with more patients—and longer, you have the perfect recipe for more injuries, which is precisely what these researchers discovered. Staffing ratios that decrease the patient load, quite literally shouldered during the workday, coupled with reductions in work schedule will reduce such injuries.[48]

As occupational health researchers point out, losing 6 to 11 percent of nurses from the hospital because of preventable injuries hardly makes sense when there is a nursing shortage of huge magnitude. In an era when healthcare systems are trying to cut costs, it certainly doesn't make sense to turn the nurses, who are hired to help care for patients, into patients themselves. Finally, it is certainly indefensible to ask nurses to sacrifice their own health to do a job that should enhance, not compromise, theirs.

Costs of Ratios

Although no specific number of nurses can be prescribed from the studies cited above, there is certainly an impressive body of literature that connects increased nurse staffing to improved outcomes for patients as well as better health, less burnout, and greater job satisfaction for nurses. Obviously, job satisfaction and burnout are linked to quality patient outcomes. If we know nurses are essential to quality patient care, anything that jeopardizes nurses' desire to stay in hospitals has an impact on nurse retention and recruitment. This, in turn, means patients will have a harder time accessing nursing care simply because not enough people will want to work in hospitals and other direct-care settings. Yet, even if people finally acknowledge the critical importance of nurses to patient care, some argue that ratios or additional nursing staff is simply too expensive.

When considering the wisdom of additional staffing on hospital units, it's thus crucial to analyze what we also know about their cost-effectiveness.

In 2006, Jack Needleman, Peter Buerhaus, and their colleagues used their 2002 data to ask whether there is a "business case" for increasing nurse staffing.[49] When the authors focused on the estimated cost savings/increase associated with deaths prevented as a result of nurse staffing increases they considered three hypothetical scenarios. In the first scenario, the ratio of RNs to licensed nursing personnel was increased to the seventy-fifth percentile of hospitals studied without changing licensed hours; in other words, hospitals using both LPNs and RNs did not increase staff (either RN or LPN, as in ratios) but simply increased the proportion of registered nurses and used fewer licensed practical nurses. In the second scenario, the number of hours nurses put in at work was increased to the seventy-fifth percentile without changing the ratio of RNs. In the third scenario, more RNs were added to the mix and RNs and LPNs also worked more hours.

The authors assert that there is an "unequivocal business case" for hospitals to increase the skill mix, or the ratio of RNs to licensed nursing personnel, as in scenario one. Whereas LPNs may be as effective in observing and treating patients, RNs are much better prepared to assess patients and to intervene. The second and third options produced positive outcomes that were, however, more costly. The authors note that society and hospitals will have to decide what value they place on patient safety and quality of care in order to determine if nurse-staffing levels should be increased. The authors recognize that their estimates ignore significant cost factors due to the focus on mortality, thereby ignoring aspects related to morbidity, patient satisfaction, hospital liability, and reduced turnover among nursing staff. By failing to consider ratios and only considering hours, the study could lead managers to ask nurses to work longer hours, which, in turn, would ignore the data coming out of both nursing and medicine that indicate significant increases in error if nurses and doctors work longer hours.

Another article on the cost-effectiveness of nurse-staffing ratios published in the journal *Medical Care* was written by three physicians and a nurse-researcher. Michael Rothberg and his team conducted a cost analysis of patient-to-nurse ratios while distinguishing between labor costs solely, labor costs and decreased length of patient stay at the hospital, and total costs related to the ratio, including higher nurse wages.[50] To do their study, researchers compared patient-to-nurse ratios ranging from 8:1 to 4:1.

In making their analysis, the investigators reviewed literature that shows how much money nurses save the system by preventing complications. For example, according to one study, when nurses saved patients from pneumonia, they saved the system a complication that "added 5.1–5.4 days to length of stay and $22,390–$28,505 to hospital costs or $4,225 to $5,279 per additional day." Or when nurses prevent an adverse drug event, according to another study, they saved patients from events that "added 2.2 hospital days at a cost of $3,344 ($1,520 per day)." When they prevent complications after surgery, they potentially prevent stays "8.1 day longer and costs $10,700 higher than patients without ($1,321/day)."

When they ran the numbers, the researchers found that as the ratio of patients to nurse went down, mortality also went down but costs went up: "We can prevent additional hospital deaths at a labor cost of $64,000 per life saved by decreasing the average PTN ratio from 7:1 to 6:1. Including all hospital costs, even if implementing lower ratios requires an increase in nursing wages, decreasing the PTN ratio from 5 to 4 would save additional lives at a cost of $136,000 per life saved."[51] According to the authors' calculations, increasing the number of nurses so that 4:1 ratios would be filled would not increase hospitalization costs by more than a few percentage points. More important, other measures that are routinely taken to save lives in hospitals—thrombolytic therapy in acute myocardial infarction and routine cervical cancer screening with PAP tests—cost more than decreasing the patient-to-nurse ratio from five to four. Theomobolytic therapy costs $182,000 per life saved, while PAP tests cost $432,000 per life saved.

The authors conclude that this expenditure is cost effective. And they leave us with several important questions: Where are the voices of American doctors when it comes to this patient safety issue? How can hospitals routinely deliver measures like those discussed above and refuse to deliver safe nursing care?

> Considered as a patient safety intervention, improved nurse staffing has a cost-effectiveness that falls comfortably within the range of other widely accepted interventions. If a hospital decided, for economic reasons, not to provide thrombolytic therapy in acute myocardial infarction, physicians would likely refuse to admit to that hospital, and patients would fear to go there. Physicians, hospital administrators and the public must now begin to see safe nurse staffing levels in the same light as other patient safety measures.[52]

In the United States the potential impact of safer nurse-to-patient ratios has just become far more relevant as the Centers for Medicare and Medicaid

Services announced new reimbursement policies that will be implemented in October 2008. If patients in hospitals suffer from any of eight different medical errors or injuries, hospitals will not be paid for the cost of the patient's care due to that error or injury. The eight categories include: objects left in patients during surgery; air embolism; blood incompatibility; catheter-associated urinary tract infection; pressure ulcer; vascular catheter–associated infections; falls; and mediastinitis, an infection of the mediastinus following coronary artery bypass graft surgery.[53]

According to the studies mentioned above there is a significant correlation between nurse staffing and the prevention of many of the complications Medicare is trying to prevent. Following the implementation of these rules, the costs of decreased nurse staffing may significantly outweigh any short-term financial benefits.

A Real Research Agenda

There is no doubt from the literature on nurse staffing that there is indeed safety in numbers and that higher nurse-to-patient ratios have a positive impact on quality of care. There does not seem to be any dispute about this matter. What is in dispute is the actual ratio—that elusive perfect number—of patients to nurses and its impact on both patients' and nurses' health. Although they would require effort, studies that would solve the ratio riddle could be conducted. Sean Clarke notes the difficulties in assessing the link between staffing and patient outcomes using conventional methods. Tools that are currently used to measure staffing, he explains, "obliterate differences across the nurses, the units and shifts where they were assigned."[54] According to Clarke, nurses of differing experience and educational levels are equated with one another. Patients too are flattened out, incorporated into patient-days so that patients with diverse needs are all rendered equal.[55] To capture enough data with enough sophistication will require the kind of intense effort that is now routinely devoted to delivering high-quality medical treatments. If hospital associations believe that patient care is not compromised with 1:10 ratios, they can prove it in their very own hospitals by asking serious workforce researchers to study the link between 1:10 staffing ratios and patient outcomes. Sean Clarke points out that such a study probably wouldn't pass any hospital's institutional review board. This is because randomly allocating patients to such a low standard of nursing staffing, the one the California Hospital Association promoted, could be considered unethical.

If hospitals insist that 1:4 or 1:3 or 1:5 is an absurd, unscientific nurse-to-patient ratio, then they can prove their case by giving researchers access to hospital units and assigning 1:3, 1:4, or 1:5 ratios and analyzing the outcomes on a variety of parameters. If nurses argue that these lower ratios will reduce stress and musculoskeletal injuries, this is also measurable. Research studies should also consider nurses' opinions about the kinds of workloads they can handle. If surveys of nurses on medical/surgical units, for example, reveal that most nurses insist that they can only safely care for four patients, their estimates of a safe workload should be incorporated into staffing research. Studies should also consider the impact of ratios on nurses' health. If it is proved that a 1:4 ratio only marginally enhances patient safety but significantly improves nurses' health, that should be factored into workforce allocations.

In the United States and Australia and other developed nations, both brainpower and funding should be made available to support this effort. What is lacking is the political and social will.

In Victoria, the government has not funded a single study to assess the connection between nurse-to-patient ratios and patient outcomes or nurses' health. Lisa Fitzpatrick, state secretary of the Victorian Branch of the ANF, believes that this is because the government simply doesn't want to document that connection because it would legitimate nurses' refusal to accept patient acuity systems.

In the United States, nurse workforce researcher Sean Clarke has explained some of the reasons researchers have not produced the scientific data needed to ascertain the appropriate nurse-to-patient ratios. It is not only because the variables outlined above are far more complex than those involved in evaluating the appropriate dose of a pharmaceutical medication. It is also because workforce researchers as well as hospitals simply don't study it. As Clarke bluntly states:

> Whereas intense research activity in medicine is devoted to developing and testing interventions for use at the front lines of patient-care delivery, comparatively little attention in nursing research is devoted to direct bedside care. Even though front-line illness care is the type of work most nurses are engaged in, academic nursing has all but turned away from studying it. Much research in nursing examines aspects of health not normally handled by the bedside generalist nurse.[56]

Another problem is that hospitals have little incentive to help in this research effort because they have little incentive to invest in nursing care. Hospitals have few incentives to invest in nursing staff, and to improve patient safety and health care quality. They are reimbursed for the nursing care provided in their institutions through patient bed-and-board charges. In other words, they are paid the same whether their medical/surgical nurse-to-patient ratios are 1:4 or 1:10. There are no incentives or even expectations built into the payment system—either through public or private payers—that encourage an optimal number of nurses or even safe care. How will such incentives materialize without effective government regulation that protects health-care workers as well as the public?

10

Arguments against and
Alternatives to Ratios

In its almost twelve-year journey through the Massachusetts legislature, the minimum nurse-to-patient staffing-ratio bill has attracted numerous opponents, of which the most powerful and prominent is the Massachusetts Hospital Association. In the spring of 2006, the MHA ran several quarter-page ads in the *Boston Globe*. One was captioned "Bad Rx for Health Care." It featured two women gazing down at a patient. In front was a trim, short-haired woman in a white coat with a stethoscope around her neck. She was, presumably, a doctor. Standing behind her was a blond, heavyset woman in a dark uniform covered by a peculiar apronlike apparatus. She too had a stethoscope draped around her neck. Presumably she was a nurse. Underneath this picture was the following commentary:

> You live in Massachusetts. You expect world-class health care. Our hospitals deliver it every day.
>
> When you go to the hospital, you trust your nurse to lead a specialized team assembled to meet your unique needs, 24/7.
>
> That is what Massachusetts hospitals and nurse leaders strive to achieve: the right care for every patient. Because of it, our hospitals have an international reputation for excellence.
>
> But now our world-class health care system is threatened by a union that represents only 1-in-5 registered nurses in the Commonwealth. They want to micromanage care in our hospitals by using government mandated nurse ratios. It's the wrong approach.

The ad claimed that ratios will "wreak havoc":

> Look what happened in California. . . . Emergency room diversions are up. Nurses' salaries are up. Nurse shortages are severe. But patient care has not improved.
>
> Bureaucrats micromanaging your care? That's bad medicine.

198

In a few short lines, we find most of the arguments against staffing ratios. Ratios will create health-care chaos. Emergency rooms will close as will entire hospitals. Hospitals now deliver individualized care, designed specifically to meet the unique needs of each patient. The blunt instrument of ratios (as they are often called) will produce an inflexible, one-size-fits-all system of nursing care delivery. Government bureaucrats will prevent nurse managers and directors of nursing from providing more nursing care to patients who desperately need it. Ratios will also cost more and even raise nurses' salaries. In spite of their high costs, they will not improve patient care.

Adding to these arguments critics contend that implementing a minimum level of nursing care on hospital units will deprofessionalize nursing. If the unions that sponsor ratio bills win, adversarial relationships will replace the more professional or familylike relationships that now, some critics suggest, prevail in hospitals. Besides, given the nursing shortage, where will hospitals find enough nurses to fill ratios, should they be mandated?

Arguments against Ratios

A one-size-fits-all system will replace individualized nursing care

Patients in hospitals are all different. Although they may have the same disease, no two patients will respond to it in precisely the same way. That's why, if possible, those making patient assignments should not only consider nurses' qualifications but should consider the emotional rapport between nurse and patient. To assure quality care, continuity of care is also essential. High-quality nursing care thus depends on institutional flexibility in staffing matters. How much flexibility do managers and nurses have without ratios? Do ratios eliminate or increase flexibility?

In the 1990s, before ratios were passed in Victoria and California, managers had considerable flexibility when making patient assignments. No government regulations intruded on their managerial prerogatives. In most hospitals throughout the industrialized world that kind of flexibility is still the norm. With unlimited flexibility, many nursing managers seem to have continuously cut, not added, nursing staff on their units. Hospitals that are adding more staff voluntarily are only doing so because nurses have complained so vociferously about hospital short staffing. One can conclude from both scientific and anecdotal data that this "flexible" system of unregulated nurse staffing has not produced much flexibility in staffing. It has not produced a system that delivers "the right care for every patient" but rather one that delivers the right head count for every cost-cutting budget.

Indeed, the kind of individualized patient care the Massachusetts Hospital Association referred to in its antiratio ad has been a casualty—to the extent that it has ever existed—of the cost-cutting work overload described in this book. In most hospitals, shortened length of stay, the difficulties of nurse scheduling, and increased patient throughput have made it very difficult to individualize patient care.

Under even the best of circumstances, it is difficult to individualize patient care. Because nurses are scheduled weeks in advance (in Australia, nurses receive their shift assignments six weeks in advance), it has always been difficult to predict which patient will be on a particular unit at which time so that the nurse who is uniquely suited to meet that patient's needs is on duty during the patient's hospital admission. Today, when scheduling, managers usually hope for the best—that nurses will not be sick, have a sick child or relative, or take a personal day, and that they will show up for work.

Continuity of care is a crucial part of individualizing care. Today, however, continuity of care is often sacrificed to another new phenomenon—shifts of twelve or more hours, as well as the shortened length of hospital stay. As more nurses work three shifts of twelve hours or more per week, fewer can stick with a patient for more than a day. Similarly, if patients are moved from unit to unit, hospital to rehabilitation facility, or to home more quickly, there will be less individual attention because the nurses caring for the patient will have less opportunity to get to know and understand their physical responses and emotional concerns. These barriers to flexibility—a product of cost cutting, restructuring, and other strategies deployed to make the hospital more efficient in purely business terms—are now built in to many contemporary hospital systems.

Staffing ratios did not create this problem. Indeed, they may help to temper it by giving nurses more time to individualize care. Staffing ratios, it must be remembered, do not establish maximum nurse-to-patient ratios but, rather, minimums below which hospitals cannot staff their units. AB 394 specifically mandates that hospitals add more staff if patient acuity system data suggests patients needs more care. Legislation proposed in Massachusetts and other states includes implementation of a system that requires hospitals to provide more nurses if a patient needs more care. The 50 percent rule in Victoria does not prohibit managers from adding more nurses if needed.

In their attacks on ratios, many opponents imply that staff nurses, unions, or government regulators will try to prevent patients from getting more nursing care. It is hard to imagine staff nurses balking if they were assigned a less arduous patient load or government regulators storming into a hospital to penalize a manager who assigned fewer patients per nurse. The history of the implementation of ratios in both Australia and California indicates that precisely the opposite is true. We have heard managers in California complain that their nurses get complacent when they have three or fewer patients or adamantly argue that no hospital will staff above ratios, even though the law mandates them to do so under certain circumstances. In Australia the debate has not been about the lack of nurses to fill ratios but about managers' refusal to add more staff when the 50 percent rule comes into play.

Concerns about flexibility can be addressed by considering the more flexible Australian model of staffing ratios that do not put into place 1:4 ratios but five nurses to twenty patients. This model allows for more flexibility in the assignment of staff. It does not, however, allow any flexibility in the overburdening of nurses with extra patients. Those considering staffing ratios would do well to consider the pros and cons of the Victoria versus the California model.

Finally, when considering the wisdom of statutory minimums, it's useful to consider the history of statutory minimum wages. When minimum wage laws were proposed in the United States, employers insisted such wages would drive them out of business and drive all wages down. No one who deserved it would be able to earn more than the minimum wage, critics intoned. The passage of minimum wage legislation has not hampered business profitability and has not pushed all wages down but has, in fact, helped to drive some wages up. Just as workers with more skill and education argue for wages and benefits that are far above minimum wages, so too, patients whose acuity and illness demand more nursing care hours should get it.

Ratios cannot help provide high-quality patient care because nurses' skill and education levels are not stipulated

Ratio legislation or regulations do not stipulate the precise skill mix, that is, educational qualifications, years of experience, or certifications that nurses must have to fill them. To many critics this reproduces a long-standing problem that has plagued the profession: the idea that there are no useful distinctions to be made between one nurse and another. This is often referred to as the "a nurse is a nurse is a nurse," problem. As a former chief nurse in Australia put it, "Ratios are insulting. They're saying any warm body in a storm."

In California, state regulations require that nurses be hired on the basis of their proven competency to do a particular job. If they are not qualified, they must be appropriately trained before they can undertake their duties. Unfortunately, hospitals often violate this regulation when they hire agency nurses or when they float nurses from units on which they have gained expertise to units where they have little experience. Hospitals can't easily check up on these nurses; they rely on agencies to do appropriate educational and background checks. Agency nurses or traveling nurses may not have the kinds of experience and qualifications as do veteran nurses whom the hospital has both trained and observed on the job. In Victoria, the ANF asked the government to more precisely specify the education and experience of nurses on units—one-third graduates, one-third experienced nurses, one-third division 2 nurses—and the government refused to do so.

With the laws or regulations lacking any language about a nurse's qualifications, management judgment and moral responsibility come into play. If nurse managers want their units and patients to be safe, then it is their professional and moral obligation to fill the ratios with the appropriate mix of experienced nurses, nurses who are certified in the technology and techniques of the unit (say, in giving chemotherapy on a cancer floor), novice nurses, new grads, and LVNs. They may also consider a growing literature exploring the relationship between nursing education and quality care, in which some researchers argue that nurses with baccalaureate of science in nursing degrees provide safer care than two-year associate degree (or enrolled) nurses or LPNs.[1]

The data on RN education is complex. What is clear is that nurses, no matter what their educational level, are complaining about patient loads; nurses with two-year degrees are not complaining twice as much as those who have a bachelor's in nursing. The point is that no nurse—not even an advanced-practice super nurse—can provide safe care if he or she is responsible for too many patients. Education may help when it comes to patient safety, but education cannot vanquish serious systemic problems.

It is also worth noting that no ratio bill prevents managers from staffing units with the appropriate mix of newly graduated nurses, veteran nurses, nurses with higher educational qualifications, or nurses who are certified in different fields. As we have seen, some hospitals, like Western Health in Victoria, have used the ratio bill as a rationale for encouraging nurses to gain more specialty training and have created programs to mentor not only new graduates but undergraduate nursing students who might be candidates for recruitment.

Nurse-to-patient ratios deprofessionalize nursing

Nurse executives, educators, and some nurse workforce researchers, among others, believe that a legislatively or legally mandated system will deprofessionalize nursing. Government bureaucrats, opponents argue, will make decisions about patient care that should be left to the professional judgment of nurse unit managers, directors of nursing, or staff nurses themselves. Nurses certainly deserve to be respected as professionals and treated in a professional manner. The question is: Do ratios deprofessionalize nursing or does deprofessionalization result from the kind of policies that produced the push for ratios?

One of the major problems that has long plagued nursing is that staff nurses lack authority over their work and control over patient-care decisions as well as decisions about the institutional organization of care and nursing practice. As Linda Aiken so aptly points out, nursing is an organized institutional intervention. Unfortunately, the nurses who deliver that intervention often have the least to say about how it is organized.

Many commentators on ratios, like James Buchan, have pointed out that the ratio solution has arisen because nurses no longer trust their managers to provide them with the conditions of professional employment. As various forms of cost cutting are implemented, nurses are subjected to conditions that few professionals would tolerate. How many oncologists, for example, would agree to be floated onto a nephrology service? How many corporate lawyers would pinch hit for a colleague in divorce court? Similarly, how many stockbrokers, or tenured professors, or physicians would tolerate arriving at work only to be told that they should go home and take a vacation day because there aren't enough students in class, patients in the waiting room, or clients looking at the ticker tape? It is assumed that a professional has some thinking to do, planning to undertake, or team building to engage in if they do not have a class to teach, a patient to examine, or a sell order to place. Nurses, on the other hand, are conceptualized, as one nurse manager commented, as "electric blankets"—if a patient is not in the bed, the nurse is not needed on the unit, so send her home and save some money on the electricity bill.

What is interesting is that the "professionalizers" who fear ratios and government micromanagment instead promote a different kind deprofessionalization, giving control over nurses' work to computerized patient acuity systems (and their corporate creators), which, as we have seen, do not work to give nurses greater control but often further deprive them of control over their work.

If the deprofessionalization of nursing were caused by ratios, it would be a far easier problem to solve. The deprofessionalization of nursing is not created by ratios. Whether at the bidding of insurance companies, hospital chief executive officers, expensive health care consultants, or government bureaucrats, the attempt to replace nurses with lower-level health-care workers seems to be a constant today. So are the technological tools that are supposed to measure nursing work and give nurses more control over it while actually Taylorizing, routinizing, and taking all individual judgment out of it.

The final straw in the deprofessionalizing dynamic is workload, which can turn even the most accomplished expert into the equivalent of a novice at the bedside. This kind of deprofessionalization has, tragically, been implemented by nursing administrators and managers who have found it difficult, if not impossible, to protect bedside nurses—and patients—from the cost-cutter's axe or physicians who choose to take money from the nursing budget to enhance the profile of medicine. In debates about the nursing budget, as researcher Joanne Spetz has commented, when a manager comes up against a physician who wants to purchase a new technological gizmo and tries to poach money from the nursing budget, the nurse executive who complains almost invariably loses.

Nurse managers fear they will be deprofessionalized because traditional management prerogatives will be taken out of their hands. Again, it is ironic that this charge is associated with ratios. Over the past decade, cost cutting has led to deprofessionalization and overwork among nurse managers. The ranks of nurse managers, at least in the United States, have been decimated by hospital restructuring and cost cutting. Managers have been laid off in droves. Like bedside nurses, those managers remaining have seen workloads skyrocket as they are assigned to oversee multiple units.[2]

Their relations with the nurses they supervise have become more strained as they are asked to implement the plans of management consultants whose schemes have led to much of the chaos we see today. In our view, ratios would make their lives easier, not harder. That is, in fact, why many managers in Australia—and some, albeit silently, in California—support ratios. For that reason, we advocate expansion of ratios to managerial work in ways that would limit nurse managers' workloads and allow them to serve as clinical leaders rather than bed shufflers or budget allocators.

*Nurses are divided about ratios, which would
exacerbate these divisions and create an intolerable
work environment*

In a recent article in the *Times*, a web-based publication from Illinois, the headline of a posting proclaimed in bold letters "Nurses Oppose New Bill to Mandate Staffing." The article detailed why "nurses" have lined up against an Illinois bill on staffing ratios. Interviews with "nurses" in the article suggested a unanimity of opinion against the ratios, which, these "nurses" contend would immeasurably hamper the ability of hospitals to deliver quality patient care in the state.

When one looks closely at the article, one discovers that the only nurses interviewed for the article are in fact not the bedside nurses whom the ratios would directly affect but management nurses who, as we have said before, at least in the United States, almost always oppose ratios or any other government mandates. Nurses interviewed for the article included one director of nursing, an assistant director of nursing, and an assistant director of nursing in a community college. The author then cited opposition by five directors of nursing. The only reference to staff nurses appeared when one of the directors of nursing said that she'd talked to a nurse from California who, she related, felt the ratios were a disaster. The reporter never tracked down that nurse. The directors of nursing quoted in the story also related the same stories about California hospital closures that the California Superior Court debunked in its 2005 decision.[3]

This depiction of staffing ratios as a catfight within nursing ignores a salient fact. Debates about ratios within nursing are usually conflicts between staff nurses many of whom are represented by unions and representatives of hospital management. This point is worth emphasizing. Although they may have RN licenses, believe that they have the best interests of the profession at heart, and consider themselves to be leaders of the profession as a whole, nurse executives are primarily employed as members of the highest level of the executive team in a hospital. As Gordon documented in *Nursing against the Odds*, some nurse executives may feel powerless to affect critical hospital decisions that relate to the nursing budget and nursing practice.[4] Nonetheless, they are hired to represent the hospital hierarchy and to manage the nursing workforce. Part of their job is to implement the priorities and policies of the hospital.

Without in any way meaning to dismiss the importance or motives of nurse executives or frontline nurse managers, it is simply a statement of fact to point out that they are paid to carry out institutional policies and insure institutional survival. Nurse executives, as many now admit today, were the ones who implemented and oversaw the hospital restructuring that helped to create and perpetuate the current nursing shortage. As Spetz has written, no matter what their personal beliefs about ratios, they are often encouraged to testify against ratios in legislative hearings or to speak out against them in public forums. Similarly, some nurse managers have confided to Gordon that no matter what their personal feelings about ratios, hospital chief executive officers often make such testimony a condition of employment. They also make it clear to nurse managers that their job is to dissuade staff nurses from evincing support for ratios and encourage staff to reach out to legislators to oppose them.

Hospital managers may counter that unions also pressure their members to support ratios. This is undoubtedly true. The kind of pressure a union can bring to bear on a member, particularly in the United States, however, bears no relationship to the kind of pressure a hospital employer can exert over those that he or she can hire and fire. For example, as one clinical nurse at the Massachusetts General Hospital in Boston explained:

> When the staffing-ratio issue was hot in 2006, they sent out information about how staffing ratios wouldn't be a good idea. Their rationale was that nurses wouldn't control nursing practice, which of course we have never done, and that there was a shortage, which is because of crappy staffing. Managers would come

on the floors and say, "Now make sure you call your legislator to tell them that you don't support ratios." There was a big antiratio march and they also came around and reminded people to go.

This nurse said that if you weren't clear about the ratios, and didn't have any exposure to an alternative point of view, the constant pressure could definitely prove influential. The message was pretty clear: if you openly show your support for the antiratio position, management will be quite pleased.

Nursing ratios will create adversarial relationships in the workplace

In its *Boston Globe* ad the Massachusetts Hospital Association criticizes ratios because they have been put forth "by a union that represents only 1-in-5 registered nurses in the Commonwealth." According to the MHA this unrepresentative group is "threatening" the health-care system of the entire state. Unions are also criticized because they are too wedded to conflict, in an era when, according to many management consultants, shared common interest is the order of the day in modern working life.

Are unions unrepresentative institutions? Certainly not in Australia, Japan, and other countries where ratios have either been enacted or are being debated. In Victoria, the ANF represents 75 percent of nurses in public-sector hospitals. In California, unions represent thousands of nurses in the state. Unions that fought for staffing ratios were clearly able to mobilize nonunion nurses as well as those in other unions. They obtained vast public support throughout their battles to pass and then implement AB 394.

The idea that unions fight for the narrow economic self-interest of their members is also commonly argued. Although some unions are narrowly self-interested, many have campaigned around a broad range of issues of concern to member and nonmembers alike and have played a leadership role in advancing the rights of workers as citizens. In the United States, a clever bumper sticker illustrates the point: "The Labor Movement: The Folks Who Brought You the Weekend." In many countries, including the United States and Australia, union nurses have been some of the only ones to blow the whistle on problems with patient care because they have protection against employer retaliation and sufficient numbers to make a difference. They have lobbied for solutions that have protected union members and the patients they care for.

The idea that unions are wedded to, and thus consistently create, destructive conflicts that are no longer needed in this era of labor-management cooperation in the hospital workplace ignores the reality of contemporary labor-management relations as well as the ways in which unions and their members cooperate with employers every day.

As the history of staffing ratios amply demonstrates, the days of conflict are not over in most workplaces. In all relationships, especially labor-management relationships, there are inherent tensions that result in periods of conflict. Cooperation and trust can be reestablished, as happened in Victoria, when both parties not only recognize that they both share mutual interests but that they have the ability to exercise power to improve working conditions as well as to enhance quality care and patient safety.

Nursing ratios will force hospitals to lay off ancillary staff

In a system that does not adequately fund hospital nursing or other hospital personnel, ratios can easily be misused. In order to fill ratios, hospitals may lay off other staff. This argues not for no ratios but for adequate funding for ratios as well as adequate funding for other hospital personnel who are just as critical to patient care as are nurses and doctors. Obviously, if a hospital hires more nurses and fires more housekeepers, the nurses' workload will either increase or the hospital will be filthy. Either way patients will suffer as will nurses' morale. The solution to this problem is adequate funding and perhaps even ratios for other hospital personnel. In the state of Victoria, ratios have not resulted in layoffs of ancillary staff because ratios were funded. In California, the Donaldson study found that some ancillary staff had been laid off, but this does not seem to be a major problem in most hospitals. If hospitals deal with staffing ratios by laying off ancillary staff this is obviously a serious problem that will need to be addressed.

Nurse-staffing ratios will force hospitals to close entirely or to close emergency rooms and curtail other services

As we've seen in the first section of this book, when the California Hospital Association and other critics argue against ratios, they contend that ratios have generated the closure of hospitals and of emergency room services. As the California Superior Court stated, this argument is erroneous. Alan Sager, of the Boston University School of Public Health, is one of the nation's foremost authorities on hospital closures. Sager explains that "it is simply inaccurate to blame hospital closings in California on the state's RN-staffing-ratio legislation and regulations."

For a variety of reasons, Sager explains, California hospitals were closing before the legislation went into effect, and they continue to do so to this day. California has a very low rate of spending on hospitals. In 2004, it ranked as the eleventh lowest in the nation in terms of spending and was 15 percent below the national per-person average. By the time the ratio bill passed, California hospitals were already in short supply. There were only 2.01 beds per 1,000 people in 2004, giving the state the sixth lowest hospital capacity in the nation—27 percent below the national rate of 2.75 per 1,000 people. Plus, California hospitals have had to contend with the high costs of earthquake proofing many of the older hospitals. As Sager explained:

> All of these problems antedated the passage of the RN staffing ratio legislation. The fact is that in comparison to national average levels of spending and care provision, hospital care in California appears to be underfinanced. To complicate matters further, no party—insurers, HMOs, state government, or the federal government—has been willing or able to take responsibility for identifying which hospitals, in which locations, are essential to protecting the health of the people of California. At the same time, there is nothing close to a functioning free market to identify and support needed hospitals. Since efficiency is never correlated with hospital closings, so this is not a case of the survival of the fittest.

Blaming problems in emergency rooms on the staffing legislation—which has become a staple of the argument against ratios—is equally suspect. In fact, emergency room closures, diversions, and long waits have been produced by the same phenomena that have led nurses to lobby for staffing regulations. As a 2006 report by the Institute of Medicine explains, emergency rooms all over the United States are having difficulty accommodating the patients lining up for their services. Rather than being a product of staffing ratios, the ER crisis is a product of the same forces that have pushed nurses to lobby for staffing ratios. As the IOM put it:

> Between 1993 and 2003, the population of the United States grew by 12 percent, hospital admissions increased by 13 percent, and ED visits rose by more than 2 million per year from 90.3 to 113.9 million—a 26 percent increase. Not only is ED volume increasing, but also patients coming to the ED are older and sicker, and require more complex and time-consuming workups and treatments. Moreover, during this same period the United States experienced a net loss of 703 hospitals, 198,000 hospital beds, and 425 hospital EDs, mainly in response to cost-cutting measures and lower reimbursement by managed care, Medicare, and other payers. By 2001, 60 percent of hospitals were operating at or over capacity.[5]

In the United States, there were about five thousand emergency rooms in 1999. Now there are roughly four thousand—a loss of one fifth of the ER capacity.[6]

Finally, an increase in the number of uninsured patients has added to the ER crisis. Lacking access to primary care, the uninsured use emergency rooms for both emergent and less urgent problems. The United States has added millions to the rolls of the uninsured each year for the past decade or more. In 2004, the last year for which government data were available, about 46 million, or 15.7 percent of the population, lacked health insurance in the United States. The number of uninsured rose 800,000 between 2003 and 2004 and has increased by 6 million since 2000.[7] In California 21 percent of the population—or over 6.3 million people—lacked health insurance at some point in 2001.[8] "In 2003–2004, California had the fifth-highest rate of lack of insurance coverage in the nation and a Medicaid program that is inadequately financed," Sager tersely commented.

Robert L. Wears, professor of emergency medicine at the University of Florida in Jacksonville, gives a picture of how these interconnected factors work on the front lines. During the 1990s, the same economically driven hospital restructuring and reengineering that produced the nursing crisis resulted in the closures or mergers of a number of hospitals. In Jacksonville, for example, two hospitals closed and two merged. When hospitals close, their ERs close with them.

If a stable or increasing number of sick people flow into fewer ERs, overcrowding inevitably leads to declining services. Add to this the fact that, as the nation ages, more of the sick people using ERs are older. "Seeing one hundred forty-year-olds is a lot less work than seeing one hundred seventy-year olds," Wears explained. "Elderly patients are more complex. They have more things wrong with them and require more tests and things done to them. They thus stay in the ER longer, contributing to overcrowding."

Then there is the problem of individuals who are poor and uninsured. "Because these people have no primary care they come to the ER sicker," Wears continued. "Because they have less resources to rely on, ER doctors and nurses tend to do more for them in the ER."

The third—and for the purposes of this discussion—most interesting factor in the ER crisis is hospital bed closures and nursing layoffs. When insurers and employers began the cycle of cost cutting in the 1990s, hospitals eliminated many beds and laid off nurses. This has produced a serious problem for the emergency room. If patients who come to the ER need to be admitted to the hospital, they need beds to lie in and—most important—nurses to take care of them. If hospitals have closed beds, patients will be held in the ER. Wears explained:

> The lack of staffed beds is what most people feel really tipped a precarious balance over into a crisis. In our ER, our treatment unit for the most seriously ill has actually twenty-two beds and four resuscitation bays, twenty-six treatment spaces. It wouldn't be unusual for us to have most or all filled with admitted patients and to have seven to ten patients stored in the hallway outside of the treatment area because all those spaces filled up.

All of this creates a crisis for patients, as well as doctors and nurses, and can add to the financial woes of a hospital. If more patients need charity care and burden the hospital with debt, a hospital in a precarious financial condition can sink while others may reduce services or deliver poorer services. One cannot blame these problems on nurse-staffing ratios, Wears adamantly insisted. For a financially strapped hospital, paying more for nursing may exacerbate a preexisting condition, but it won't cause that condition. Moreover, Wears added, this is happening in practically every ER in the country, and only a fraction of those emergency departments are in California.[9]

Given the problems of hospital nursing, many RNs who favor ratios believe that improved working conditions will help to alleviate the nursing shortage in ERs and on other floors of the hospital.

Similar claims are often made in critiques of staffing ratios in Australia. In a widely publicized article in the journal *Health Affairs*, "Minimum Nurse-to-Patient Ratios in Acute Care Hospitals in California," Janet M. Coffman, Jean Ann Seago, and Joanne Spetz also discussed staffing ratios in Victoria. They ended on a discussion of its failures:

> The experience of hospitals in Victoria, Australia, one of the few jurisdictions to implement minimum-nurse-to-patient ratios in hospitals, is instructive. Large numbers of nurses returned to the nursing profession after minimum ratios were established. However, hospitals continued to face a shortage of nurses, because there were not enough returning nurses to meet demand. Some hospitals have been forced to close hospital beds.[10]

Joanne Spetz continued to highlight the problems of the Victoria ratios in a 2004 article in the *Journal of Nursing Administration* (*JONA*). Spetz accurately described the history of the ratios and then went on to discuss the results:

> The ANF claims that the ratios and a corresponding recruitment drive conducted by the government brought 2,650 inactive nurses into the public health system. However, recent action by the union closed 1 in 4 hospital beds, canceled 1 in 4 elective surgeries, because the government sought to eliminate the fixed ratios in favor of a flexible system in its most recent union negotiations. A continuing shortage of nurses has made it difficult for the government to staff all available hospital units. Nonetheless, the union prevailed in the 2004 negotiations, and thus the fixed ratios will persist.[11]

There are several major problems with these assessments of the Victoria experience with the ratios. First, in her article Coffman and her coauthors seem to connect the shortage of nurses with the advent of ratios. This shortage of nurses is, however, a national phenomenon, not a product of ratios. Bed closures occur just as frequently in states without ratios—such as New South Wales—as they do in Victoria. In fact, the ratios in Victoria ensure that beds remain open and that quality staffing levels prevail.

Spetz's assessment of ratios confuses the closure of "one bed in four" due to a temporary period of upheaval with permanent bed closures due to ratios. The bed closures she mentions occurred only when nurses took industrial action to defend ratios when management attempted to remove the ratios in the 2004 round of collective bargaining. As soon as the negotiations were concluded and the ratios retained, nurses immediately lifted the bans on opening beds. The capacity of the public hospital system was restored to predispute levels.

Ratios are an unfunded mandate that forces unfair burdens on hospitals

Many nurse executives and hospital administrators in California complained that ratios were an unfair imposition because they represented an unfunded mandate. Where were they going to get the money to hire all these nurses if they could find them, they asked. This is a very serious concern.

In Australia, ratios were smoothly implemented because they were a funded mandate. In Japan, ratios are also funded, with government giving hospitals more money if they fulfill the ratio of one nurse to seven patients. In both cases, we are dealing with tax-supported, publicly funded national health systems in which hospitals have budgets and planning.

In the United States, there is no national or even state mechanism for funding hospital nursing. Funding nursing ratios is not, nevertheless, impossible. University of Pennsylvania nursing workforce researcher Sean Clarke suggests, for example, that it would be possible to estimate how many nurses would be necessary to fill ratios on a particular unit. At present, a committee at the Centers for Medicare and Medicaid Services meets to calculate the rates it pays certain doctors for certain services. With effort, the same could be done to calculate how much it would cost to fund nursing services if ratios were set for particular units. This cost could then be added to the cost per case. Nursing would no longer be an invisible part of the calculus, and third-party payers could make sure—just as they do for physician services—that the money allocated for those services goes to the person performing them.

"If you had a system through which you measured the nursing contribution you could get away from nickel and diming in terms of how low could you go in terms of the average number of minutes per patient that you pay for," Clarke said. Insurance companies and Medicare could insist that it would no longer tolerate a situation where "patients are looked after in hospitals in which it's physically impossible to provide the care they need because the staffing levels are too low. They could say they put their money where their mouth is and come up with adequate reimbursements that would explicitly target nursing care."

One of the lessons of the Victoria ratios is that they are far easier to implement in a country with a national health system in which hospital budgets are publicly funded. The obvious conclusion, one that is of particular interest to nurses and health policy planners in countries with national health systems, is that ratios are a useful component of any plan to recruit and retain more nurses and that their implementation in Victoria, not just the United States, should be used both as a model and analytical tool.

Nurse-patient ratios are too blunt an instrument to be effective

In discussing ratios, critics often complain that they are a blunt instrument used to solve a complex problem. James Buchan concludes his analysis of ratios, "Mandatory 'top down' nurse-patient ratios are a blunt instrument for achieving employer compliance."[12]

We couldn't agree more. Ratios are indeed a blunt instrument. They stipulate a minimum number of nurses on a unit. They don't say what kind of nurse should fill the ratios. They don't prescribe the skill mix. They don't address who will work best with whom. They aren't exquisitely tailored to the patient population. We believe, as we've said above, that they are designed to be a blunt blade that astute managers should sharpen in various ways.

To focus only on how they can be sharpened prevents us from understanding—making sense of—why nurses reached for this blunt tool in the first place. Joanne Spetz candidly commented that nursing ratios in California were not designed to address, and certainly not to reverse, the policies and practices of the 75 percent of hospitals or hospital shifts that were well staffed before ratios. Ratios were used, Spetz puts it candidly, to "kick the butts" of consistently poorly performing hospitals that were understaffed. Nurses had tried to make the ostensibly sharper tool of patient acuity systems work and had been stymied. After failing with the scalpel, they chose the blunt knife. Similarly in Australia, ratios were chosen as a very blunt but very potent tool to reverse the policies of a conservative government that had decimated nursing care in the state's hospitals.

As Buchan concludes in his assessment of staffing ratios, this blunt tool is used to replace "alternative voluntary (and often more sophisticated) methods of determining nurse staffing levels [that] have not been effectively managed or have been ignored by policy makers."[13]

Even if ratios are implemented, hospitals won't be able to find enough nurses to fill them

Here we are confronted by the typical chicken and her egg. Hospitals argue that they will not be able to fill ratios because there is a nursing shortage. Staff nurses argue that hospitals can't find nurses because heavy workloads drive RNs out of the hospital workplace. If hospitals do not overburden the nursing workforce, nurses won't leave hospital jobs; nurses who have left the workplace may return; and more new recruits will be attracted to hospital work and remain at the bedside over the long term.

The facts of the shortage speak for themselves. The nursing shortage is not an artifact of nature. It was created by policies that have for years led to cyclical shifts in demand that in turn create a kind of permanent instability in the nursing workforce. Nurses or future candidates for nursing look at the future and do not see a sustainable long-term career. The future either brings with it layoffs or work overload or both. This is created by a refusal to do long-term planning and financing for and of the nursing workforce. The tendency is, in fact, quite the opposite. When they need to cut costs, hospital administrators and government policymakers can't unbuild buildings or get a refund on the latest MRI machine. Nor can they safely attack physician reimbursement. So nurses and ancillary staff—whose work is poorly understood and often devalued—become the soft targets.

The key to ending the shortage is to address its root causes. Yes, it may take time to create a new crop of nurses, but then the issue is not whether or not to have ratios, but how to time their implementation and what to do to make sure there are enough students in the pipeline to produce new nurses. This means that we need to figure out which states, provinces, or countries are underinvesting in nursing education and remedy that problem—all the time remembering that investments in nursing education without changes in human resources policies and practices will only produce the kind of revolving door into and out of the hospital that we see today. Similarly, if investments in nursing education only produce nurses who do not want to work at the bedside at all, or for only a short period of time, they will not produce the kind of patient care we will need in the future.

With proper attention to changes in working conditions and attention to timing, we believe ratios can be helpful. In both the Victoria and California cases, timing was a critical factor. In Victoria, thousands of inactive nurses were brought back into the system and nursing was made more attractive to new recruits. In California, we can only surmise what would have happened had the hospital industry put as much time, money, and effort into recruiting new nurses—or appealing to inactive nurses to return to the system—as it did on financing lawsuits, lobbying politicians, and producing public relations material attacking the ratio law. Had the industry backed, as the Victorian government did, no-lift policies in hospitals, that would have also made an enormous difference to present and future nurses.

If industry hospitals put as much money into pay and benefits for their veteran nurses as they have into hiring travelers (nurses who travel from state to state and work in hospitals on a temporary basis) and agency nurses (in the year 2000, U.S. hospitals spent $7.2 billion on temps and travelers, some of whom earned up to $100 an hour),[14] they would become real magnets for nurses, and some of these temporary staff would actually be hired on a permanent basis. More nurses—and new recruits—might stay at the hospital bedside if hospitals addressed problems with patient lifting, hours, and patient load, for example, by adding more nurses than ratios stipulated when patient-care needs demanded such adjustments. To cite only one example, at New York Presbyterian Hospital the union won a safe-staffing clause in its contract and turnover dropped from 15.3 percent in 2000 to 10.3 percent in 2002.[15]

The question still remains: What if some hospitals—with sufficient applicants to choose from—can't attract enough nurses to fill the ratios? The answer is another question: Why can't they? Are there hospitals whose working conditions are simply incompatible with safe patient care? Since we believe that nurses are the engine of the hospital, if that were the case, then those hospitals would have to either change or close.

Alternatives to Ratios

The debate about the future of nursing has engendered countless committees, surveys, meetings, conferences, and proposals about how best to solve the global shortage of nurses and make nursing a satisfying career over the long term. Opponents of ratios insist that mandated staffing regulations are not part of the solution. So what is?

The Massachusetts Hospital Association's "Patients First" Campaign

The Massachusetts Hospital Association has put forward its solution to the crisis of nurse work overload in its Patients First campaign. "Patients First: Continuing the Commitment to Safe Care" asks hospital administrators to voluntarily sign a pledge. In it, they promise to provide "staffing that meets patient needs" with "a team of caregivers, managed by clinical leaders, to deliver care that meets the unique needs of the individual patient."

When a hospital administrator signs on to Patients First, he or she pledges that "my hospital will voluntarily make staffing plans available to patients and the public and will voluntarily submit an annual patient staffing plan to the state or to another entity with health care expertise. The plan will include information on care hours per patient day." Hospitals will also voluntarily commit to "promoting a safe and supportive working environment for all those who provide care and in which patient safety is the top priority."

Hospitals voluntarily commit to

> providing the public with the hospital performance measures they need to make informed decisions about their care. My hospital will commit to a common framework of measurement and reporting that is based on the national Hospital Quality Alliance and which includes a patient experience survey. My hospital also will commit to publicly reporting at least three common nurse-sensitive measures selected from the National Quality Forum list, including one which will be care hours per patient day. These measures will help advance patient safety while educating the public about the performance of hospitals.

Hospital administrators will also promise to deal with "the chronic problem of shortages of nurses and other caregiving professionals by building a plentiful and committed workforce through hospital-based initiatives and strategic partnerships."[16]

To help them make informed choices, patients and potential patients can access staffing plans that are posted on the Patients First website. This, the association claims, will help them easily access and understand what kind of staffing is available at a hospital to which they might be admitted. The association has also helped to craft and has lobbied for a bill sponsored by state senator Richard Moore that requires hospitals to develop staffing plans and post them with the state. If passed, the bill would financially penalize hospitals that do not prepare such annual staffing plans. There is, however, no penalty if hospitals do not adhere to those plans nor is there any standard established to which hospitals must adhere in creating their unit staffing. Patients are given no information that would help them judge the staffing that is now available nor would the law require that such information (for example, what constitutes a safe nurse-to-patient ratio) be posted should the legislation pass.

There are several problems with the MHA approach. First, who is to say that the staffing plans hospitals develop are safe? How will safety be judged? How can a patient or potential patient judge whether staffing of 1:12 is adequate for a particular unit? We may not have data that shows that 1:4 is the perfect number, but we do know that 1:12 is not. Do patients? Why won't the

MHA or the Moore bill require information that goes beyond raw numbers to help patients make their informed choices? What if hospitals don't adhere to their plans? Shouldn't they be penalized?

The most serious shortcoming of the MHA approach is the assumption that a self-correcting market can adequately guard patient safety and assure nurse retention and recruitment. If the patient—herein reincarnated as a rational consumer—has enough information about nurse staffing, the MHA assumes he or she can easily choose between hospital A and hospital B. If consumers reject hospitals with poor staffing, those hospitals will be forced to change their behavior in order to attract more consumers or they will simply fail.

Unfortunately, this approach ignores the reality of how patients make choices about hospital care. If patients go into a hospital for an elective admission or procedure, they do not usually choose a hospital, they choose a doctor. That doctor has admitting privileges or works on staff at that hospital and the patient follows the doctor into the hospital. Although most patients don't explicitly consider nursing care when they follow their doctor, most probably implicitly assume that the nursing care at this hospital is top notch. Why would their top-notch doctor choose it if it weren't? Unless the physician decides to stop admitting patients to hospital A because of poor nursing care, patients will continue to follow their physician to hospital A.

In the United States in today's world of private insurance and managed care, insurance providers add a new wrinkle to the choice calculation. Many HMOs and other insurance schemes limit a patient's choice of hospital. If, based on information like that provided on the MHA website, a patient decides he would prefer hospital Y to hospital X, his private insurer may disallow the admission. To ignore insurance dictates would mean paying out of pocket, something few can afford.

And, under this scheme, what happens to patients who have medical emergencies and simply have no time to research and choose their hospital? The reality is, whether one suffers an emergency or not, most patients are not rational choice makers. When they are sick, they go to the hospital their doctor advises or with whom their insurance company contracts. If they need emergency care, they go to the nearest hospital they can find.

Even if one agrees with the MHA approach, perusing the Patients First website is not an exercise in reassurance. The website promises patients easy-to–access-and-understand information about hospital's units and nurse staffing. When we scanned the Patient's First website, we found the data in table 2.

It is hard to understand how a layperson could make sense of this baffling array of "worked hours per patient day" without extensive explanations. Here we learn nothing about how many admissions and discharges a unit and an individual nurse have to contend with. The acuity of patients is invisible as is the

Table 2. Daily Staffing at One Hospital Unit by Shift

Shift	Direct Caregivers	Scheduled hours	Shift length	Mon.	Tues.	Wed.	Thurs.	Fri.	Sat.	Sun.
Day										
	RN	7 a.m.–3 p.m.	8	4	4	4	4	4	4	4
	Unlicensed assistive personnel	7 a.m.–3 p.m.	8	2	2	2	2	2	2	2
Evening										
	RN	3 p.m.–11 p.m.	8	3	3	3	3	3	3	3
	Unlicensed assistive personnel	3 p.m.–11 p.m.	8	1	1	1	1	1	1	1
Night										
	RN	11 p.m.–7 a.m.	8	2	2	2	2	2	2	2
	Unlicensed assistive personnel	11 p.m.–7 a.m.	8	1	1	1	1	1	1	1

Note: Data from fiscal year 2006. The average number of patients per day was 12.2. The Plan/Budgeted Direct WHPPD (worked hours per patient day) was 7.11.

Source: http://patientsfirstma.org/, accessed January 2, 2007.

actual staffing ratio shift by shift. Even if sick and frightened patients were rational choice makers who had the time to visit hospital websites and plan their hospital admissions based on the nursing care they would receive, could they make rational choices given this kind of information? We think not.

On a recent radio documentary on the nursing shortage that aired on Boston station WBUR, the chief executive officer, Alan D. Knight, and chief nursing officer, Carol A. Dilliplane, of Jordan Hospital, a 150-bed community hospital in Plymouth, Massachusetts, talked about their efforts to end a serious nursing shortage in their hospital.[17] Knight and Dilliplane touted their efforts to revamp their policies to make them more nurse friendly. They outlined changes in scheduling, greater educational opportunities, and giving nurses a greater voice in decision making. Although she works at a hospital that just attained Magnet status, Dilliplane acknowledged that without changing nurse staffing, none of these shifts would make much difference. "If we're still making nurses take care of eight patients, they're not doing nursing, they're just doing a bunch of tasks," she said. So the hospital has added 25 percent more nurses. We speculate that if nurses were taking care of eight patients at Jordan, this would effectively make the ratio 1:6, which was were California began on its ratio journey.

Although Dilliplane implicitly expressed support for such a ratio, she nonetheless staunchly opposed the mandated ratio bill in the Massachusetts legislature. "We in the hospital do not want to be mandated to have ratios. It's not ratios that people object to, it's mandating a specific ratio," she commented.

In other words, providing patients with what nursing and hospital leaders acknowledge to be the conditions of safe and effective nursing care should be voluntary, not mandatory, and could thus change on the whim of the hospital leadership. Jeanette Ives Erickson, senior vice president for patient care and chief nurse of Massachusetts General has been quite frank about the fact that hospitals just couldn't get rid of nurses fast enough in the 1990s. Now, she insists, hospitals have learned their lesson, this in spite of the fact that nurses in Massachusetts are still leaving hospitals in which they have to take care of eight or even nine patients. So what happens to the patient who isn't lucky enough to find himself or herself in a hospital with enlightened leadership and good staffing? Or what happens if hospital administrators change their tune and decide it's time to start firing nurses again? Should this be the patient's problem, not the society's?

The Hyperefficient Hospital

Another proposal that has been used to counter staffing ratios has come out of the prestigious nonprofit Institute for Healthcare Improvement whose headquarters is in Cambridge, Massachusetts. The IHI is the brainchild of patient-safety expert Dr. Donald Berwick. Berwick has launched a series of impressive initiatives to deal with the epidemic of medical errors and injuries in the United States. His suggestions have been taken up in other international health-care systems.

The IHI has also trained its sights on nursing care and, in partnership with the Robert Wood Johnson Foundation, has created a program called Transforming Care at the Bedside.[18] Inspired in part by insights gleaned from the car manufacturer Toyota, the IHI model promises to reduce complexity and waste. To do so, it has worked with thirteen U.S. hospitals. Some of the mechanisms used include bringing medications closer to the bedside so that nurses don't have to travel back and forth to central supply areas; encouraging nurses to come up with their own ways to improve the flow of work; posting the nurses' photograph in patients' rooms as well as writing the patient-care plan on a white board in the patient's room; and cutting down on paperwork. Participating hospitals also use special rapid response teams to deal with crises.

At one hospital, M. D. Anderson in Houston, the hospital created a "nurse tranquility project" by installing a recliner in a quiet space so nurses could take a quick break-time nap. The institute says hospitals that use this model have reduced turnover as well as error.[19]

To "nurture professional formation," nurses at Seton Northwest Hospital in Austin, Texas, developed a traffic light system to declare their availability for additional patient care. At four check-in times during each shift, front-line nurses indicate on a centrally located whiteboard their capacity to care for new admissions. This declaration is not based on available *beds*, but rather on available *care*. A green magnet shows they are able to take on new patients; yellow means they are nearing their capacity; and red means they cannot safely accept another patient.

Not only does this respect nurses' professional judgment, but nurses at Seton Northwest report that knowing which of their colleagues is working at full capacity at any given time enhances teamwork.[20]

This traffic light system is recommended for other hospitals.

A recent article in the *Wall Street Journal*, "Why Quota for Nurses Isn't Cure-All," hailed the model as a viable alternative to nurse-staffing ratios. "The intention of those advocating nurse-to-patient ratios is right—they want to make sure there is enough professional nursing care to intervene with their loved ones in the hospital," said Pat Rutherford, a nurse and vice president at the Institute for Healthcare Improvement. "The right solution is to get rid of the wasteful and unnecessary work nurses have to do so they have more time for patient care."[21]

As we explain when we address the Magnet hospital below, these initiatives do have the potential to help restructure care in more positive ways. In our view, they do not, however, adequately address the issue of nurse workload and the pervasive nature of the problems facing nurses. The nurses we have talked to have not mentioned that running for supplies or doing paperwork is their chief problem. Their problem is taking care of too many patients who are too sick and have too many complex needs. Similarly, installing "traffic light" systems that indicate that a nurse is maxed out does little to alter patient load or to assure nurses that they will not be subject to such intense work pressure. Nor does it allow physicians, patients, or hospitals to better plan care in advance so the red-light stage becomes a rare rather than a routine event. If the patient workload is not controlled, adjusting the amount of paperwork and figuring out how to locate supplies nearer to the bedside or putting up red, green, and yellow magnets will be nothing but window dressing that can, in fact, have unintended but pernicious consequences. Such initiatives convince legislators and policymakers that hospitals are "doing something" about their nursing problem when the fundamental nature of that problem remains unaddressed. For such experiments to succeed they should be seen as adjuncts to, not replacements for, staffing ratios or, as in the U.S. context, adjuncts to, not replacements for, more fundamental changes in the entire health-care system.

In the United States, one of the primary reasons that nurses are besieged by so much paperwork is the fragmentation of a health-care system in which there are more than fifteen hundred private insurance plans, each requiring their own labs for testing, their own complex forms to fill out, their own networks of nursing homes and rehab hospitals to which patients can be discharged, and their own requirements for home care (to mention only a few of the complexities such a fragmented system creates). Projects like that proposed by IHI, while certainly valuable, seem designed to work around these systemic obstacles to efficient and effective care rather than to address their root causes.

Magnet Hospitals

Perhaps the most popular solution to the perennial problems of nursing are what are known as Magnet hospitals. The Magnet movement began in the early 1980s when the United States was facing another of its periodic nursing shortages. The American Academy of Nursing established a task force of administrators and researchers to investigate hospital nursing. One of the task force members was Dr. Mabel Wandelt from the University of Texas at Austin. Wandelt pointed out what was to be termed the Magnet phenomenon—that some hospitals, near to or even next to hospitals that had difficulties attracting nurses, seemed to have little turnover and little difficulty recruiting and retaining nursing staff. The AAN taskforce quickly began to study these hospitals and, in 1983, published a report, *Magnet Hospitals: Attraction and Retention of Professional Nurses*.[22]

Over the years, what started as an insight and investigation has turned into a credentialing process through which hospitals pay the American Nurses Credentialing Center—a subsidiary of the American Nurses Association—for a kind of nursing seal of approval in the form of Magnet status. Hospitals that pass this extensive credentialing process are deemed to be Magnet hospitals and can advertise themselves as both magnets for nurses and places where patients can expect to get excellent nursing care—or, as the American Nurses Credentialing Center puts it, "the Magnet recognition program provides consumers with the ultimate benchmark to measure the quality of care that they can expect to receive."[23]

In its promotional material, the ANCC writes that Magnet status helps hospitals maintain a competitive advantage, recruit the best nurses, improve patient care, attract high-quality physicians and specialists, and reinforce positive collaborative relationships. To gain this competitive advantage hospitals have to pass a series of tests. The ANCC judges hospitals according to "their ability to meet fourteen standards of nursing care evaluated in a multistage process of written documentation and on-site evaluation by nurse experts." To check whether their organization is ready for Magnet status, nursing leaders can go to the website and download a five-page document that lists the requirements of a Magnet hospital. For example, the chief nursing officer must have, at a minimum, a baccalaureate in nursing. The hospital must have "patient care documentation systems that reflect interdisciplinary communication." Nurses must participate on committees, task forces, and collaborative mechanisms to formulate and approve clinical-care policies, standards, and guidelines. The Magnet movement is designed to make sure hospitals have strong nursing leadership and that nurses have some voice in shaping nursing practice. Staffing is mentioned on the Magnet website, but the Magnet movement is increasingly counterpoised to the idea of staffing regulations.

To succeed in gaining Magnet status, hospitals have to allocate a great many financial resources. The ANCC charges to appraise hospitals, which must also pay hefty application fees. These fees do not include the considerable expenditure hospitals must make in allotting staff to prepare for visits from accreditors. In-house staff have to provide reams of material to qualify for Magnet status. Nurses have to write narratives about their practice and have to help establish and participate on a shared governance council as well as a variety of other committees. If the hospital is so accredited, it can advertise itself as a certified Magnet hospital.[24]

As Gordon has written elsewhere, it is hard to argue with the idea of giving nurses a voice in their practice, encouraging a strong nursing leadership that has access to the highest levels of the hospital administration and creating an environment in which nursing practice is respected and given adequate resources. Many nurses and nurse executives report that it is indeed better to work in Magnet hospitals and that the very process of securing Magnet status gives nursing more of a profile and sometimes more clout within organizations that have long denied nurses and nursing much of an institutional voice. The central question is why the Magnet movement is so often presented as a competitor to staffing ratios rather than as a complement to them. We would argue that Magnet hospitals need minimum staffing to function. How can nurses participate on committees and governing councils, take advantage of the kind of consistent educational opportunities Magnet accreditation requires, and establish solid interdisciplinary communication and collaboration with physicians and members of other clinical disciplines, if there are too few of them to get off the ward to attend a meeting, go to an educational event, or forge collegial relationships? How can managers exert leadership if they are supervising too many units, with too many nurses, who are demoralized because they are taking care of too many patients, who are too intensely ill?

Of course, minimum staffing ratios do not stipulate the kinds of bodies—and, most important, the kinds of minds—that fill them. But, at a certain point quantity does undermine quality, and the best, most educated, most experienced nurse is reduced to functioning at almost novice status because he or she is overwhelmed with too heavy a patient load. Indeed, the National Institute for Occupational Safety and Health report on the changing organization of work that we cited in our introduction, specifically points out the potential pitfalls of such work-empowerment initiatives. If not accompanied by significant restrictions in workload, these programs can actually add to work intensification by requiring RNs to add participatory activities to their already burdensome workloads:

> Increased worker control and learning opportunities are recognized in the job stress literature as powerful antidotes to stress and illness. But concern exists that various worker participatory or involvement strategies may often be more ceremonial than substantive, having little meaningful influence on worker empowerment—or perhaps even eroding workers' means to influence job conditions through more traditional labor-management mechanisms such as collective bargaining. Concern also exists that cross-functional teamwork and job enlargement strategies may in some instances multiply the number of tasks workers perform with little net effect on worker competencies.[25]

The final problem with Magnet hospitals and other alternatives posed to staffing ratios is that they are individual rather than systemwide solutions. The problem of nursing shortages and nurse dissatisfaction and burnout is a mass problem that is occurring in hospitals all over the industrialized world. This problem demands a mass solution, not an elite solution. Since the Magnet movement began in the United States over twenty years ago, only several hundred of the nation's more than five thousand hospitals have obtained Magnet status. In the case of the IHI initiative, thirteen hospitals are working with the organization. Many of these Magnet or IHI hospitals are wealthy facilities that have the time and resources to devote to complex application and accreditation processes. These initiatives are intended to be models that spread to all hospitals. In many instances they turn into costly efforts that few can afford. Why aren't all hospitals required to implement the same kinds of policies and practices? If Magnet certifiers judge hospitals on the basis of staffing, what criteria do they use? And if nursing is, as nurses claim, the engine of a hospital, and nurse staffing is critical to making that engine run smoothly and safely, shouldn't clearly articulated staffing ratios be part of the Magnet credentialing process, and shouldn't Magnet—or for that matter IHI standards—be required of all hospitals, not only in the United States but elsewhere?

We asked Sean Clarke about a variety of innovations, such as Magnet hospitals or Transforming Care at the Bedside:

> Rapid response teams, making sure patients on ventilators get evidence-based treatments so they don't develop pneumonia, giving nurses better schedules and more educational resources—it's all great. The problem is that if you don't have

enough staff, these things are not going to have their intended effects. Why won't people simply admit that there are levels below which it's impossible to provide safe nursing care? Why is that such a dangerous idea? I don't know why people are so afraid to make that statement. Why can't we just admit it and move on?

Conclusion: Ratios and Beyond

In January 2007 the Massachusetts Coalition for the Prevention of Medical Errors held one of its monthly meetings. In the developed world thousands of groups have formed over the past decade as high-tech health-care systems confront an epidemic of medical errors and injuries, such as hospital acquired infections, ventilator acquired pneumonias, medication errors, and other potentially fatal and often preventable complications. At this particular meeting, representatives of many of the state's hospitals and health plans gathered with experts in patient safety; officials from medical, nursing, and pharmacy boards; as well as scholars and lawyers. Coalition leaders presented the group with a strategic planning report that outlined several key goals—eliminating methicillin-resistant *Staphylococcus aureus* (MRSA) in hospitals; eliminating harm due to anticoagulation management; and increased sharing and learning through educational programs and publications, as well as the implementation of national patient-safety initiatives. After a leader of the coalition presented the ambitious agenda, a prominent participant raised his hand. He just wanted to alert the group, he said, to something they had not yet considered—the nursing manpower issue. "If we don't have enough nurses, none of these efforts will succeed," he predicted. Although most participants were adamantly opposed to the nurse-staffing bill then in the Massachusetts state legislature, all nodded their heads in agreement. But there was no further discussions of how to make sure there were enough nurses in hospitals, and there was no mention of staffing as an integral part of the patient safety movement.

In his comments the speaker referred to a segment from the National Public Radio series *Nursing: A Shortage*, which had aired just the week before. The segment once again related the sorry statistics with which every hospital

224

official in the room was all too familiar. The average age of nurses in the United States will soon reach forty-seven. There will be a shortfall of almost eight hundred thousand nurses by the end of the decade. To meet the needs of the eighty million baby boomers soon to hit the hospitals, rehab facilities, nursing homes, and retirement communities with complex combinations of chronic illnesses, U.S. nursing schools will have to graduate 90 percent more RNs over the next decade, and even then it will fall short of what's needed.

The documentary also aired interviews with nurses and nursing students in the Northeast. Nursing students reported that they were eager to join the ranks of RNs, that is they were until they entered the workplace. One nurse explained that she'd left the hospital workplace after only a year because the workloads were so stressful that she believed she would do more harm than good to her patients. She then recounted the truncated work history of a fellow graduate who, after only nine months, decided to quit. This young woman, who had graduated at the top of her class, became a dog walker, where she could earn as much as a nurse with less stress.

A new study published in the *American Journal of Nursing* in 2007 confirmed these anecdotal reports. A survey was sent to a random sample of new RNs in thirty-five U.S. states and the District of Columbia, and 3,266 of those recipients returned surveys. Although most RNs said they felt relatively satisfied with their jobs, many complained about their working conditions. Thirteen percent changed jobs after only one year and 37 percent said they felt ready to change jobs.[1] Meanwhile, in American hospitals staffing ratios vary dramatically, just as they did in California before ratios were implemented. Thus on meidcal-surgical units nurses may be taking care of a low of 2.7 patients or a high of 13.8.[2]

In states that do not have nurse staffing ratios or little or no legislative action on the issue, conditions in hospitals have become dire indeed. In Alabama, a professor of nursing told us that one of her students was assigned as charge nurse on the night shift for an orthopedic floor even though she had graduated from nursing school only three months earlier. Her colleagues were, for the most part, traveling nurses who had little experience on the unit or in that particular hospital. Her professors had instructed her not to accept any unsafe staffing assignments. So she would refuse to accept more patients on the unit if she felt there were not enough nurses to safely care for them. Her managers constantly hassled her, the professor said, because she refused to be a team player. Finally, the nurse quit and now works in a physician's office.

In the radio series *Nursing: A Shortage* some hospital administrators did acknowledge that they can't recruit new nurses unless they retain the ones already in their employ. Alan Knight, chief executive officer of Jordan Hospital in Massachusetts, argued that he had to change working conditions for nurses.

If he did, the nurses employed by his hospital could be his best advertisement. If he didn't, they could be his worst. Knight claimed he was working hard to keep his nurses.

Nurses, as we have written here and elsewhere, suffer from a myriad of problems, and not only from work overload. Nurses don't have enough authority over their work. They often lack supportive nursing management. Too many physicians fail to understand their role and importance and treat them like servants rather than like colleagues. They don't get enough support as novices and lack rewards as experts. Their pay has stagnated and their pensions and health-care benefits may not be sufficient, depending on the country in which they work (the United States being a prime example). They are often asked to subsidize their hospital or health-care system with uncompensated work.

All of these problems must be addressed. Ratios alone do not address them. Yet ratios are central to any solution. If nurses believe they are harming their patients and themselves because of excessive patient loads, they will leave the hospital bedside. More than that, they will turn into the worst advertisement for both hospitals and the profession of nursing itself. The refrain "You're crazy to go into nursing" is one that too many potential new recruits have heard from veteran RNs.

That's why a number of hospital administrators are in fact implementing some innovations to retain and recruit nurses. As we have seen, they are experimenting with new ways of scheduling and giving nurses better educational opportunities. They are asking them to express their opinions about institutional policies and practices and trying to encourage interdisciplinary teamwork. As Sean Clarke noted earlier, however, all of these innovations depend on having enough bodies at the bedside. If there is not enough staff on the ward to take care of patients, nurses can't get off the ward to attend a meeting or take advantage of educational opportunities. If they can't get someone to cover for them, nurses can't go to the bathroom much less to a quiet room to take a nap. If there are not enough physical bodies, there will not be enough minds to innovate care at the bedside. Nor will there be enough voices raised to support—or suggest alternatives to—them. If they are taking care of six or seven or eight patients, nurses can't take the ten or fifteen minutes needed to do the rounds with physicians and convey the critical information on which decisions about medical treatment and nursing interventions should be made. Without this kind of interaction, it is impossible for nurses to become full participants as well as fully respected members of the interdisciplinary team. Without enough nurses, when hospitals offer RNs the means to exercise their voices and participate more fully in workplace decisions, this offer can simply intensify work and make such participation less attractive to nursing staff. Without enough nurses, both patients and nurses suffer unnecessarily.

Although there is no scientific study documenting the perfect number of nurses on particular units, the evidence that better nurse staffing improves patient health is incontrovertible. We may not know what the perfect nurse-to-patient ratio is, but we certainly know what it isn't.

The Importance of Collective Action and Support

As they talk about new innovations in their institutions, hospital administrators often argue that these improvements make nurse-staffing regulations unnecessary. These and other opponents of ratios ignore the fact that many of the solutions now proposed as an antidote to ratios were developed, in large part, because nurses voted with their feet by leaving hospital work or challenged hospital policies with their voices by campaigning for ratios. Would the hospitals or governments that, in the 1990s, couldn't cut nurses fast enough, as Jeanette Ives Erickson of the Massachusetts General Hospital so candidly expressed it, be seeking Magnet status; would they be offering nurses better salaries and benefits as well as more of a voice in policy decisions if nurses hadn't lobbied for ratios, become active in unions, or expressed their disaffection in a decade's worth of rallies, marches, media, and whistle-blowing activities?

One of the many lessons learned from the example of ratios in Victoria and California is that a noxious status quo will not change without collective advocacy and public campaigning.

Work intensification has become one of the major problems in advanced market economies. It is an especially serious problem in health care. At a time of increased preoccupation with cost control and profit maximization, demand for health-care services is growing dramatically. In such a context the pressure for doing more with less becomes overwhelming and irresistible. Nurses have learned that managers who might otherwise have fought to give patients more nursing care and nurses more support on the job find it impossible to resist the pressure to cut, cut, cut.[3]

Although nurses in Victoria and California have not "solved" the problem of cost cutting and work intensification, in both places they have achieved major success because they engaged in collective action and launched a public campaign to connect the problem of quality patient care, as well as that of professionalism and clinical competence, with workplace policies and practices.

"Nurses built a movement," said Rose Ann DeMoro, executive director of the California Nurses Association. "The campaign for ratios was not an easy campaign. It was a hard fought campaign with a lot of behind-the-scenes power plays. But nurses in California were in motion; there was a drum beat around ratios that was unstoppable. We didn't find that having a Democratic majority and Democratic governor made a difference with a lot of issues in the state but when it came to nursing and patient care issues, because nurses were in motion and because they were so powerful and articulate, we passed every piece of legislation introduced."

In their campaign against Governor Arnold Schwarzenegger's attempt to derail the ratios and temper union political activism, DeMoro says that nurses were up against tough odds. "Everyone said it wasn't viable to take on such a popular governor." Because nurses are so humanisitic and had a clear vision, DeMoro said, they were able to humble even the Terminator. "It just shows the power of activism," she concluded.

The nurses we have heard from mobilized a variety of tactics to protect their patients and their professional integrity and personal health. Prominent among the tactics was using scientific data—research studies, surveys, and polling data—as the basis for proposals to regulate nursing-staffing levels. Both the California and Victoria nurses' unions devoted considerable resources to conducting or collecting research and translating it into lay terms. Through this effort they tried to empirically identify the most appropriate ratios for the various domains of nursing practice. Nurses' unions in both states recognized, however, that adoption of evidence-based policy required active mobilization. Employers in the 1990s had achieved major cost savings by imposing new regimes of cost control. They would not walk away from these gains willingly.

The nurses' success, however, was not simply determined by the formulation of clear ideas supported by an effective campaign. In both cases the nurses were successful because they articulated their concern in terms of patient safety and a sustainable health system (as opposed to simply protecting nurses). From the outset the California nurses connected understaffing to patient safety. Understaffing, they argued, compromised patient care. We recall the newspaper advertisements that proclaimed that nurses do have a special interest—an interest in patient care. This was a simple but effective message that ensured a high degree of public support. It also elicited practical support from members of the public who wrote letters and op-ed pieces in the press about harm they or a loved one had experienced in a hospital.

Nurses in Victoria used a similar but slightly different campaign theme. The goal of nurse-patient ratios was couched in terms of "nursing the system back to health." For them the challenge was to revitalize the public health system—the dominant provider of hospital-based health care in Australia. Their demand for ratios was part of a wider range of initiatives aimed at achieving sustainability, not only in their profession but in the health-care system as a whole. That is why their campaign included proposals to strictly limit the number, use, and organization of agency nurses. This proposal directly targeted the amount of money hospitals were wasting—money that could be put to use serving the public health—by paying huge fees to temporary staffing agencies. Private agencies' ability to operate was severely limited as a result of creating "nurse banks" at each hospital. Other demands included the need for greater education for nurses and the reorganization of shifts to ensure better flows of knowledge and information on the job on a daily basis.

In both cases, nurses' actions proved to the public that unions, which many probusiness groups portray as an antiquated artifact of a long-ago past (or as a group of selfish workers out to exploit the public to advance a set of narrow interests), could serve as a guardian of the public good. This is why the ratio story is of interest to anyone interested in the revitalization of the labor movement.

Changing the System Not Just the Hospital

Nurses in Victoria and California also succeeded because they understood that only systemwide change could improve a systemwide problem. Critics of nurse-patient ratios have argued that the problem is best solved at the hospital level. They insist that those workplaces that offer superior working conditions will attract the nurses they need. This will, in turn, create a virtuous cycle of a "race to the top" as all hospitals seek to become "employers of choice." This is an attractive story that, unfortunately for nurses as well as many other workers, seems more like a fairy tale when examined in actual practice. There will always be islands of excellence in a sea of mediocrity. Some Magnet hospitals, for example, do indeed offer superior employment conditions, including good nurse-patient ratios. But such hospitals have been around since the health system began. They remain the exception—not the rule. When the underlying system of health care is itself dysfunctional, change in any one unit within it will not change the system at large. As the nineteenth-century economist and philosopher John Stuart Mill noted, under conditions of competition, standards are set by the morally least reputable agent. In other words, in spite of so-called pioneering businesses, the race to the bottom generally continues.

An understanding of these realities informed the California and Victoria campaigns. This was why they pitched their call for change at the level of the health sector at large, not just for particular hospitals within it. Through hard experience they understood that their managers were unable to resist systemic pressures for increased cost cutting and productivity on a workplace-by-workplace basis. Moreover, the political energy nurses would have to expend to fight for better staffing on a hospital-by-hospital basis would overwhelm individual professionals who were already depleted by the demands of their daily work. Even more important, they recognized that patients who had the misfortune to be hospitalized in institutions where nurses either lacked the energy or will to fight—or where they lost their battles—would inevitably suffer. Because they recognized these facts, nurses fought for and won minimum ratios that apply to an entire sector. They did not expect their members at the level of site or business unit to solve the problem on their own.

Nurses also fought for systemic change because they understood how changes in the system were affecting their integrity as professionals and the integrity of their profession. The common refrain of nurses who have suffered from cost cutting and work intensification has not been "you're crazy to work at General Hospital," it's "you're crazy to go into nursing." Rather than blaming the system or discouraging people from working in particular hospitals, many nurses have expressed a blanket condemnation of the profession as a whole. To counter this, a strong tacit assumption informing both campaigns has been the renewal of the nursing profession. Instead of continuing to accept whatever role or flavor-of-the-month scheme is put forth by hospital managers, accountants, or consultants, ratios have provided a way for nurses to assert a pride in their profession and get the basic resources necessary to do their job properly. Issues of quality care and support take center stage when ratios are set and implemented. This creates a very different environment in which to work. We recall the comment of the reluctantly supportive California nurse manager who acknowledged that ratios forced hospitals and even doctors to take nursing seriously.

Industrial Relations and Policy

Another lesson from the implementation of ratios in Victoria and California is that the structure of industrial relations and health policy influences, but does not determine, the success of such campaigns. One of the most striking differences we note in the stories of the Victoria and California campaigns has been how smoothly and effectively Victorian ratios were implemented—even though California won ratios almost a year before Victoria did. The different industrial relations and health-policy settings of the two states help explain the difference. In California bargaining units are fragmented. There are different, often feuding, unions representing registered and licensed nurses. None of them can legally represent executive or even supervisory nurses. Employers in California were thus able to mobilize managers and administrators to oppose the nurse union campaign. In Victoria, on the other hand, that state's branch of the Australian Nursing Federation covered registered and enrolled nurses as well as supervisory and executive-level nurse managers. The ANF also bargained for all nurses in the public health care system regardless of whether they were ANF members. This meant that the ANF Victoria spoke for all nurses and did not have to contend with a formalized split in the profession. These industrial-relations arrangements were the legacy of an industrial-relations system that has, until recent times, encouraged unified employee representation and actively discouraged breakaway unions. In the Australian industrial-relations system, management has, until recent times, also accepted the role of arbitration. Both legacies gave Victoria's nurses powerful institutional resources to formulate clear demands and have them endorsed quickly within the industrial-relations system. The downside of the Australian model is that ratios may be—and have been—challenged in each bargaining round. The government challenged them in 2004. Once again in 2007, the government of Victoria tried to eliminate them, but the ANF succeeded in fending off that attempt and in actually improving them. One advantage of the California ratios over the Victorian is that once they are legislated the only dispute is over how to implement them.

The structure of health-care funding also helped nurses in Victoria. The ratios there were applied only to the largest single group of hospital nurses—those employed in the public sector, the flywheel of the Australian health system. The Labor government responsible for this system indicated from the outset that if ratios were adopted, supplementary funding would be provided to make them work. Nothing of this nature assisted nurses in California.

Despite the lack of the institutional supports their Victoria colleagues enjoyed, the California nurses eventually succeeded. Although it has taken longer to implement ratios in California, the achievement is in fact more far reaching because it prevents subsequent challenges in bargaining and because it affects all nurses, not only those in the public sector. A key basis for the success of the California nurses' unions in a more hostile institutional environment has been their ability to build alliances with patients. While the ANF in Victoria could rely on a solid power base of a relatively united profession, the California nurses have had to place greater emphasis on mass mobilization. This leads to yet another lesson.

Government Intervention Plays a Positive Role

The support of the government and other public agencies is ultimately decisive in achieving success. In Victoria, nurses had the great fortune to negotiate with a newly elected Labor government that was at least prepared to let a state-based "umpire"—the Australian Industrial Relations Commission—adjudicate the dispute between labor and management. Backing from a quasi-judicial member of this state agency gave them immense legitimacy as well as enforceable rights to carry their claim forward. Moreover, in Australia the state government's attitude was that the referee had called the play and they would abide by his judgment.

The role of government and public agencies was also central to success in California. The ratios ultimately became law when the newly elected Democratic California legislature passed AB 394 and a newly elected Democratic governor signed the bill. The California Department of Health Services then thoroughly worked out the details of their implementation. When an incoming Republican governor, Arnold Schwarzenegger, attempted to suspend their implementation, the judicial arm of the state moved decisively against what was determined to be an abuse of executive power.

At crucial moments in the disputes leading up the adoption of the ratios in both settings, judicial and quasi-judicial bodies played a critical role in scrutinizing the evidence and asserting the rights of workers and the public. This highlights the importance of having third parties who can carefully assess the evidence in situations where managers, government officials, and employees are locked into a cycle of rancor that is unsustainable. In both cases judicial or quasi-judicial bodies willingly took on this role once the evidence was presented to them and broke the vicious cycle.

Ratios Are Not Enough and Must Be Constantly Recalibrated

One of the final lessons of the California and Victoria stories is that ratios, once set either through an arbitrated or legislative process must constantly be reevaluated and recalibrated. Because of the ever-changing nature of patient requirements, technological innovation, emerging diseases, and the complexities associated with an aging and, in some places increasingly multicultural population, ratios that are appropriate at one period of time would not be adequate at another.

The latest study of the Victorian ratios conducted in 2007 revealed that many nurses felt that the ratios determined in 2000 were no longer adequate given the changing nature of the population and medical and nursing practice.[4] Nurses in Victoria argued that jettisoning the 50 percent rule would provide them with immediate relief. Instead of the ratios being rounded down, extra staff would be recruited where patient numbers were slightly below the threshold required for another nurse on the unit. This is what they won in their fall 2007 bargaining. An evaluation of the California ratios, which was mandated for five years after their implementation, may similarly reveal the need to adjust the ratios and give nurses fewer patients to care for.

Even though staffing ratios can enhance patient outcomes, improve nurses' health, and interrupt the cycle of demoralization in the nursing workforce, it is important to recognize, as we said earlier, that the ratios have not solved the nursing shortage or the labor problem in either Victoria or California. This informs our final conclusion: ratios are a necessary but not sufficient condition for ending the nursing shortage. The nurse-to-patient ratios in Victoria and California have been a remarkable achievement. In an era in which unions are in decline and the development of new, progressive workplace standards is rare, these ratios represent a significant advance. Ratios also represent an advance in patient safety. Even those managers and administrators who seem unalterably opposed to trade unionism and the idea that government can perform a positive public role benefit from the control of work intensification.

Indeed, we believe that the story of ratios in Victoria and California has a great deal to teach other health-care workers—professionals as well as so-called lower-level workers—as well as workers who experience work overload in non–health-care settings. Social workers, respiratory therapists, physical therapists, and even physicians are experiencing an explosion of work overload in the health-care system.

In considering this phenomenon it is worth exploring briefly the stake physicians have in nurse-staffing ratios. Physicians who used to be in control of their schedules now find themselves reduced in status by the pressure to see more patients more quickly. In the United States, surgeons are pushed—or push themselves—to do more operations. Many internists and family practice doctors now have panels of between three thousand and five thousand patients. This means they have little time to take a thorough history, perform an exam, give preventive education, explain how to follow complex medication regimens, consult with other physicians, or answer phone calls. One 2007 study published in the *Archives of Internal Medicine* found that patients had a higher risk of mortality when graduate physicians in training who are responsible for frontline care are forced to take on more patients.[5]

In one of the first cases of its kind, Robert K. Greene, a physician on the staff of Westmoreland Regional Hospital near Pittsburgh, was recently sued for negligence after the birth of a stillborn child. The hospital was also sued because it forced the physician to work too long and hard. According to the report in *American Medical News*:

> Rose and James Thompson accuse Westmoreland Regional Hospital of "maintaining a health care practice with an unmanageable number of patients" and referring too many patients to the obstetrician-gynecologist. The lawsuit also contends the hospital did not address the doctor's concerns about his work schedule. . . . During his deposition, Dr. Greene testified he typically saw about 85 patients per day, delivered more than 400 babies per year, and performed between 450 and 500 surgeries annually, according to the complaint against the hospital.

The idea of a physician out of his residency working such a hectic schedule was startling, said Harry S. Cohen, a Pittsburgh attorney who represents the Thompsons in both cases.[6]

Physicians also have a stake in the ratio debate because their patients will suffer if there are not enough nurses to take care of them. In many health-care systems, the physician, not the hospital or the nurse, will get blamed for the results if their patient dies or suffers from a preventable complication. Many physicians we have spoken to have told us that they often complain about nurse staffing to hospital higher-ups. One physician we spoke with at a major Massachusetts teaching hospital lamented the differences in nursing care that he sees at three different institutions to which he admits his patients. The Brigham and Women's Hospital, he said, had the best nursing because it had the best staffing. Although he didn't quite understand the reason for this, it was because the hospital is represented by the Massachusetts Nurses Association, which has continuously made staffing an issue at the hospital.

A cardiac-surgery critical care nurse practitioner at another nearby teaching hospital, whose nurses do not benefit from the same kind of union contract, told us a very different story. Cardiologists, surgeons, and nurse practitioners, he said, have frequently expressed their concern that patients who leave the ICU for other hospital floors may not do as well because of short staffing. When they complain to nurse managers and the director of nursing, they are told that staffing is fine. "It's not," this nurse practitioner said, "but they do nothing about it." He said that the physicians can't do anything to solve the problem because only nursing controls the nursing budget.

This nurse practitioner insisted that, research or no research, physicians understand the connection between nurse staffing and patient outcomes. Unfortunately, few physicians have launched the kind of public discussion and protest over these issues that might result in changes at the state and federal level. In fact, medical societies tend not to support staffing ratios. The Massachusetts Medical Society remained neutral regarding the state's nurse staffing bill. This public silence, or even opposition, on the part of physicians is a cause for concern. It's worth recalling that, in their article in *Medical Care*, Michael Rothberg and his colleagues observed that: "If a hospital decided, for economic reasons, not to provide thrombolytic therapy in acute myocardial infarction, physicians would likely refuse to admit to that hospital, and patients would fear to go there."[7] Why aren't physicians refusing to admit patients to hospitals where understaffing is an equally imposing threat to their patients' lives and recovery?

Not the Whole Solution

In spite of the success of ratios, it is important to keep their accomplishments in perspective. Staffing levels are but one part of the challenge of managing the workforce in the health-care system. Issues of pay, hours of work, possibilities for career advancement, authority over work and participation in decisions affecting it, plus the ever increasing problems of documentation and underlying funding levels, pose serious challenges for all involved in health care, not just nurses. Ratios can make a major contribution to solving some of these problems, but on their own they are not enough.

When we consider the heated debate about the wisdom of ratios, we are reminded of a recent cartoon in the *New Yorker*, a publication famous for its witty political and social commentary. In this particular cartoon—whose caption reads "Good Shrink, Bad Shrink"—a man lies on a classic psychiatrist's couch. He is flanked by two chairs. A woman sits in one, a man in the other. The man, with beard and glasses, arms crossed firmly over his chest advises, "Face your Demons." The woman sits with her legs crossed and counsels, "Take a Pill." This conflicting advice reflects an intense debate in psychiatry. Some psychiatrists insist that people dealing with mental problems should engage in the kind of talk therapy that will allow them to excavate and confront their "demons." Others insist that this approach is not useful. Mental problems, they argue, are the result of biochemical imbalances that can be remedied by an evolving pharmacopoeia of psychiatric medications. Each side marshals its own scientific evidence to refute the other.

The truth almost undoubtedly lies, as it usually does, somewhere in the middle, in a combination of talk therapy and pharmacology. The same is true of the nursing crisis. In fact, the comparison is particularly apt when it comes to nursing. As the studies show, the nursing workload itself generates depression, or at least demoralization. Depressed nurses, like depressed patients, become overwhelmed by the challenges of their environment. Their body chemistry, and with it the chemistry of their brains, is affected by a cascade of stress-related chemicals. Their professional chemistry is equally affected. Feeling powerless and lacking any control over their daily work, they become defeatist, irritable, and sometimes irascible. They don't have the energy to fight to improve things. They retreat from friends and family—even from their patients—and then feel unsupported and undervalued. Indeed, a few even engage in a version of professional suicide. They leave the ranks of nursing to become dog walkers. Or if they stay on the wards, they greet new recruits with a hostile assault—inquiring of the new graduate why on earth he or she has chosen such a profession. New recruits, not surprisingly, begin to wonder whether the veteran nurse isn't on to something and act accordingly.

Thus nurses discourage and push away the very people who could help ease their workload. (Imagine, if soldiers at the front greeted new troops by telling them they ought to desert—immediately?)

In such an environment, ratios act like antidepressants. They alter the chemistry of the unit as well as the responses of the individual nurse. They give nurses more energy and a sense of control. The very struggle for ratios has helped nurses gain a recognition of their own importance. To win ratios, they have had to support one another and have received support from politicians, the media, and the public. This, in turn, enhances their self-esteem. From addressing patient loads, this more hopeful and professionally invigorated nurse can move on to tackle the other problems he or she faces in the workplace or the wider society. Deprived of a concrete way to deal with the daily reality of patient care, the depressed nurse is like the depressed patient. She or he simply does not have the emotional and physical energy to initiate or participate in the other innovations—the talk therapy if you will—that is also necessary to change the clinical environment for the better.

This is why we believe that ratios can play a critical role in solving the broader nursing crisis by providing a new reference point for thinking about health-care reform. The great power of ratios is that they put issues of quality of service and quality of working life at center stage. Having these issues, and not just cost control, figure in debates about the future of nursing and health care is a major advance on the recent past. It is one that could—and should—also be considered by other health-care workers. Indeed, any workers overwhelmed by the injunction to do more with less can consider the lessons learned by these nurses and reflect on how they might be relevant to their workplace concerns.

Many health-care observers are heartened that some hospital administrators are seeking Magnet status, paying nurses more, and trying to woo nurses back into the workforce. They are encouraged by corporate advertising campaigns that tout nursing's importance and also by the fact that there has been a spike in admissions to nursing schools worldwide. We are too. But we also become disheartened when we hear about more cost cutting, layoffs in the midst of shortage (the UK National Health Service springs to mind), and efforts in the United States and elsewhere to cut hospital nurses' pensions and benefits. We began this book with a discussion of trust. When nurses stop trusting hospital managers to make practical, concrete changes that allow them to do their work without risk of harm to patients or to themselves, they either use their voices to change things for the better or choose to exit from the hospital and even from the profession.

In his testimony in a private arbitration concerning the Victoria nurses dispute in August 2000, a prominent hospital chief executive officer argued:

When management failed to listen [to] nurses' concerns, nurses were left with no option other than to take strong industrial action. It is my belief that hospitals' management across [the state] are still not capable of listening to nurses' concerns, particularly relating to workload and addressing those issues as they arise. It is only the existence of mandatory minimum staffing levels and automatic closure of beds when the minimum staffing levels are not in place that will force management to consider nurses' concern.[8]

Nurses in Victoria and California have led the way with mandatory nurse-to-patient ratios. It will be interesting to see how many others—nurses, medical professionals, and patients alike—learn and benefit from their hard-won achievements.

APPENDIX

Decision of the Australian Industrial Relations Commission on Nurse-to-Patient Ratios

Note: What follows is derived from the decision of the Australian Industrial Relations Commission on nurse-to-patient ratios. The description of ratios presented is not a word-for-word reproduction of the ratios as they appear in the official industrial relations ruling but has been compacted for the purposes of this book.

The methodology used to apply the nurse patient ratio needs to be consistent with the principle of ensuring that the number of nurses available is commensurate with the number of patients requiring care. It is noted that average occupancy may not reflect variations in patient numbers, and therefore may not match staff to periods of peak demand.

Consequently, the nurse patient ratios should be calculated on actual patient numbers in a given ward/unit. Obviously, if a hospital has a particular ward of 30 beds and only 26 beds are usually occupied, then the four "unused" beds can only be used when additional staff are available to meet the ratio requirements.

The word "nurse" refers to:

- Division 1 registered nurse—undertakes a 3-year degree course prior to registration
- Division 2 registered nurse—(sometimes referred to as "state enrolled nurse")—undertakes a 12–month certificate level course prior to registration

In the major acute hospitals no more than one Division 2 nurse per ward per shift can be rostered to meet the ratios.

In aged care and smaller rural hospitals more Division 2 nurses may be rostered on to meet the ratios but this must be determined by local agreement with the nursing staff in individual wards.

General Medical/Surgical Wards

Hospital categories are listed below into amended hospital groups. The rationale for hospital categories includes bed numbers and service provision.

Level 1 Hospital

(Mainly leading teaching, research and referral hospitals, general and specialist services for trauma, transplant, oncology, neurosciences, cardiac, obstetrics, paediatrics and acute surgical and medical services.)

am shift	1:4 + in charge
pm shift	1:4 + in charge
night duty	1:8

Level 2 Hospital

(Large metropolitan and country base hospitals.)

am shift	1:4 + in charge
pm shift	1:5 + in charge
night duty	1:8

Level 3 Hospital

(Small to medium metropolitan and country base hospitals.)

am shift	1:5 + in charge
pm shift	1:6 + in charge
night duty	1:10

Level 3a Hospital

(Medium country hospitals.)

am shift	1:6 + in charge
pm shift	1:6 + in charge
night duty	1:10

Hospitals other than levels 1, 2, 3, and 3a

(Generally small country hospitals with less than 30 beds and limited theatre sessions.)

am shift	1:6 + in charge
pm shift	1:7 + in charge
night duty	1:10

All Aged Care Wards

(Where aged care patients generally occupy beds designated as acute, "aged care ward" ratios shall apply for these patients.)

am shift	1:7 + in charge
pm shift	1:8 + in charge
night duty	1:15

Acute Wards

am shift	1:6 + in charge
pm shift	1:7 + in charge
night duty	1:10

Ante/Postnatal Wards

(All hospital levels.)

am shift	1:5 + in charge
pm shift	1:6 + in charge
night duty°	1:8

° Night duty staff may assist in Levels 1 and 2 nurseries where geography and workload allows.

Delivery Suites Levels 1, 2, and 3

All shifts 2 midwives to 3 delivery suites.
- If the ward/unit believes that there is not the same requirement for staffing levels on night duty as for am and pm, then a local agreement will be entered into.

- In hospitals with less than 2 births per day, rosters should ensure that where possible two midwives are rostered on in the hospital. If this is not possible, one may be on-call.
- If other parts of the hospital are not busy, midwives may be relocated to work in delivery suites.
- Where hospitals have introduced different models of care such as Box Hill, Werribee and Sunshine, agreements on staffing will be developed and agreed between hospital management and ANF.

NICU (Neonatal Intensive Care Unit)

(Four major units that contain "special nursery" and NICU babies: Mercy Hospital for Women, Royal Women's Hospital, Monash Medical Centre, and Royal Children's Hospital.)

all shifts   1:2 + in charge.

Discrete Level 2 Special Care Units

(a) where 10 or more cots: 1:3 on all shifts
(b) where less than 10 cots: 1:4 on all shifts

The general rounding principles, as determined, shall apply, provided that two nurses shall be required in respect of six cots. To illustrate in respect of the 1:3 ratio:

- 10 cots = 3
- 11 cots = 4
- 12 cots = 4
- 13 cots = 4
- 14 cots = 5
- 15 cots = 5
- 16 cots = 5

Level 1 Nurseries

Given the ratios in acute and postnatal wards these babies will be cared for by ward staff.

Accident and Emergency

Group 1 Accident and Emergency Departments

(The Alfred, Austin and Repatriation Medical Centre, Monash Medical Centre, Royal Melbourne Hospital, Clayton Campus, Angliss Health Service, St Vincent's Hospital [Melbourne] Ltd., Royal Children's Hospital, Box Hill Hospital, Frankston Hospital, Geelong Hospital, The Northern Hospital, Dandenong Hospital, Western Hospital [Footscray], Ballarat Health Services [Hospital], Bendigo Health Care Group [Hospital], Goulburn Valley Health [Hospital], New Latrobe Regional Hospital, Maroondah Hospital, Mercy Hospital Inc., Werribee Campus.)

am shift	1:3 + in charge + triage
pm shift	1:3 + in charge + triage
night duty	1:3 + in charge + triage

These night duty ratios should not to be based on all cubicles but rather adjusted for presentations and cubicle occupancy for the previous 12 months. The number of cubicles used for determining night duty staffing ratios is reduced in proportion to the average number of presentations at night compared with the day shifts.

Group 2 Accident and Emergency Departments

(Accident and Emergency departments not in Group 1 with over 5000 presentations per annum.)

am shift	1:3 + in charge
pm shift	1:3 + in charge
night duty	1:3 + in charge

Where these units have previously had a triage nurse these positions remain. Ratios refer to nurses required for the average number of patients in the unit at any one time. To be based on previous 12-month history of presentations and total number of patient hours per shift.

Group 3 Accident and Emergency Departments

(Less than 5000 presentations per annum.)

There should be 2 Division 1 Registered Nurses plus 1 "floater" (Division 1 or Division 2) per shift as staffing for the facility including Accident and Emergency. There are no dedicated staff rostered in Accident and Emergency Departments.

Designated Coronary Care Unit

am shift	1:2 + in charge
pm shift	1:2 + in charge
night duty	1:3

High Dependency Unit

(Stand alone units in Level 1 Hospitals.)

am shift	1:2 + in charge
pm shift	1:2 + in charge
night duty	1:2

Where HDU is part of an Intensive Care Unit, the "in charge" position is to cover both HDU and ICU.

Palliative Care

am shift	1:4 + in charge
pm shift	1:5 + in charge
night duty	1:8

Rehabilitation and Geriatric Evaluation Management

Category 1 Rehabilitation (amputees, acquired brain injury, spinal injury)

am shift	1:5 + in charge
pm shift	1:5 + in charge
night duty	1:10

Category 2 Rehabilitation

am shift	1:5 + in charge
pm shift	1:7 + in charge
night duty	1:10

Geriatric Evaluation Management Beds

am shift	1:5 + in charge
pm shift	1:6 + in charge
night duty	1:10

Where Rehabilitation and GEM beds are less than 25 per cent of a ward or unit, the ratios according to the dominant clinical description shall apply. Where a ward or unit has combined GEM and Rehabilitation only one in charge nurse is required.

Operating Theatre

3 per theatre

Operating Theatres will normally have three nurses, one scrub nurse, one scout nurse, and one anaesthetic nurse. This may be varied up or down, depending on the following circumstances:
1. Complexity of the surgery or procedure;
2. Pre-existing condition of the patient;
3. Number of operations on the list;
4. Experience and skill mix of staff;
5. Type of equipment used;
6. Number of students requiring supervision;
7. Temporary fluctuations in demand across the whole theatre suite during a session; and
8. Layout and number of operating suites.

Post-Anaesthetic Care Unit/Recovery Room (PACU)

All shifts 1:1 for unconscious patients.

Notes

Introduction

1. www.MHA.org.

2. http://www2.rcn.org.uk/congress/2007/2007_agenda/right_numbers_right_care, accessed June 5, 2007.

3. http://news.bbc.co.uk/2/hi/uk_news/scotland/4323971.stm., accessed June 5, 2007.

4. Center for Disease Control and Prevention, Estimates of Healthcare-Associated Infections. http://www.cdc.gov/ncidod/dhqp/hai.html, accessed August 22, 2007.

5. Suzanne Gordon and Timothy McCall, "Healing in a Hurry: Hospitals in the Managed Care Age," *Nation* 268 (March 1, 1999): 11–15.

6. Roy J. Lewicki and Carolyn Wiethoff, "Trust, Trust Development, and Trust Repair," in *The Handbook of Conflict Resolution: Theory and Practice*, ed. Morton Deutsch and Peter T. Coleman (San Francisco: Jossey Bass, 2000), 86–90.

7. Linda H. Aiken et al., "Nurses' Reports on Hospital Care in Five Countries," *Health Affairs* (May–June 2001): 43–53.

8. Ibid., 48.

9. Ibid., 51.

10. Julie Sochalski, "Nursing Shortage Redux: Turning the Corner on an Enduring Problem," *Health Affairs* 21, no. 5 (2002): 159.

11. Christopher Hood, "A Public Management for All Seasons?" *Public Administration* 69, no. 1 (Spring 1991): 3–19; and C. Hood, "Emerging Issues in Public Management," *Public Administration* 73 (1995): 165–83.

12. E. J. Schumacher, *The Earnings and Employment of Nurses in an Era of Cost Containment* (East Carolina University: Department of Economics, 1999).

13. E. Ferlie, L. Ashburner, L. Fitzgerald, and A. Pettigrew, *A New Public Management in Action* (Oxford: Oxford University Press, 1996).

14. David Osborne and Ted Gaebler, *Reinventing Government: How the Entrepreneurial Spirit Is Transforming the Public Sector* (New York: Penguin, 1993).

15. S. C. Bolton, "A Simple Matter of Control? NHS Hospital Nurses and New Management," *Journal of Management Studies* 1 (2004): 317–33.

16. Simon Head, *The New Ruthless Economy: Work and Power in the Digital Age* (Oxford: Oxford University Press, 2003), 23.

17. European Agency for Safety and Health at Work, *Working on Stress: Prevention of Psychosocial Risks and Stress at Work in Practice*, 2002; http://osha.europa.eu/publications/reports/104/stress_en.pdf, accessed January 25, 2007.

18. Health and Safety Executive, "Occupational Stress Statistics," Information Sheet 1/03/EMSU, September 2003, http://products.ihs.com/Ohsis-SEO/590062.html, accessed January 25, 2007; J. T. Bond et al., *The National Study of the Changing Workforce* (New York: Families and Work Institute, 1998), 1–176.

19. National Institute for Occupational Safety and Health, *The Changing Organization of Work and the Safety and Health of Working People: Knowledge Gaps and Research Directions* (Cincinnati: Centers for Disease Control and Prevention, 2002), 14–16.

20. L. R. Murphy et al., "The USA Perspective: Current Issues and Trends in the Management of Work Stress," *Australian Psychologist* 38, no. 2 (2003): 151–57.

21. Ibid.

22. J. H. Silber et al., "Hospital and Patient Characteristics Associated with Death after Surgery: A Study of Adverse Occurrence and Failure to Rescue," *Medical Care* 30 (1992): 615–29.

23. American Hospital Association, *Hospital Statistics*, 2007 ed. (Chicago: AHA, 2007).

24. http://blog.aflcio.org/2006/10/03/labor-board-ruling-may-bar-millions-of-workers-from-forming-unions/, accessed June 5, 2007.

25. Michael Silverstein, "Ergonomics and Regulatory Politics: The Washington State Case," *American Journal of Industrial Medicine* 50, no. 5 (May 2007): 391–401 at 396.

1. Hospital Restructuring and the Erosion of Nursing Care in California and the United States

1. Julie Sochalski, "Nursing Shortage Redux: Turning the Corner on an Enduring Problem," *Health Affairs* 21 (2002): 159.

2. WBUR (Boston) radio, "Nursing a Shortage: Inside Out," January 17, 19, 20, 2007.

3. California Code of Regulations, Licensing and Certification of Health Facilities and Referral Agencies, Title 22, Register 75, no. 24, 6-14-75, 1844.

4. Ibid., 1882, 1884, 1885, 1886, 1901.

5. For a fuller discussion of this phenomenon, see Suzanne Gordon, *Nursing against the Odds: How Health Care Cost-Cutting, Media Stereotypes, and Medical Hubris Undermine Nurses and Patient Care* (Ithaca: Cornell University Press, 2005).

6. Suzanne Gordon, *Life Support: Three Nurses on the Front Lines* (Ithaca: Cornell University Press, 2007), 260.

7. Board of Registered Nursing, State of California, Licenses Issued 1994–2005/2006.

8. H. S. Luft, "How Do Health Maintenance Organizations Achieve Their 'Savings?' " *New England Journal of Medicine* 298 (1978): 1336–43.

9. Uwe Reinhardt, "Spending More through 'Cost Control': Our Obsessive Quest to Gut the Hospital," *Health Affairs* 15 (1996): 145–54.

10. Suzanne Gordon and Timothy McCall, "Healing in a Hurry: Hospitals in the Managed Care Age," *Nation* 268 (March 1, 1999): 11–15.

11. Institute of Medicine, *Nursing Staff in Hospitals and Nursing Homes: Is It Adequate?* (Washington, D.C.: National Academies Press, 1996), 20.

12. Ibid.

13. Tim Porter-O'Grady, "Working with Consultants on a Redesign," *American Journal of Nursing* 94, no. 10 (October 1994): 33, 34.

14. Judith Shindul-Rothschild and Marry Duffy, "The Impact of Restructuring on Nursing Practice and Patient Care," *Best Practices and Benchmarking in Health Care* (November–December 1996): 271–82.

15. Bernice Buresh and Suzanne Gordon, *From Silence to Voice: What Nurses Know and Must Communicate to the Public*, 2nd ed. (Ithaca: Cornell University Press, 2006), 181–182.

16. Ibid., 182.

17. California Department of Health Services, "Final Statement of Reasons," August 25, 2003, 1–2.

18. James Buchan, "A Certain Ratio? Minimum Staffing Ratios in Nursing: A Report for the Royal College of Nursing," April 2004, http://www.rcn.org.uk/news/display.php?ID=1172, 7, accessed September 20, 2006.

19. Hearing on petition for writ of mandamus, California Superior Court's ruling under submission, March 27, 2005: 4, in case of California Nurses Association v. Schwarzenegger, Cal. Super. Ct., No. 04CS01725.

20. Institute for Health and Socio-Economic Policy, "California Health Care: Sicker Patients, Fewer RNs, Fewer Staffed Beds" (September 1999), report prepared for the California Nurses Association, www.calnurses.org/research/pdfs/Fewer-RNs-to-More-Patients.pdf, accessed July 20, 2007.

21. Judith Shindul-Rothschild, "Where Have All the Nurses Gone? Final Results of Our Patient Care Survey," *American Journal of Nursing* 96, no. 11 (November 1996): 25–39.

22. Institute of Medicine, *Nursing Staff*, 5.

23. Ibid., 102.

24. Ibid., 15 and 16.

25. Ibid., 9–10.

26. Ibid., 17.

27. Dick Davidson, *Reality Check: Public Perceptions of Health Care and Hospitals* (Chicago: American Hospital Association, 1996), 8.

28. Ibid., 10.

29. Mary A. Blegen, Colleen J. Goode, and Laura Reed, "Nurse Staffing and Patient Outcomes," *Nursing Research* 47, no. 1 (1998): 43–50. Mary Blegen and Tom Vaughn, "A Multisite Study of Nurse Staffing and Patient Occurrences," *Nursing Economics* 16, no. 4 (1998): 196–203.

30. Christine Kovner and Peter J. Gergen, "Nurse Staffing Levels and Adverse Events Following Surgery in U.S. Hospitals," *Image: The Journal of Nursing Scholarship* 30, no. 4 (1998): 315–21.

31. Kenneth K. Westbrook, *Tenet*, September 13, 1999; and Thomas B. Mackey, September 23, 1999.

32. Janet M. Carter, California Association of Catholic Hospitals, September 20, 1999.

33. Barbara Glaser, Association of California Healthcare Districts, September 22, 1999.

34. Patricia Lenihan McFarland, Association of California Nurse Leaders, no date.

35. C. Duane Dauner, California Healthcare Association, September 20, 1999.

36. California Department of Health Services, Final Statement of Reasons, 1.

37. Assembly Bill No. 394, Chapter 945, 1999, p. 2.

38. Superior Court 2005, 2.

39. California Superior Court 2005, 6.

40. Ibid., 14.

41. California Legislature, Assembly Bill No. 394 (approved by governor October 10, 1999, filed with the secretary of state October 10, 1999).

42. California Department of Health Services. Final Statement of Reasons. R-37-01, 08/25/03, P12.

43. Board of Registered Nursing, State of California, Licenses Issued 1994–2005/2006.

2. Not Out of Thin Air

1. Linda H. Aiken, Sean P. Clarke, Douglas M. Sloane, Julie Sochalski, and Jeffrey Silber, "Hospital Nurse Staffing and Patient Mortality, Nurse Burnout, and Job Dissatisfaction," *Journal of the American Medical Association* 288, no. 16 (2002): 1987–93.

2. Ann E. Rogers et al., "The Working Hours of Hospital Staff, Nurses, and Patient Safety," *Health Affairs* 23 (2004): 202–12.

3. California Department of Health Services, "Statement of Reasons," R-37-01, 08/25/03, 4.

4. Ibid., 6–12.

5. Institute for Health and Socio-Economic Policy, AB 394, "California and the Demand for Safe and Effective Nurse to Patient Staffing Ratios," March 2001, 26.

6. CDHS, "Statement of Reasons," 12.

7. Ibid., 14.

8. For further information on the concept of cumulative workload, see Barbara R. Norrish and Thomas G. Rundall, "Hospital Restructuring and the Work of Registered Nurses," *Milbank Quarterly* 79 (2001): 55–79.

9. CDHS, "Statement of Reasons," 15.

10. Ibid., 15.

11. Ibid., 15–17.

12. UC Davis Center for Health Services Research in Primary Care and UC Davis Center for Nursing Research, "Hospital Nursing Staff Ratios and Quality of Care: Final Report on Evidence, Administrative Data, an Expert Panel Process, and a Hospital Staffing Survey," May 2002, 2.

13. Ibid.

14. Joanne Spetz, Jordan Rickles, and Paul M. Ong, "California's Nursing Labor Force: Demand, Supply, and Shortages," *California Nurse Workforce Initiative* (Sacramento: Employment Development Department, California Health and Human Services Agency, January 2004), 16.

15. CDHS, "Statement of Reasons," 22.

16. Ibid., 20.

17. Ibid., 21.

18. Ibid., 21.

19. Ibid., 25–28.

20. Ibid., 28–29.

21. Ibid., 29–30.

22. Ibid., 31–32.

23. Ibid., 32.

24. Ibid., 33–34.

25. Ibid., 35.

3. The Hospital Industry Response

1. California Healthcare Association, "Nurse Staff Ratios," Powerpoint presentation, 2003, slide 1.

2. Superior Court of California, County of Sacramento, *California Healthcare Association vs. California Department of Health Services*, May 24, 2004, 3.

3. Ibid., 3.

4. Superior Court of California, County of Sacramento, *California Healthcare Association vs. California Department of Health Services*, Ruling on Submitted Matter, May 24, 2004, 4–5.

5. Ibid., 8.

6. Ibid., 3, 4.

7. Ibid., 4.

8. Ibid., 8.

9. Ibid., 5.

10. California Legislature, 2003–04 Regular Session, Assembly Bill No. 2963, February 20, 2004.

11. Superior Court of California, *California Nurses Association v. Schwarzenegger, et al.*, Case No. 04CSO1725, Hearing on Petition for Writ of Mandamus, 05/27/2005, 11.

12. Ibid., 12.

13. Dan Glaister, "Schwarzenegger Meets His Match," *Guardian*, April 15, 2005.

14. Superior Court, March 2005, 15.

15. Ibid., 15, 16.

16. Ibid., 20.

17. Ibid., 23.

18. Ibid., 24.

19. Ibid., 22.

20. Ibid., 25.

21. Ibid., 25–27.

22. Ibid., 27, 28.

23. Ibid., 29.

24. Ibid., 31.

25. Ibid., 32.

4. Ratios Redux

1. Nancy Donaldson, et al., "Impact of California's Licensed Nurse-Patient Ratios on Unit-Level Nurse Staffing and Patient Outcomes," *Policy, Politics, and Nursing Practice* 6, no. 3 (2005): 198–210.

2. David Keepnews, "Reading from Ratios," *Policy, Politics, and Nursing Practice* 6, no. 3 (2005): 165–67.

3. Peter I. Buerhaus, Douglas O. Staiger, and David I. Auerbach, "New Signs of a Strengthening U.S. Nurse Labor Market?" *Health Affairs* W4-528 (Web exclusive), November 2004.

4. Joanne Spetz, "California's Minimum Nurse-to-Patient Ratios: The First Few Months," *Journal of Nursing Administration* 34, no. 12 (2004): 575.

5. Ibid.

6. Ibid., 576.

7. California Board of Registration of Nursing, "Registered Nursing Licenses Issued."

8. California Board of Registration of Nursing, "Number of Licensed Registered Nurses 1985–86 through 2005–06."

9. California Healthcare Association, press release, "CNA and Ratios—A Campaign of Misinformation," January 18, 2005, http://www.calhealth.org/public/press/node1.asp?ID=1.

10. Spetz, "California's Minimum Nurse-to-Patient Ratios," 574.

11. Ibid., 573.

5. Working Life for Nurses in the Late 1990s in Australia: A Snapshot

1. G. Considine and J. Buchanan, *The Hidden Costs of Understaffing: A Report for the Australian Nursing Federation (Victorian Branch)* (Sydney: Australian Centre for Industrial Relations Research and Training, University of Sydney, 1999).

2. Statistical Office of the European Communities, "Using a Labor Market Framework to Aid a Structured Assessment of the Factors Affecting the Quality of Employment," Joint UNECE Eurostat ILO Seminar on the Measurement of the Quality of Employment, May 27–29, 2002, Geneva; M. Beatson, "Job Quality and Job Security," *Labour Market Trends* (October 2000): 441–51; F. Green, "It's Been a Hard Day's Night: The Concentration and Intensification of Work in the Late Twentieth Century in Britain," *British Journal of Industrial Relations* 3 (March 2001): 53–80; F. Green, *Demanding Work: The Paradox of Job Quality in the Affluent Economy* (Princeton: Princeton University Press, 2007).

3. National Institute for Occupational Health and Safety, *Stress at Work*, publication 99–101 (Washington, D.C.: 1999). See also VicHealth, *Workplace Stress in Victoria: Developing a Systems Approach* (Melbourne: VicHealth, 2006), 5.

4. M. Dollard and A. Winefield, "Mental Health: Overemployment, Underemployment, Unemployment, and Healthy Jobs," in *Mental Health and Work*, ed. L. Morrow, I. Verins, and E. Willis (Adelaide: Auseinet, 2002); I. Steven and E. M. Shanahan, "Work-Related Stress: Care and Compensation," *Medical Journal of Australia* 176 (2002): 363.

5. Considine and Buchanan, *Hidden Costs of Understaffing*, 20.

6. Ibid., 22.

7. Ibid.

8. Ibid., 23.

9. J. Buchanan and G. Considine, *Stop Telling Us to Cope! New South Wales Nurses Explain Why They Are Leaving the Profession*, report prepared for the NSW Nurses Association (Sydney: University of Sydney, Australian Centre for Industrial Relations Research and Training, 2002), 45.

6. How Did It Come to This?

1. Productivity Commission, *Report on Government Services* (Canberra: Productivity Commission, 2001).

2. Commonwealth Senate, *The Patient Profession: Time for Action—Final Report on the Inquiry into Nursing* (Canberra: Commonwealth of Australia, 2002).

3. Department of Premier and Cabinet, *Victorian Government Population Policy Statements* (Melbourne, 2006).

4. Australian Centre for Industrial Relations Research and Training (ACIRRT), *The Hidden Costs of Understaffing in Victoria*, unpublished data from commissioned report (Sydney: University of Sydney, 1999).

5. Australian Institute of Health and Welfare, *Nursing Labour Force 1998* (Canberra: AIHW 1999).

6. E. M. Chiarella, *The Legal and Professional Status of Nursing* (Edinburgh: Churchill Livingstone, 2002), 282.

7. Ibid., 283, 285.

8. J. Buchanan and G. Considine, *Stop Telling Us to Cope! New South Wales Nurses Explain Why They Are Leaving the Profession*, report prepared for the NSW Nurses Association (Sydney: University of Sydney, Australian Centre for Industrial Relations Research and Training, 2002).

9. Australian College of Nurse Management and Victorian Australian Nursing Federation, *Nursing Workforce Survey 1999* (Melbourne: 2000).

10. C. Hood, "Emerging Issues in Public Management," *Public Administration* 73 (1995): 165–83.

11. "More Permanent Nurses for Victorian Hospitals," media release from the Minister for Health, March 3, 2002.

12. B. Norrish and T. Rundall, "Hospital Restructuring and the Work of Registered Nurses," *Milbank Memorial Fund* 7 (2001): 55–79.

13. Senate Hansard Community Affairs Reference Committee, "Patient Profession Inquiry," Melbourne hearings, February 28 (Canberra: Australian Parliament Hansard, 2002), 7.

14. M. Carter, "Case Studies of Public Hospital Privatisation," *Health Issues Centre Journal* (September 1999).

15. "Hospitals Struggle as Cash Dries Up," *The Age*, May 27, 1999.

16. ABC Television, *Hospitals: An Unhealthy Business*, June 17, 1997, Melbourne; "Deadly Bugs Are Infesting Hospitals," *The Age*, November 9, 1999.

17. P. W. Stone, S. Clarke, J. Cimiotti, and R. Correa-de-Araujo, "Nurses' Working Conditions: Implications for Infectious Disease," *Emerging Infectious Diseases* 10 (2004): 253.

18. L. Aiken, S. P. Clarke, D. M. Sloane, J. Sochalski, and J. Silber, "Hospital Nurse Staffing and Patient Mortality, Nurse Burnout, and Job Dissatisfaction," *JAMA: Journal of the American Medical Association* 16 (2002): 1987–93.

19. Victorian Advisory Committee on Infection Control, *1998 Infection Control Task Force Reports*, Department of Human Services, Victoria.

20. D. W. Spelman, "Hospital-Acquired Infections," *MJA: Medical Journal of Australia Practice Essentials* 176 (2002): 286–91.

21. Ibid.

22. Gastroenterological Nurse Society of Australia, *Standards for Endoscopic Facilities and Services*, 1998.

23. See Suzanne Gordon, *Nursing against the Odds: How Health Care Cost-Cutting, Media Stereotypes, and Medical Hubris Undermine Nurses and Patient Care* (Ithaca: Cornell University Press, 2005), 347.

7. Winning Ratios in Victoria

1. W. Madsen, "Learning To Be a Nurse: The Culture of Training in a Regional Queensland Hospital 1930–1950," *Transformations* 1 (September 2000).

2. J. Bloomfield, "The Changing Image of Australian Nursing," *CIAP* (Sydney: NSW Health St Vincents, 1999): 1–6; http:www.ciap.health.nsw.gov.au/hospolic/stvincents/stvin99/jacqui .htm.

3. J. Barber, "A Gentle Hand on the Tiller? Nurses' Lives of the 1930s," *Proceedings of the Second National Nursing History Conference, Royal College of Nursing* (Melbourne, Royal College of Nursing, 1995).

4. Madsen, "Learning To Be a Nurse."

5. A. Bessant, "Good Women and Good Nurses: Conflicting Identities in the Victorian Nurses' Strikes 1985–1986," *Labour History* 63 (1992): 155–73.

6. P. L. Chinn and C. Wheeler, "Feminism and Nursing: Can Nurses Afford to Remain Aloof from the Women's Movement?" *Nursing Outlook* 33 (1985): 74–77; M. Sandelowski, *Devices and Desires: Gender, Technology, and American Nursing* (Chapel Hill: University of North Carolina Press, 2000).

7. This means staff would en masse walk off the job and refuse to attend work until employers agree to demands or agree to renegotiate the terms of a deal.

8. I. Colson, *More Than Just the Money* (Melbourne: Prowling Tiger Press, 2001), 110.

9. L. Ross, "Sisters Are Doin' It for Themselves . . . and Us," *Hecate* 13 (1987).

10. Ibid.

11. P. Gahan, "The Future of State Industrial Regulation: Can We Learn from Victoria?" *Australian Review of Public Affairs*, November 14, 2005; http://www.australianreview.net/digest/ 2005/11/gahan.html.

12. Wages boards did not operate Australia wide. Victoria and Tasmania were the only states to use this system of regulation to handle industrial concerns.

13. L. Walker, "Beers, Bed and Board: Industrial Behaviour around the Gender, Age and Class in the Hospitality Industry, Victoria 1900–1914," honors thesis, Monash University Department of History, Melbourne, 1995.

14. "Determination of the Hospital Nurses' Board," *Victoria Government Gazette* 756 (1948).

15. Gahan, "Future of State Industrial Regulation."

16. Ross, "Sisters Are Doin' It."

17. The clause was narrow in scope and dealt with nursing homes and hostels. The ratio for these nurses stipulated a ratio of one nurse to ten patients for day shift and one nurse to fifteen patients for night shift. Australian Industrial Relations Commission, Nurses Victorian Health Services Award 1992, Print K6359 [N0175].

18. A "full bench" means a case is heard by a panel of three or more residing members of the Commission, with at least two presidential (senior) members composing part of the team of judges. Australian Industrial Relations Commission, Workplace Relations Act 1996 s.33, Action on the Commission's own motion 107, reference to Full Bench, Review of awards pursuant to

item 51 of the Workplace Relations and Other Legislation Amendment Act 1996, Victorian Health Services Award 1992, Print K 6359 [N0175], August 30, 1999.

19. J. Buchanan, I. Watson, and C. Briggs, "Skill and the Renewal of Labour: The Classical Wage Earner Model and Left Productivism in Australia," in *The Skills That Matter*, ed. C. Warhurst, I. Grugulis, and E. Keep (Basingstoke: Palgrave Macmillan, 2004).

20. A. Hodgkinson, "Productivity Measurement and Enterprise Bargaining—The Local Government Perspective," *International Journal of Public Sector Management* 12 (1999): 470.

21. J. Buchanan and G. Considine, *Stop Telling Us to Cope!* (Sydney: NSW branch of the Australian Nursing Federation, 1998).

22. J. Buchanan and C. Briggs, "Unions and the Restructuring of Work: Contrasting Experiences in the Old and New Heartlands," *Labour and Industry* 16, no. 1 (2005): 10.

23. S. Kitto, "Negotiating Medical Dominance: The Social Construction of the Care Coordinator within the Tasmanian Coordinated Care Trials," *Australian Journal of Primary Health—Interchange* 7 (2001): 62–74.

24. C. Allan, "Work Intensification: A Lacuna in the Labour Utilisation Literature," *AIRAANZ Annual Conference Papers* (Brisbane: Association of Industrial Relations Academies of Australia and New Zealand, 1997).

25. E. Willis, "Enterprise Bargaining and Work Intensification: An Atypical Case Study from the South Australian Public Hospital Sector," *New Zealand Journal of Industrial Relations* 27 (2002): 221–32.

26. Since 2006, however, the authority of the AIRC's decision-making powers with regard to pay and conditions has been significantly diminished with the establishment of an alternative body (the Fair Pay Commission).

27. Evidence given by Shane Solomon, executive director, Metropolitan Health and Aged Care Services, Department of Human Services, to Commonwealth Senate Hansard Community Affairs Reference Committee, "Patient Profession Inquiry," Melbourne hearings, February 28 (Canberra: Australian Parliament Hansard, 2002), 185.

28. J. Iliffe, "Editorial: Aged Care Nurse-Wage Impasse," *Australian Nursing Journal* (February 2004): 1.

29. Victorian Hospitals Industrial Association documents submitted to the Commission, August 2000, labeled VHIA exhibit 5.

30. Evidence given by Dr. Michael Walsh, Alfred Hospital, official transcript of Commission proceedings in the matter C no. 35605 of 2000 s. 99, Notification of industrial dispute, Victorian Hospitals Industrial Association and Australian Nursing Federation, August 28, 2000: 208.

31. Sworn statement provided by Dr. Michael Walsh, chief executive officer at Alfred Hospital, Melbourne, in the matter of C no. 35605 of 2000. Exhibit VHIA no 5.

32. Alec Djoneff, chief executive officer, Victorian Hospitals Industrial Association, official transcript of presentation of evidence, August 28, 2000: 200.

33. An ambulance bypass occurs when an ambulance (carrying a not–time critical patient) bypasses a specific emergency department (even though this hospital may be geographically closer to the place where the patient has been collected) because the hospital has reached its maximum capacity. Bypass occurs at the request of the emergency department.

34. Transcript of Commission proceedings in the matter C no. 35605 of 2000 s. 99, Notification of industrial dispute, Victorian Hospitals Industrial Association and Australian Nursing Federation, August 28, 2000: 211.

35. Ibid., 213–14.

36. Ibid., 217.

37. Ibid., 213–14.

38. Ibid., 268–70.

39. Ibid., 322.

40. Ibid., August 28, 2000: 232–33.

41. Ibid., 233.

42. Australian Industrial Relations Commission (AIRC), Matter C no. 35605 of 2000, Industrial dispute by the Victorian Hospitals Industrial Association (VHIA) against the Australian Nursing Federation (ANF), Print Decision S9958 (Melbourne: AIRC, 2000).

43. Ibid.

44. It is important to note that overlap occurs between a.m. and p.m. shifts, for example, the 7 a.m. to 3:30 p.m. shift and the 1 p.m. to 9:30 p.m. shift.

45. Australian Industrial Relations Commission, Victorian Hospitals Industrial Association and Australian Nursing Federation (Victorian Health Services) Award 1992, NO175 Dec 1079/00 M Print 59958, Melbourne, August 2000.

46. Over the last ten years, the Federal Government led by John Howard has significantly reduced the power of the Australian Industrial Relations Commission to set wages and conditions of employment in legally binding instruments (also known as awards).

47. Previously this organization was known as the Arbitration Inspectorate and then Awards Management Branch of the Federal Labour Department.

48. "Nurse Jobs Secure Thwaites," media release from the Minister for Health, July 16, 2001.

49. Australian Industrial Relations Commission (AIRC), Matter C no. 35605 of 2000 s. 99, Notification of industrial dispute Victorian Hospitals Industrial Association and Australian Nursing Federation, Print Decision AW790805 PR 902692, Commissioner Blair (Melbourne: AIRC, March 27, 2001).

50. Ibid.

51. Australian Industrial Relations Commission (AIRC), Matter C no. 35605 of 2000 s. 99, Notification of industrial dispute Victorian Hospitals Industrial Association and Australian Nursing Federation, Print Decision AW790805 PR 906762, Commissioner Blair (Melbourne: AIRC, July 20, 2001).

52. Ibid.

53. Ibid.

54. P. Stanton, "Enterprise Bargaining in the Victorian Public Hospital System 1992–1999," *AIRAANZ Annual Conference Papers*, ed. D. Kelly (Wollongong: Association of Industrial Relations Academies of Australia and New Zealand, 2000), 311–19.

55. See, for example, "Stateline Nurse Reveals Hospital Working Conditions," August 11, reporter Kathy Bowlen (Melbourne: ABC TV, 2000). Transcript available at www.abc.net.au/stateline/vic.

56. NSW Health, *Nursing Recruitment and Retention Taskforce Final Report* (Sydney: NSW Health, 1996); Queensland Health, *Nursing Recruitment and Retention Ministerial Taskforce Final Report* (Brisbane: Queensland Health, 1999); Human Services Victoria, *Nurse Recruitment and Retention Committee Final Report* (Melbourne: DHS Victoria, May 2001).

57. Queensland Nursing Council Senate Committee Affairs, *Inquiry into Recruitment and Retention of Nurses Submission no 887* (Brisbane: QNC, 2001), 8.

58. Commonwealth Senate, *The Patient Profession: Time for Action—Final Report on the Inquiry into Nursing* (Canberra: Commonwealth of Australia, 2002), 13.

59. Roy Morgan Research Gallup International Association, *Roy Morgan Special Poll Report 24*, finding number 3938 (Roy Morgan, 2005). Available at www.roymorgan.com.

60. "Members Vote to Work to Nurse Patient Ratios," *Guardian*, August 15, 2001.

61. Department of Training, Education and Youth Affairs, *Job Futures* (Canberra: Australian Government Publishing Service, 1998).

62. Buchanan and Briggs, "Unions and the Restructuring of Work," 10.

63. "Victorian Nurses Feel Betrayed by the Bracks Government," Victorian ANF media release, April 27, 2004.

8. Evaluating the Impact of Ratios

1. Some of the findings of this survey remain unpublished; however, a summarized account of the key results is provided in J. Buchanan, T. Bretherton, S. Bearfield, and S. Jackson, *Stable, but*

Critical, report prepared for the ANF Victoria on the impact of nurse-to-patient ratios (University of Sydney, 2004): 36.

2. Research by Bartram and Stanton indicates that ANF Victoria continues to represent the majority of nurses employed in the state's public sector and that this representation has been on the rise over the last fourteen years. See T. Bartram and P. Stanton, "How to Make Your Union Grow: The Experience of Officials and Organisations ANF Victoria Branch," Association of Industrial Relations Academies of Australia and New Zealand Conference, February 3–6 (Brisbane: AIRAANZ Conference Papers, 2004): 42–52.

3. Full copies of the reports relating to the ratio evaluations are available on the Workplace Research Centre website, www.wrc.org.au.

4. Conclusions generated by analysis of survey questions 73 and 81, "Which of the following best describes your workload as a nurse?" Population: all ANF (Victorian Branch) public-sector members. Sample: ratios n = 1,159; nonratios n = 366.

5. Conclusions generated by analysis of survey question 66: "In your opinion, are nurse-to-patient ratios essential for ensuring that nurses have manageable workloads?" Population: All ANF (Victorian Branch) members in the Victoria public sector. Sample size: nurses with ratios = 1,168.

6. Conclusions generated by analysis of survey question 59: "Please state how nurse-to-patient ratios have improved the working conditions in your work area? Please tick more than one box if necessary." Population: ANF (Victorian Branch) public-sector members with ratios who have been in same work area for three or more years who indicated working conditions would be worse without the ratios, that is, 33% of the survey population. Sample: n = 574.

7. http://www.trendcare.com.au/patient_nurse_dependency.html, accessed June 6, 2007.

8. Response to an open-ended question included in the 2003 ANF Victoria survey.

9. J. Buchanan, T. Bretherton, S. Bearfield, and S. Jackson, *Stable, But Critical*, report prepared for the ANF Victoria on the impact of nurse-patient ratios (University of Sydney, 2004): 36.

10. An acute ward typically admits patients suffering from severe conditions which have rapid onset.

11. Conclusions generated by analysis of survey question 53, "Please give examples of the major changes in this work area since 2000," and question 59, "Please state how nurse-to-patient ratios have improved the working conditions in your work area? Please tick more than one box if necessary." Population: ANF (Victorian Branch) public-sector members with ratios who have been in same work area for three or more years who indicated working conditions would be worse without the ratios, that is, 33% of the survey population. Sample: n = 574.

12. Conclusions generated by analysis of findings from survey question 63: "If the nurse-patient ratios were abolished, which of the following responses would you be most likely to make? Please give *one* response only." Population: ANF (Victorian Branch) public-sector members currently working in areas covered by the ratios, that is, 70.4% of the survey population. Sample: n = 1,222.

13. See Minister for Health, "Nurses Return to Work in Their Thousands," media release, July 12, 2001, and Victorian Auditor General's Office, *Nurse Workforce Planning: Performance Audit Report* (Melbourne, 2002).

14. Evidence given by Shane Solomon, executive director, Metropolitan Health and Aged Care Services, Department of Human Services, to Commonwealth Senate Hansard Community Affairs Reference Committee, "Patient Profession Inquiry," Melbourne hearings, February 28 (Canberra: Australian Parliament Hansard, 2002), 179.

15. ANF Victoria, "What Nurses Have Achieved over the Last Decade," media release, April 3, 2007.

16. A dearth of national data means that it is not possible to closely track nurse migration among all states. However, an interstate drainage effect is possible because Australia has a single entry-level qualification for RNs and there is mutual recognition between the states and territories for these professional classifications.

17. V. Plummer, "An Analysis of Patient Dependency Data Utilizing the TrendCare System," Ph.D. diss., School of Nursing, Monash University, 2005.

18. Buchanan, Bretherton, Bearfield, and Jackson, *Stable but Critical*.

19. It is important to note that this situation would arise when an ANUM (Associate Nurse Unit Manager) was in charge of a shift where a NUM (Nurse Unit Manager) was not rostered. This would typically occur on afternoon and night duty shifts and on weekends.

20. Source: 2003 Nurses survey; overtime incidence; population: All public-sector ANF Victoria nurses; sample: n=1,711. 1999 Nurses survey; overtime incidence; population: 11,859; sample: n=1,149.

21. Conclusions generated by analysis of survey question 35: "What is the main reason you work overtime?" Population: ANF (Victorian Branch) public-sector nurses working overtime. Sample: n = 1,025.

22. Conclusions generated by analysis of survey question 36: "How is your overtime reimbursed?" Population: ANF (Victorian Branch) public-sector nurses who work overtime, either paid or unpaid. Sample: n = 1,070.

23. Buchanan, Bretherton, Bearfield, and Jackson, *Stable, but Critical*.

24. Despite the persistence of some problems, hospital closures have never been caused by ratios. A number of U.S. commentators have asserted that ratios in Victoria have resulted in the closures of up to one in four public-hospital beds. They appear to have confused widespread temporary bed closure taken as industrial action by nurses as part of their campaign in support of the ratios with permanent bed closures by management as part of their ongoing decision making in running the health system. The widespread bed closures ended as soon as their relevance to the industrial campaign was over. They did not trigger any ongoing closure of beds throughout the health-care system.

25. Conclusions generated by analysis of survey question 53: "Please give examples of the major changes in this work area since 2000." Population: ANF (Victorian Branch) public-sector members in work areas with ratios who have been there for three or more years and who reported there had been a change in their day-to-day work as nurses caring for patients, that is, 30% of the total survey population. Sample size: n =512.

26. For full details, see Sarah Wise's report on the Workplace Research Centre/Australian Nursing Federation (ANF Victoria) 2006 survey of nurses' working conditions.

27. ANF Victoria website, citing ABC news, 25 October 2007. Available at http://www.anfvic.asn.au.

28. Ibid.

29. John Buchanan, "Recasting Australian Employment Law: Implications for the Health Sector," *Australian Health Review* 29, no. 3 (2005): 264–69.

30. Wise 2007.

31. "Nurses Dispute Heading to the Courts," *The Age*, 22 October 2007.

32. Ibid.

33. "Nurses' Agreement Reached," ABC News Service, 25 October 2007. Available at http://www.abc.net.au/news/stories/2007/10/25/2070252.htm.

34. Department of Human Services Victoria, "Victoria Records Biggest Increase in Hospital Doctors," media release, December 20, 2006.

9. What We Know about Nurse Staffing

1. G. S. Wunderlich, F. A. Sloan, C. K. Davis, eds., *Nurse Staff in Hospitals and Nursing Homes: Is It Adequate?* (Washington, D.C.: Institute of Medicine, National Academy Press, 1996).

2. Sean Clarke, "Research on Nurse Staffing and Its Outcomes," in *The Complexities of Care: Nursing Reconsidered*, ed. Sioban Nelson and Suzanne Gordon (Ithaca: Cornell University Press, 2006), 161–84.

3. Jeffrey H. Silber, S. V. Williams, H. Krakauer, and J. S. Swartz, "Hospital and Patient Characteristics Associated with Death after Surgery: A Study of Adverse Occurrence and Failure to Rescue," *Medical Care* 30 (1992): 615–29.

4. Ibid.

5. Jeffrey H. Silber, Paul R. Rosenbaum, and Richard N. Ross, "Comparing the Contributions of Groups of Predictors: Which Outcomes Vary with Hospital Rather Than Patient Characteristics," *Journal of the American Statistical Association* 90, no. 429 (1995): 7–18.

6. Ibid.; Jeffrey H. Silber, Sean K. Kennedy, Orit Even-Shoshan, et al., "Anesthesiologist Direction and Patient Outcomes," *Anesthesiology* 93 (2000): 152–63; Sharina D. Person et al., "Nurse Staffing and Mortality for Medicare Patients with Acute Myocardial Infarction," *Medical Care* 42, no. 1 (2004): 4–12; Linda H. Aiken, Sean P. Clarke, Douglas M. Sloane, et al., "Hospital Nurse Staffing and Patient Mortality, Nurse Burnout, and Job Dissatisfaction," *Journal of the American Medical Association* 288, no. 16 (2002): 1987–93; Linda H. Aiken, Sean P. Clarke, Robyn B. Cheung, et al., "Educational Levels of Hospital Nurses and Surgical Patient Mortality," *Journal of the American Medical Association* 290, no. 12 (2003): 1617–23.

7. Aiken, Clarke, Sloane, et al., "Hospital Nurse Staffing and Patient Mortality"; Aiken, Clarke, Cheung, et al., "Educational Levels of Hospital Nurses"; Silber, Rosenbaum, and Ross, "Comparing the Contributions of Groups of Predictors"; Silber, Kennedy, Even-Shoshan, et al., "Anesthesiologist Direction and Patient Outcomes"; Jack Needleman, Peter Buerhaus, Soeren Mattke, et al., "Nurse-Staffing Levels and the Quality of Care in Hospitals," *New England Journal of Medicine* 346, no. 22 (2002): 1715–22.

8. Sung-Hyun Cho, Shake Ketefian, Violet H. Barkauskas, and Dean G. Smith, "The Effects of Nurse Staffing on Adverse Events, Morbidity, Mortality, and Medical Costs," *Nursing Research* 52 (2003): 71–79; Needleman, Buerhaus, Mattke, et al., "Nurse-Staffing Levels and the Quality of Care"; Christine Kovner and Peter J. Gergen, "Nurse Staffing Levels and Adverse Events Following Surgery in U.S. Hospitals," *Image: Journal of Nursing Scholarship* 30, no. 4 (1998): 315–21; Christine Kovner, Cheryl Jones, et al., "Nurse Staffing and Postsurgical Adverse Events: An Analysis of Administrative Data from a Sample of U.S. Hospitals, 1990–1996," *Health Services Research* 37, no. 3 (2002): 611–29.

9. Kovner and Gergen, "Nurse Staffing Levels and Adverse Events."

10. Ibid.; Needleman, Buerhaus, Mattke, et al., "Nurse-Staffing Levels and the Quality of Care."

11. Mary Blegen and Tom Vaughn, "A Multisite Study of Nurse Staffing and Patient Occurrences," *Nursing Economics* 16, no. 4 (1998): 196–203; Margaret D. Sovie and Abbas F. Jawad, "Hospital Restructuring and Its Impact on Outcomes," *Journal of Nursing Administration* 31, no. 12 (2001): 588–600.

12. Blegen and Vaughn, "A Multisite Study of Nurse Staffing."

13. Sovie and Jawad, "Hospital Restructuring and Its Impact on Outcomes."

14. Kovner and Gergen, "Nurse Staffing Levels and Adverse Events."

15. Needleman, Buerhaus, Mattke, et al., "Nurse-Staffing Levels and the Quality of Care."

16. Ibid.

17. Silber, Rosenbaum, and Ross, "Comparing the Contributions of Groups of Predictors."

18. Silber, Kennedy, Even-Shoshan, et al., "Anesthesiologist Direction and Patient Outcomes."

19. Aiken, Clarke, Sloane, et al., "Hospital Nurse Staffing and Patient Mortality."

20. Ibid.

21. Kovner and Gergen, "Nurse Staffing Levels and Adverse Events."

22. Ibid.

23. Needleman, Buerhaus, Mattke et al., "Nurse-Staffing Levels and the Quality of Care."

24. Ibid.

25. Cho, Ketefian, Barkauskas, and Smith, "Effects of Nurse Staffing on Adverse Events, Morbidity, Mortality, and Medical Costs."

26. Mary A. Blegen, Colleen J. Goode, and Laura Reed, "Nurse Staffing and Patient Outcomes," *Nursing Research* 47, no. 1 (1998): 43–50.

27. Cho, Ketefian, Barkauskas, and Smith, "Effects of Nurse Staffing on Adverse Events."

28. Blegen, Goode, and Reed, "Nurse Staffing and Patient Outcomes."

29. Blegen and Vaughn, "A Multisite Study of Nurse Staffing."

30. Thomas A. Lang et al., "Nurse-Patient Ratios: A Systematic Review on the Effects of Nurse Staffing on Patient, Nurse Employee, and Hospital Outcomes." *Journal of Nursing Administration* 34, no. 7/8 (2004): 326.

31. Bruce E. Landon, Sharon-Lise T. Normand, et al., "Quality of Care for the Treatment of Acute Medical Conditions in U.S. Hospitals," *Archives of Internal Medicine* 166 (2006): 2511–17.

32. Ann E. Tourangeau et al., "Impact of Hospital Nursing Care on 30–Day Mortality for Acute Medical Patients," *Journal of Advanced Nursing* 57, no. 1 (2006): 41.

33. Agency for Healthcare Research and Quality, "Nurse Staffing and Quality Patient Care," Evidence Report/Technology Assessment, Number 151 (Publication No. 07–E005), March 2007.

34. Anne Marie Rafferty et al., "Outcomes Variation in Hospital Nurse Staffing in English Hospitals: Cross-sectional Analysis of Survey Data and Discharge Records," *International Journal of Nursing Studies* 44 (2007): 175.

35. Joel J. Hillhouse and Christine M. Adler, "Investigating Stress Effect Patterns in Hospital Staff Nurses: Result of a Cluster Analysis," *Sociology of Science and Medicine* 45 (1997): 1781.

36. Ibid.

37. C. Maslach, W. B. Schaufeli, and M. P Leiter, "Job Burnout," *Annual Review of Psychology* 52 (2001): 397–422.

38. Aiken et al., "Hospital Nurse Staffing and Patient Mortality."

39. Louisa Sheward et al., "The Relationship between UK Hospital Nurse Staffing and Emotional Exhaustion and Job Dissatisfaction," *Journal of Nursing Management* 13 (2005): 53.

40. Ibid., 57.

41. Rafferty et al., "Outcomes Variation in Hospital Nurse Staffing," 175.

42. Ann P. Rogers, "The Working Hours of Hospital Staff Nurses and Patient Safety," *Health Affairs* 23, no. 4 (2004): 2092–2112.

43. Alison M. Trinkoff et al., "Workplace Access, Negative Proscriptions, Job Strain, and Substance Use in Registered Nurses," *Nursing Research* 49, no. 2 (2000): 83–90; Trinkoff et al., "Physically Demanding Work and Inadequate Sleep, Pain Medication Use, and Absenteeism in Registered Nurses," *Journal of Occupational and Environmental Medicine* 43, no. 2 (2001): 355–63.

44. Sean P. Clarke, Douglas M. Sloane, and Linda H. Aiken, "Effects of Hospital Staffing and Organizational Climate on Needlestick Injuries to Nurses," *American Journal of Public Health* 92, no. 7 (2002): 1115–19.

45. Ibid.; Sean P. Clarke et al., "Organizational Climate, Staffing, and Safety Equipment as Predictors of Needlestick Injuries and Near-Misses in Hospital Nurses," *American Journal of Infection Control* 30, no. 4 (2002): 207–16.

46. Alison M. Trinkoff et al., "Perceived Physical Demands and Reported Musculoskeletal Problems of Registered Nurses," *American Journal of Preventive Medicine* 24, no. 3 (2003): 270.

47. Alison M. Trinkoff et al., "Workplace Prevention and Musculoskeletal Injuries in Nurses," *Journal of Nursing Administration* 33 (2003): 153; Trinkoff et al., "Physically Demanding Work and Inadequate Sleep, Pain Medication Use, and Absenteeism in Registered Nurses."

48. Alison M. Trinkoff et al., "Longitudinal Relationships of Work Hours, Mandatory Overtime, and On-call to Musculoskeletal Problems in Nurses," *American Journal of Industrial Medicine* 49 (2006): 964–71.

49. Jack Needleman, Peter I. Buerhaus, Maureen Stewart, et al., "Nurse Staffing in Hospitals: Is There a Business Case for Quality?" *Health Affairs* 25, no. 1 (2006): 204–11.

50. Michael B. Rothberg et al., "Improving Nurse-to-Patient Staffing Ratios as a Cost-Effective Safety Intervention," *Medical Care* 43, no. 8 (August 2005): 785–91.

51. This focus on patient mortality only and not on patient mortality and morbidity is a weakness of the study, because it underestimates the effect of nurse staffing and does not consider relevant factors such as quality of life adjustments associated with morbidity. In addition, its design is such that no direct relationship between nurse staffing and hospitalization costs can be established. The optimal nurse-staffing level remains unknown, as do effective ratios for specific units.

This would require a large randomized trial and a commitment to recognize adequate nurse staffing levels as central to patient safety like other interventions.

52. Ibid., 791.

53. http://www.bizjournals.com/milwaukee/stories/2007/08/27/story13.html?t=printable, accessed September 1, 2007.

54. Sean P. Clarke, "Research on Nurse Staffing and Its Outcomes," in *Complexities of Care: Nursing Reconsidered*, ed. Sioban Nelson and Suzanne Gordon (Ithaca: Cornell University Press, 2006), 164–65.

55. Ibid.

56. Ibid., 176–77.

10. Arguments against and Alternatives to Ratios

1. Linda H. Aiken, et al., "Educational Levels of Hospital Nurses and Surgical Patient Mortality," *Journal of the American Medical Association* 290 (2003): 1617–23; Sean P. Clarke and Charlene Connolly, "Nurse Education and Patient Outcomes: A Commentary," *Policy, Politics & Nursing Practice* 5, no. 1 (February 2004): 12–20; Sharina D. Person et al., "Nurse Staffing and Mortality for Medicare Patients with Acute Myocardial Infarction," *Medical Care* 42, no. 1 (2004): 4–12.

2. For a fuller discussion of the impact of cost cutting on nursing management, see Suzanne Gordon, *Nursing against the Odds: How Cost-Cutting, Media Stereotypes, and Medical Hubris Undermine Nurses and Patient Care* (Ithaca: Cornell University Press, 2005), 318–28.

3. "Nurses Oppose New Bill to Mandate Staffing," http://mywebtimes.com/ottnews/archives/ottawa/display.php?id=293987, accessed April 7, 2007.

4. Gordon, *Nursing against the Odds*.

5. Institute of Medicine, *Hospital-Based Emergency Care: At the Breaking Point* (Washington, D.C.: National Academies Press, 2006), 1.

6. Interview with Robert L. Wears, professor of emergency medicine at the University of Florida in Jacksonville.

7. C. DeNavas-Walt, B. D. Proctor, and C. H. Lee, *Income, Poverty, and Health Insurance Coverage in the United States: 2004* (U.S. Census Bureau, August 2005). From National Coalition on Health Care, http://www.nchc.org/facts/coverage.shtml, accessed November 14, 2006.

8. Spetz et al., 2004, 13.

9. A recent example illustrates that nurse-staffing ratios have not produced the ER crisis. During one of our talks at a major northeastern teaching hospital, Gordon meet with nurses in the ER. The hospital was applying for Magnet status and nurses were thus supposed to be as if magnetized to their hospital and to be thrilled to be working on every unit in the institution. The ER nurses were, however, almost apoplectic. They were taking care of seven or eight patients or more on every shift. Patients were stacked up in the hallways. The place was a mess, sometimes filthy even. Nurses and doctors were beyond frazzled. They had asked—begged, pleaded, implored—the administration to do something. "No one is listening to us," one nurse told me almost in tears. "We ask for extra staff and they tell us they are $100,000 over their nursing budget." The hospital nursing department had money to pay for Magnet accreditation but apparently not to provide more nurses to patients in the ER.

10. Janet M. Coffman, Jean Ann Seago, and Joanne Spetz, "Minimum Nurse-to-Patient Ratios in Acute Care Hospitals in California," *Health Affairs* 21, no. 5 (2002): 60; http://content.healthaffairs.org/cgi/content/full/21/5/53.

11. Joanne Spetz, "California's Minimum Nurse-to-Patient Ratios: The First Few Months," *JONA* 34 (2004): 574.

12. James Buchan, "A Certain Ratio? The Policy Implications of Minimum Staffing Ratios in Nursing," *Journal of Health Services Research Policy* 10 (2005): 243–44.

13. Ibid., 244.

14. California Nurses Association, "CNA Blasts Study on Alleged Costs of Safe Staffing, Implementing Ratios May Be Cost Neutral, RNs Say," press release, July 26, 2001.

15. Diane Cadrain, "An Acute Condition: Too Few Nurses," *HR Magazine* 47, no. 12 (December 2002).

16. http://www.patientsfirstma.org/, accessed January 2, 2007.

17. WBUR, "Nursing a Shortage: Inside Out," January 19, 2007.

18. http://www.ihi.org/IHI/Programs/TransformingCareAtTheBedside/ TransformingCareAtTheBedside.htm?TabId=3, accessed January 2, 2006.

19. Christopher Rowland, "Cambridge Nonprofit Cuts Nursing Turnover," *Boston Globe*, November 27, 2006, A1.

20. Institute for Healthcare Improvement, Transforming Care at the Bedside, Innovation Series, 2004, 8.

21. Laura Landro, "Why Quota for Nurses Isn't Cure-All," *Wall Street Journal*, December 13, 2006, http://online.wsj.com/article/SB116596592537648199–search.html?KEYWORDS= Hospital+nursing+care&COLLECTION=wsjie/6month.

22. Margaret L. McClure and Ada Sue Hinshaw, *Magnet Hospitals Revisited: Attraction and Retention of Professional Nurses* (Washington, D.C.: American Nurses Publishing, 2002).

23. American Nurses Credentialing Center, "What Is the Magnet Recognition Program?" http://www.nursecredentialing.org/magnet/index.html, accessed March 2, 2007.

24. Ibid., http://www.nursecredentialing.org/magnet/apply/eligibility_org.html and http://www .nursecredentialing.org/magnet/goals.html.

25. Department of Health and Human Services, Centers for Disease Control and Prevention, National Institute for Occupational Health and Safety, "The Changing Organization of Work and the Safety and Health of Working People," April 2002, Publication No. 2002-116, chap. 3, 15–16.

Conclusion: Ratios and Beyond

1. Christine T. Kovner et al., "Newly Licensed RNs' Characteristics, Work Attitudes, and Intentions to Work," *American Journal of Nursing* 107, no. 9 (2007): 58–70.

2. Institute for Healthcare Improvement and the Robert Wood Johnson Foundation, M21: Transforming Care at the Bedside, the 18th Annual National Forum on Quality Improvement in Health Care, final handout, December 11, 2006, 5.

3. For a fuller discussion of the pressures on managers and nurse executives, see Suzanne Gordon, *Nursing against the Odds: How Health Care Cost-Cutting, Media Stereotypes, and Medical Hubris Undermine Nurses and Patient Care* (Ithaca: Cornell University Press, 2005), 318–28.

4. Sarah Wise, "Undermining the Ratios: Nurses under Pressure in Victoria," 2006 ANF Victoria Survey of Public Sector Nurses' Working Conditions, prepared by the Workplace Research Centre, University of Sydney, October 2007.

5. Michael Ong, et al., "House Staff Team Workload and Organization Effects on Patient Outcome in an Academic General Internal Inpatient Service," *Archives of Internal Medicine* 167 (2007): 47–52.

6. Mike Norbut, "Lawsuit Accuses Hospital of Overworking Doctor," *American Medical News*, October 3, 2005.

7. Michael B. Rothberg, Ivo Abraham, Peter K. Lindenauer, and David N. Rose, "Improving Nurse-to-Patient Staffing Ratios as a Cost-Effective Safety Intervention," *Medical Care* 43, no. 8 (2005): 791.

8. Australian Industrial Relations Commission, Victorian Hospitals' Industrial Association and Australian Nursing Federation—Nurses (Victorian Health Services) Award 1992, N0175 Dec 1079/00 M Print S9958, Melbourne, August 2000, 47.

Index

Italic page numbers refer to tables and figures.

About the Authors

Suzanne Gordon is an award winning journalist who has been writing about nursing and health care for the past two decades. Her articles have appeared in the *Atlantic Monthly*, the *Nation*, the *New York Times*, the *Washington Post*, the *Boston Globe*, the Toronto *Globe and Mail*, and the *Los Angeles Times*, among other places. She has been a radio commentator on health care for public radio's Marketplace and served on the Robert Wood Johnson's national advisory committee on the nursing shortage. Her books include *Life Support: Three Nurses on the Front Lines*; *From Silence to Voice: What Nurses Know and Must Communicate to the Public*, 2nd ed., written with Bernice Buresh; *Nursing against the Odds: How Health Care Cost Cutting, Media Stereotypes, and Medical Hubris Undermine Nurses and Patient Care*; and *The Complexities of Care: Nursing Reconsidered*, edited with Sioban Nelson. Gordon is Visiting Professor at the University of Maryland School of Nursing and Assistant Adjunct Professor at the University of California at San Francisco School of Nursing. She lectures nationally and internationally on health care issues.

John Buchanan is the director of the Workplace Research Centre at the University of Sydney. In the 1990s Buchanan was part of the team that undertook the first Australian Workplace Industrial Relations Survey (AWIRS). Since the early 1990s Buchanan has lead a large number of research teams and significant national projects on the changing nature of work in Australia. He was one of the authors of Workplace Research Centre's 1999 book, *Australia at Work: Just Managing?* and a coauthor of *Fragmented Futures: New Challenges in Working Life*. Building on this research, he is now devoting special attention to the implications of the changing nature of work for trust relations between workers and their employers and changing trust relations between different occupational groups.

Tanya Bretherton is a sociologist and a senior research analyst at the Workplace Research Centre at the University of Sydney. Her research interests include workload management, women and work, and qualitative analysis of atypical forms of employment. In the 1990s, Bretherton worked as a labor market policy researcher for the federal government and has worked as a researcher and teacher in the academic sector for more than ten years.